PUBLICATIONS OF
THE WELLCOME INSTITUTE OF THE HISTORY OF MEDICINE

(*General Editor:* F. N. L. Poynter, Ph.D., D.Litt., Hon.M.D.(Kiel))

New Series, Volume XVIII

THE HISTORY OF CORONARY HEART DISEASE

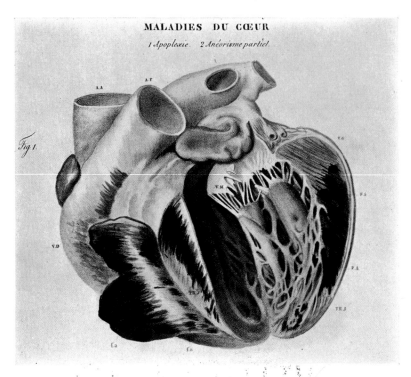

Plate I 'Apopléxie du coeur.' Myocardial infarction, faithfully depicted, but not named as such. Jean Cruveilhier (1791–1874), *Anatomie pathologique du corps humain*, Paris, 1829–42; t. II, 22° livraison, planche 3, figure 1.

THE HISTORY
OF
CORONARY
HEART DISEASE

J. O. LEIBOWITZ

UNIVERSITY OF CALIFORNIA PRESS

Berkeley and Los Angeles · 1970

UNIVERSITY OF CALIFORNIA PRESS
Berkeley and Los Angeles, California

ISBN 0-520-01769-2

Library of Congress Catalog Card Number : 78-122931

This work is also published in the United Kingdom
by The Wellcome Institute of the History of Medicine

Printed in Great Britain

For Hannah
her help and encouragement

The first, and one may say the most necessary, task for writers of any kind of history is to choose a noble subject and one pleasing to their readers.

DIONYSIUS OF HALICARNASSUS

The Three Literary Letters, edited and translated by W. Rhys Roberts, Cambridge University Press, 1901, *Letter to Pompeius,* chapter 3, p. 105).

Table of Contents

		Page
Preface		xv
Chapter I	Introductory survey	1
Chapter II	Antiquity and the Middle Ages	15
	1. Ancient Egypt:	
	a. Pathological evidence	15
	b. Literary sources	19
	2. Ancient Greece and Rome: The notion of impeded blood flow, first mention of the coronary vessels, and description of cardio-genic shock	25
	3. Bible and Talmud	39
	4. The Middle Ages: The elaboration of Greek ideas in coronary symptomatology	41
Chapter III	From the Renaissance to the End of the Seventeenth Century	49
	1. The Sixteenth Century: Case histories with early pathology	49
	2. The Seventeenth Century: The beginning of physiological studies	61
Chapter IV	The Eighteenth Century	73
	1. The search for pathological evidence in coronary disease. The diagnosis of angina established	
	2. Heberden and his followers	83

Page

Chapter V   The Nineteenth Century: The Development
of the Concept of Infarction   104

1. Burns' ischaemic theory—Early studies of
arteriosclerosis — Scarpa — Lobstein —
Myocardial involvement: Adams — Cruveilhier — Laënnec — Hodgson — Williams — Quain — Erichsen — Peacock —
Malmsten and Düben — Latham: Thomas
Arnold's case-history

2. Vascular pathology — Tiedemann —
Rokitansky — Virchow: thrombosis and
embolism — Weigert: myocardial infarct — Cohnheim — Vulpian — Radcliffe — Payne — Hammer: first clinical
diagnosis of coronary thrombosis — Leyden's classification — Kernig — Allbutt's
aortic theory   123

Chapter VI   The Twentieth Century: The Recognition of
Coronary Heart Disease   146

1. Krehl — Obrastzow and Straschesko —
Hochhaus — Herrick — coronary anas-
tomoses: Gross — Electrocardiography —
Einthoven and subsequent developments
— Mackenzie — Lewis' physiological
approach

2. Diagnostic Aids — Sphygmomanometry
— temperature rise — leucocytosis —
erythrocyte sedimentation rate — serum
transaminase   160

3. Etiological factors — emotions — diet and
arteriosclerosis — social and occupational
factors — age   163

4. Therapy — early attempts — amyl nitrite,
nitroglycerine — intensive care — surgery
— anticoagulants   169

5. Conclusion: The antiquity of coronary
heart disease, its changing manifestations
and incidence   172

Appendix   Select texts:
                Galen   177
                Froissart (The death of the Count de Foix)   179
                Heberden   180
                Vulpian   184

Bibliography   1. Historical surveys   187
                2. General   191

Index   215

List of Illustrations

PLATE I   'Apopléxie du coeur'. Myocardial infarction, *Frontis-* faithfully depicted, but not named as such. Jean   *piece* Cruveilhier (1791–1874), *Anatomie pathologique du corps humain*, Paris, 1829–42; t.II, 22° livraison, planche 3, figure 1.

PLATE II   First depiction of the origin of the coronary vessels from the coronary sinus. Leonardo da Vinci (1452–1519), *Quaderni d'anatomia*, 1911–18, vol. II, folio 9 verso, figures 4–9.

PLATE III   William Harvey, *Exercitationes duae anatomicae de circulatione sanguinis. Ad Johannem Riolanum filium* (etc.), Rotterdam: A. Leers, 1649; pp. 34–35.

PLATE IV   Death of Count Gaston de Foix (1391). MS Harl. 4379 fol. 126 in the British Museum.

PLATE V   Heart injected with red wax showing the finest ramifications of the coronary vessels. Frederik Ruysch (1638–1731), *Thesaurus anatomicus quartus*, Amsterdam, 1704 (Tab. III). On page 45 Ruysch remarks: 'English magnates preserve the embalmed hearts of deceased members of their families in golden or silver boxes, and thus my art flourishes (et sic ars mea vigeret)'.

PLATE VI   Portrait of Adam Christian Thebesius (1686–1732). Engraved by A. Hoger after M. Tyrnoff. From a copy in the Royal College of Physicians of London.

PLATE VII   Dissected heart. A. C. Thebesius, *Dissertatio medica de circulo sanguinis in corde*, Leyden, 1716 (1st edition 1708).

PLATE VIII   Ruptured heart of King George II 'having the orifice in the right ventricle, and the extravasation covering the fissure in the aorta'. Frank Nicholls, 'Observations concerning the Body of his late Majesty, October 26, 1760.' *Phil. Trans. R. Soc. Lond.*, vol. 52, pt. I, 1761, pp. 265–275.

PLATE IX   First page of William Heberden's autograph manuscript *Pectoris dolor*, in the Royal College of Physicians of London, conforming to his paper published in English in 1772.

PLATE X   Antonio Scarpa (1747–1832), *Sull' aneurisma. Riflessioni ed osservazioni anatomico-chirurgiche*, atlas folio, Pavia, 1804. Title-page.

PLATE XI   Five small figures from Tabula IX showing coagulated material within an aneurysmal sac. Antonio Scarpa, *Sull' aneurisma*, Pavia, 1804.

PLATE XII   Albrecht v. Haller (1708–1777), *Disputationes ad morborum historiam et curationem facientes. Tomus secundus: Ad morbos pectoris*, Lausanne, 1757. Title-page. The volume consists of a collection of tracts and medical theses on diseases of the chest from the earlier 18th century.

PLATE XIII   Heart and vessels showing multiple aortic aneurysms and thrombi removed from the aneurysmal sacs. Christian Gottfried Stenzel (1698–1748), *Dissertatio de steatomatibus aortae*, 1723. In: Albrecht v. Haller, *Disputationes ad morborum historiam et curationem facientes. Tomus secundus: Ad morbos pectoris*, Lausanne, 1757, facing page 562.

PLATE XIV Partial aneurysm of the heart occupying the apex of the left ventricle. Jean Cruveilhier (1791–1874), *Anatomie pathologique du corps humain*, Paris, 1829–42, t. II, 22° livraison, planche 3, figure 2.

PLATE XV String galvanometer, 1903, of William Einthoven (1860–1927). From: *Some Dutch contributions to the development of physiology*. (Souvenir of the 22nd International Congress of Physiological Sciences.) 1962, p. 35.

Preface

In presenting this first monograph on the history of coronary heart disease I have tried to fill a gap strongly felt in historical literature. In view of the importance and prevalence of this disease, such a history may be regarded as a necessary task. I hope to have satisfied the demand of the ancient Greek historian from whom the motto for this volume is taken, at least insofar as I have chosen a subject of some quality.

This book concerns the development of knowledge about a disease with changing manifestations, some of which have been clearly defined only in recent times. Much thought has been given to tracing the beginnings of our knowledge to primary sources, so as to establish a long and respectable pedigree. Not only facts leading to the ultimate recognition of the condition, but also ideas, such as that of 'obstruction', of ancient fame, have been thoroughly investigated.

Likewise, much attention has been paid to the historical publications which bear on our subject, as far as they were available. Whenever these deal with a particular author or item they are mentioned in the text and listed in the bibliography. Surveys or chapters in books, even when devoted to a special period or geographical area, have been listed separately in order to give due credit to previous writers.

To keep the book as concise as possible, I have tried to avoid digressions into the general history of cardiology, however enticing this might have been. On the other hand, I have dealt with developments in cardiology which emerged or prevailed at a particular period and influenced progress in our subject. The history of arteriosclerosis and thrombosis in general have therefore been given special consideration.

The term coronary heart disease, as used in the title, is meant to include the older notion of angina pectoris, as well as the more recent terms: coronary thrombosis and myocardial infarction. It has been chosen as most nearly expressing the manifold effects of coronary arterial disease on the heart. Much of the contents of this book has been devoted to an often dramatic struggle for clarification which resulted in a separation of the different manifestations of the disease. The proposed name reconciles the divergent views. The historian of today, no less than the clinician, is called upon 'to demand the consideration of basic definitions

and nomenclature' (P. D. White, *Heart Diseases*, 1951, pp. 517–18).
I decided to retain the title adopted by this author for his chapter on
the subject, in which he discusses the problem of nomenclature at some
length.

The decision to embark on the present study came about in the year
1959, when I supervised a thesis written by Dr. Joseph Danon for the
Hebrew University Medical School, Jerusalem (see List of Surveys).
This was a fruitful collaboration, including an extensive search for
source material. Then came the elaboration of this study, chiefly at the
Wellcome Historical Medical Library, with all its facilities for scholarly endeavour, under the stimulating directorship of Dr. F. N. L.
Poynter. Here I was aided by a grant from the Wellcome Trustees, for
which I wish to express my most sincere appreciation.

The section on Ancient Greece and Rome was completed in 1966
at the Johns Hopkins Institute of the History of Medicine, where I
enjoyed the counsel of Dr. O. Temkin, who later read the final manuscript. I wish to thank him for his valuable help.

The conclusion of the work was advanced by Dr. Poynter, who not
only made available the facilities of the Wellcome Institute but person-
ally provided the most competent advice whenever requested. He
extended his kindness to reading the whole typescript and watching over
the production of the volume, including style and arrangement. I wish
to express my warm thanks for all his help and encouragement.

During this phase of the work, I had the benefit of discussing several
items which needed clarification with Dr. K. D. Keele, to whom goes
my sincere appreciation for his interest and suggestions and for reading
the typescript.

I also wish to acknowledge assistance and advice from many other
quarters. In the body of this volume I have mentioned a number of
persons to whom I am indebted and who readily and generously
gave their advice. Among these are Mr. E. Gaskell, the librarian, and
the staff of the Wellcome Institute; the Jewish National and University
Library, as well as the libraries of the Royal College of Physicians, the
Royal Society of Medicine, and the many libraries in different countries
which I visited for shorter periods.

To my wife I am indebted not only for her help in the technical
preparation of the book, but also for her sound advice and encouragement over the years.

In the earlier stages of this work I had the benefit of the secretarial
help of Miss Pauline Donbrow and in the final version I was helped by
Dr. Elinor Lieber. To both of them I extend my thanks and appreciation.

Aided by all these persons and institutions, I hope to have produced a work, rooted in the sources of historical scholarship, which provides a fairly accurate account of a disease regarded by past investigators as both a riddle and an inspiration.

J. O. LEIBOWITZ

Division of the History of Medicine,
Hebrew University,
Jerusalem.
March 1969

CHAPTER I

Introductory Survey

While the syndrome of anginal pain became recognized as a well-defined entity in the second half of the eighteenth century, and that of myocardial infarction early in the twentieth, some knowledge of the underlying conditions can be traced in the earlier records. The belated recognition of infarction of the myocardium especially, has puzzled most historians in this field and invites particular consideration.

The facts and notions which could have led to earlier recognition may now be briefly surveyed, while details and documentation will be relegated to later chapters. One question, however, whether coronary artery disease existed at all in earlier recorded history, requires special attention. Some morbid conditions, though very rarely, have only a brief existence. Two examples at least are known: the Sweating Sickness (*sudor anglicus*) prevailing for a short time during the sixteenth century, and the Epidemic Encephalitis Economo at the end of the first world war. However, these were infectious diseases, which flared up and then practically disappeared, although there was no way of treating them. Coronary degenerative disease does not belong to this small group, though historically it has possibly shown changes in its manifestations. Coronary sclerosis may occur without marked involvement of the aorta and vice versa. However, arteriosclerosis in Egyptian mummies has been demonstrated histologically. Since 1852 it has been found in the aorta, in peripheral arteries, and, at least in one instance (1931), also in a coronary artery. Thus the antiquity of degenerative vascular disease has been established.

In the literary sources difficulties are met with which require for their solution a precise knowledge of language and the correct interpretation of terms. Some older translations and appraisals of the Ebers papyrus, for instance, have been criticized by more recent Egyptologists such as H. Grapow and J. A. Wilson. The word 'heart' in Egyptian, Greek, Hebrew and Arabic has not only the meaning of the viscus responsible for the circulation of the blood, but also of the stomach. This has been perpetuated even in modern usage ('heartburn', cardia). Thus the Greek 'kardialgia' in the sources may be precordial pain as much as a gastric condition, and already Galen pointed to this ambiguity in his Commentaries on Hippocrates and Plato. Only the context reveals the correct significance.

In spite of all the limitations of understanding and judgement imposed on us, facts and concepts which led ultimately to the recognition of anginal and myocardial disease can be set out: in ancient Egypt, apart from archaeological evidence, the occasional notion of precordial pain with 'death that threatens him'; many Biblical references to a sore heart, the vast majority of them poetical, but some also of medical implication; and Talmudical references to heart pain as meaning disease; the Hippocratic concept of obstruction, which includes vascular obstruction, and the Hippocratic mention of sudden death probably due to an anginal episode; then we come to Galen with his clear anatomical description of the coronary vessels along with their nutrient function; the Graeco-Roman syndrome of 'morbus cardiacus' seems to include the later notion of shock, (the full and beautiful description of this latter condition by Caelius Aurelianus mentions many precipitating factors, but none involving the heart and its vessels); there is the clinical picture that survived for so long representing syndromes of collapse and its less severe form of 'lipothymia', some of the descriptions of which are strongly suggestive of coronary disease. And to the genius of Leonardo da Vinci we owe the pictorial representation of narrow and tortuous peripheral vessels in the aged and the idea of the harmful influence of this condition on the tissues. But he made no reference to coronary narrowing in spite of his interest in the coronary vessels, which he depicted so artistically.

The next steps, far from a 'steep ascent from unknown to the known' were made in the sixteenth century. Benivieni's (1507) often-quoted case 35 is a well-described and early clinical case of pain in the heart while the pathological findings are not significant. Amatus Lusitanus' (1560) classical description of 'Sudden Death due to an Obstruction in the Heart', is outstanding, but devoid of anatomical verification. The ideas of Petrus Salius Diversus (1586) on cardiac syncope and sudden death through obstruction of the vessels are remarkable, though arrived at apparently more by reasoning than by actual observation. The seventeenth century brought the insight of William Harvey's (1649) description of a 'third and extremely short circulation' through the coronary arteries and veins, in the first letter to Riolan, and of two cases strongly suggestive of myocardial infarction in the second letter. But this information was to have no great influence on medical thought and practice in general, although a century and a half later the same ideas were to gain currency. However, individual contributions accumulated speedily. To name only a few of them, Bellini (1683) described calcification of the coronary vessels along with occlusion and appropriate clinical signs; and Thebesius (1708) not only referred to calcification of the coronaries in his refreshingly brief book, but also provided one of the earliest illustrations of the condition.

With the advent of the eighteenth century, which was to prove momentous in the history of anginal and allied diseases, a considerable body of facts and concepts had already been accumulated, and were awaiting further elaboration. There was, first, the classical idea of blood 'coalescence', stemming from Galen and Caelius, supplemented by Malpighi's (1666) observations on the coagulation of the blood and foreshadowing the recognition of vascular obstruction in the modern sense; there was also an increasing knowledge of syncopal events and occasional descriptions of precordial pain. Harvey's epochal discovery of the circulation of the blood had been acknowledged in the meantime, but did not lead immediately to any better understanding of pathological processes in the circulatory system.

The technique of history-taking and recording reached high perfection, though often marred by mannerism and verbosity. Bonet's *Sepulchretum* (1679) with its approximately 3,000 (all too brief) case histories and anatomical findings contained much material on ossified vessels, cartilaginous degeneration of the heart muscle and aneurysms, many of the findings being suggestive of myocardial infarction. Dissection of human bodies, especially in Italy, became more common, often supported, and sometimes even requested, by the highest dignitaries of the Church. The early reports of dissections, however, dealt with such gross changes of the heart as pericardial effusion, calcareous plaques and rupture of the myocardium, while neglecting the small structure of the coronaries. Even Harvey (1649) paid attention mainly to the ruptured hearts of his two anginal patients. It is also true with regard to descriptions of other diseases, that the more dramatic signs and symptoms are first recorded. For instance, peptic ulcer in its manifestation of complete pyloric stenosis had been described as early as 1586, while its associated symptom of hunger pain was noted only as late as 1832. Thus, Lancisi presented two books, one *On Sudden Deaths* (1707) and the other *On Aneurysms* (posthumously published in 1728) with much clinical data and detailed autopsy reports. Here again, the more conspicuous anatomical deviations, such as enormous dilatation and hypertrophy ('ox-heart') and fatal case-histories were predominant. It is remarkable that in Lancisi's books coronary vessels are more frequently mentioned than in older post-mortem reports; however, instead of narrowing of the coronary arteries, Lancisi refers more often to dilatation of coronary veins as part of the general cardiac insufficiency of his patients.

A new feature of the first half of the eighteenth century is the increased interest in cardiology and the appearance of textbooks on the heart and its diseases (Vieussens, 1715; Sénac, 1749). In comparison with the timid beginnings in the foregoing century, the eighteenth-century cardiological texts are more detailed and that by Senac also well planned and organized. Their common pattern was threefold: clinical data of different degrees of information, Lancisi's case-histories being the most detailed; correlation with post-mortem pathological findings which began long before Morgagni, though not on his large scale; and an obligatory modicum of theoretical reasoning in a more modernized form, but at least leaning on ancient medical authors, particularly Galen.

Great progress in correlating clinical and pathological data was made by Morgagni (1761). It is not easy to overrate his *De sedibus* in the development of morbid anatomy. Its shortcomings—lengthy references to ancient and 'modern' authors and numerous digressions—are often welcome to the historian, these parts of the book providing useful, though not too easily readable, information. As to ischaemic heart disease, Morgagni described many findings, such as ruptured heart-aneurysms, scars of the myocardium, even 'ulcers', along with clinical signs of precordial pain, but he does not correlate the signs with a pathological condition in the coronary vessels. His most important contribution in this field is his patho-physiological approach culminating in the dictum: 'The force of the heart decreases so much more in proportion as the greater number of its parts becomes tendinous instead of being fleshy'(Epistle 27, Article 18).

Then, nine pages, printed in rather tall characters, the lines generously spaced, stirred up the medical world. This was Heberden's *Some Account of a Disorder of the Breast*, read at the College 21st on July, 1768, and published in the second volume of the *Medical Transactions* by the College of Physicians in London, in 1772. This short paper, so often reproduced and eulogized, is still a starting-point for historical appraisal. The data he adduced were later to be integrated with the developing facts and concepts of ischaemic heart disease. Quite unique in nosological sagacity and straightforwardness, this paper was equally so in its formal composition. Of the three constituents of an eighteenth-century cardiological book or paper, Heberden chose but one: an unsurpassed outline of the clinical data. He abstained from referring to morbid anatomy, not even mentioning the heart and its vessels; no more than a vague hint (only in the first paper, 1772) to an 'ulcer', which cannot be interpreted as a sign of angina pectoris proper, but rather of cardiac failure ('spit up matter and blood') due to late, but not explicitly stated, sequelae of an anginal attack. The third obligatory constituent, theoretical reasoning and reference to the ancients, is totally absent from the original paper (1772), while in the final version, in the *Commentaries*, it is relegated to one short reference to Caelius Aurelianus, in a footnote at the end of the paper. The credit for identifying a morbid entity not hitherto named in the history of diseases must go to Heberden largely because of his quite exclusive approach to a clinical syndrome, characteristic of only one phase in the course of ischaemic heart disease. To find this entity in the absence of pulse anomalies, dyspnoea, and heart failure, was a privilege of Heberden's genius, though the signs and symptoms of a failing heart were definitely included in his description as belonging to later phases of this disease. As to pain in the heart and its possible fatal outcome, they had been clearly mentioned by earlier authors, among them Harvey (1649), but always as being associated with other clinical and anatomical findings. Heberden's originality, in historical perspective and in his own view, is understood in picturing the disease in its first phase, when clinical symptoms drew his attention before death intervened, or before the already known, if not yet scientifically explained, signs of heart failure became apparent.

It seems that some similarity in the formal approach links Heberden with the greater genius of Harvey: the exclusiveness with which both looked at their target. Harvey concentrated exclusively on the mechanism of the blood-flow. In the same way Heberden's study of the disease became exclusively focused on those manifestations which he could readily delineate, not disturbed by the magnitude of the myocardial lesions, which he may have had in mind. Two words are striking in Heberden's original (1772) version: time and attention. He left the task of elucidating the complexities of the disease bearing his name to those who came after him, while concentrating his own endeavour on calling attention to them.

With precordial pain established as a working diagnosis along with the notion of a usually serious prognosis, a group of Heberden's younger colleagues and countrymen embarked on a brilliant though short phase of research in ischaemic heart disease, which was only resumed a hundred years later (*c.* 1880) by pathologists and clinicians. To this group (Fothergill, 1776; Black and others) belonged Edward Jenner, and it seems that his was the leadership in the endeavour to recognize more fully the disease described by Heberden and to correlate it with an impairment of coronary circulation. This is testified by Parry in the introduction[1] to his book (1799):

> 'It was suggested by Dr. Jenner, that the angina pectoris arose from some morbid change in the structure of the heart, which change was probably ossification, or some similar disease, of the coronary arteries.'

Jenner, in his letter addressed to Heberden, mentions what may have been a thrombus in the coronary artery in a person who had died of angina pectoris. This was done with the collaboration of the surgeon, Mr. Paytherus, who drew his attention to this structure. This important finding preceded the concept of thrombosis inaugurated by Virchow some seventy years later, but as it lacked conceptual clarity, its etiological significance could not be fully appreciated.

The best literary production leading to the coronary theory of the disease was C. H. Parry's book: *An Inquiry into the Symptoms and Causes of the Syncope Anginosa, commonly called Angina Pectoris; Illustrated by Dissection*, Bath, 1799. It was preceded by Parry's paper read in July 1788, 'Angina pectoris, a disease of the heart, connected with malorganization of the coronary arteries'. All of the cases were of a more protracted type, though sudden death occurred eventually. The post-mortem findings were 'ossification' and partial obstruction of the coronaries and gross pathology of the aorta, but no conspicuous pathology of the myocardium was reported. However, the description of the clinical features was extraordinarily well done. In proposing the new name 'Syncope Anginosa', along with clinical signs of collapse, Parry revived the old notion of the 'lipothymia' and, on the other hand, came nearer to the later notion of myocardial infarction. These ideas of the vital importance of the coronary circulation were extended by Allan Burns in his book *Observations on Diseases of the Heart* (1809). Burns added more material to the differentiation of the consecutive stages of the disease: the early stage without dyspnoea, and the terminal outcome, often, but not necessarily, connected with heart failure. Moreover, he promoted the ischaemic theory by experimental ligation of the limbs and he inserted a chapter on consequences resulting from change in the structure of the substance of the heart, without,

---

[1] Pp. 3–5, letter by Jenner.

however, progressing to a notion of infarction of this organ, again for lack of conceptual support yet to come.

During the early part of the nineteenth century the coronary theory of the disease, so vigorously expounded by the British school late in the eighteenth century, gained widespread, but not unanimous, international acknowledgment. This theory, although the best to explain the disease, when taken too literally, did not always prove satisfactory. Some autopsies, for instance, failed to demonstrate 'ossification' or any other gross changes of the coronaries in persons who had suffered from angina. On the other hand, ossification was sometimes found without a clinical history of angina pectoris. An early criticism was expressed by J. Warren (1812). With 'no intention of controverting the principal doctrine of Dr. Parry', Warren felt that the ossification theory is 'apt to simplify too much'. From its inception angina pectoris was regarded as a disease not too easy to explain; hence Heberden's wording: '*Some* account', 'peculiar symptoms'.

This state of affairs in the struggle to understand the anginal syndrome called for a new ally which was found in the concept of arteriosclerosis (Scarpa, 1804; Lobstein, 1833). In his *Sull' Aneurisma*, a large but slim folio, Scarpa produced fine illustrations, based on dissection, giving evidence of a process now named atherosclerosis. His explanation is cautious and lucid: '. . . especially the internal coat is subject, from slow internal cause, to an ulcerated and steatomatous disorganization, as well as to a squamous and earthy rigidity and brittleness' (translation by Wishart, 1819). Scarpa refers to 'cases of ulcerated corrosions of the heart,' again 'from internal unknown causes'. Even now, in spite of the progress in clinical, pathological, and biochemical research, the last cause is not firmly established. With Scarpa the concept of arteriosclerosis was introduced, later to become the ruling principle in the practice and research of coronary artery disease.

On the other hand it was Lobstein who coined the name arteriosclerosis, which he described in a brief chapter of the second and last volume of his *Traité d'Anatomie pathologique*. Lobstein gives credit to, and amplifies, Scarpa's findings. The concomitant processes of hardening and softening, which in modern medicine eventually provoked a preferential use of the word atherosclerosis, are clearly implicated in the old descriptions of ossification and 'atheroma' of the arteries and in Scarpa's report. However, Lobstein seems to be more explicit when he devotes a special chapter to 'arteriomalacia'. He was an eager namegiver, using Greek and Latin roots as more likely to be perpetuated than the vernacular. This is evidenced from his 'cardiomalacia', a name which was revived at the end of the nineteenth century by Ziegler (myomalacia cordis, 1881). The finding was referred to as 'ramollisse-ment de la substance musculaire du coeur' by Laënnec who even mentioned the yellow colour, now understood as necrosis[2] while Sénac and many previous authors mentioned only softening.

Thus the pathological notion of arteriosclerosis was born. Both Scarpa and Lobstein understood that this is a process of its own, not connected with the old notion of inflammation, but arising from a 'slow internal cause', and being a result of an 'abnormal state of nutrition' of the tissues (Lobstein, II, 1078). The tissues involved were the coats of the arteries, where concomitant hardening and softening led to their destruction and the beginning of clot formation. Again this concept was soon forgotten. Even Rudolf Virchow, the greatest contributor to the notion of thrombosis, did not expressly stress the concept of arteriosclerosis as an autonomic non-inflammatory entity and called the condition 'chronic endarteritis deformans' in his paper 'The atheromatous process of the arteries' (1856).

It is hardly possible to overrate Virchow's great contribution to the concept and study of thrombosis. His publications began in 1846 when he described a clot in the pulmonary artery. He referred repeatedly to this item at great length. Virchow coined the name after an old Galenic pattern.[3] Clotted blood was also called *thrombus* from the Greek, by Caelius Aurelianus.[4] The classic usage did not, however, exclusively involve localization of the obstruction in a vessel. The contemporary usage was introduced by Virchow, along with the concept of embolization. However, the mechanism as described in the cases of pulmonary embolism, often arising from a thrombus in a large vein of the leg and its being carried to the right heart, has no features common with coronary thrombosis. Virchow was a very industrious writer; his bibliography (1843–1901) fills a volume of 183 pages. However, the index does not list myocardial infarction. In his numer-ous publications one can find only scattered information on it or on allied subjects. It seems that Virchow was not much interested in coronary artery disease, but his concept of thrombosis gave the start to further developments in this field of cardiac pathology.

Experimental studies of coronary function began as early as 1698 when Chirac reported the tying-off of these vessels in a dog, thus

[2] *De l'Auscultation*, 2nd ed. 1826, vol. II, 533–43.
[3] E.g. Kühn VII, 726; XVIIIB, 496.
[4] Drabkin, 573.

producing cardiac arrest. This was an isolated and primitive experiment. The ligation effects were then studied with greater refinement during the nineteenth century by Erichsen (1842), Panum (1862), Bezold (1867), and others, the most conspicuous study of this kind being that by Cohnheim (1881). This pathologist clearly stated that many conditions, such as the so-called 'fibrous myocarditis' or 'heart aneurysm' are due to coronary obstruction and that oxygen lack is responsible for the myocardial damage. However, it seems that he too did not pay much attention to myocardial infarction proper as a precise clinico-pathological entity. One of his contributions to the problem rested on his view that a myocardial disturbance may exist *intra vitam*, even when *post mortem* findings are non-conclusive. Cohnheim's error of describing the coronary arteries as 'end-arteries'—*Endarterien*—which in the event of obstruction could receive no help from anastomosing branches, was soon corrected by other investigators. They found out that a collateral circulation does exist; the greatest help and solace to the victims of myocardial infarction.

Almost at the same time (1880) Weigert described the classical signs of myocardial infarction, both its gross and microscopic pathology. He seems to have been the first to note the loss of nuclei in the infarcted area, but in a general description of myocardial necrosis he was preceded by the Swedish pathologist Düben (1859) who anatomized Malmsten's case. Again Huber (1882) added quite a number of dissections, thus implying that 'the influence of coronary disease on the heart' was no longer a rare occurrence.

On the clinical side of the arena stood keen physicians who added their observations bearing on many of the later-accepted features of myocardial infarction. According to the nineteenth-century practice, these observations were backed by more or less adequate post-mortem findings. Latham's case (1846) of Thomas Arnold is a full-fledged description of a rapidly recurring and ultimately lethal coronary event, even when the autopsy is not elaborate, and only 'softening' of the heart-muscle is reported. Malmsten–Düben's (1859) report is less spectacular clinically, but is a masterpiece of pathological description. Hammer's (1878) is bold and forceful from the inception, the title being 'A Case of thrombotic occlusion of one of the coronary arteries'. The case is remarkable in spite of later doubts whether this was in fact a manifestation of coronary disease (W. Dock, 1962). Finally came Leyden's (1884) detailed and balanced paper. More than any other clinician of the period preceding the diagnostic acceptance of myocardial infarction, Leyden came nearest to the goal. However, even

his paper ('On sclerosis of the coronary arteries and the morbid conditions dependent on it') failed to give a final touch to the diagnosis
of myocardial infarction, to which he often referred, without distinguishing it from the rich additional content of the paper. In fact
Leyden was able to outline different types of anatomical lesions:

1. Coronary sclerosis without heart pathology;
2. Acute thrombotic softening or haemorrhagic infarction;
3. Chronic fibrous degeneration of the myocardium; and
4. Combined forms of old fibrotic changes with acute recent softening.

The clinical types he established were: acute, with sudden death;
sub-acute with repeated thrombotic events, often relieved by collateral
blood supply; and chronic, with later appearance of congestive heart
failure, reminding us of the earlier description given by Parry in
1799.

The end of the nineteenth century saw a great deal of publication
on almost every kind of coronary disease. Medical theses on this
subject, mostly French, were painstakingly scrutinized and abstracted
by Huchard in his famous textbook (3 volumes, 2168 pages in the 3rd
edition). The second volume is very rich in historical information,
the last chapter containing 185 case-reports, beginning with the
year 1703 and ending in 1899. Huchard supports vigorously the
coronary theory, and in this chapter all references to the coronaries
have been italicized, but not those concerning the myocardium. The
doctoral thesis by R. Marie, *L'Infarctus du Myocarde et ses Conséquences*,
in 1896, must be singled out for its completeness and exclusive adherence to the topic. Finally, Dock's publication of 1896 is a classic
description of myocardial infarction both clinically and anatomically,
case IV having been correctly diagnosed during the life of the patient.
These are a few of the highlights in the recognition of coronary artery
disease with myocardial changes. The medical profession at large was,
however, not yet prepared to accept and absorb these discoveries
which ultimately led to the diagnosis of myocardial infarction.

Looking back to the main trends during the nineteenth century, it
appears that research in cardiac pathology was instrumental in producing a gradual shift of interest from the coronary vessels to the
myocardium. In this changed atmosphere many of the facets of myocardial infarction were detected. This movement was also felt in the
clinical approach, as evidenced by beautiful and striking descriptions.
It is true that nobody dared to give the diagnosis the required promi-
nence until the beginning of the twentieth century. However, a

diagnosis of 'angina pectoris' seemed no longer comprehensive, and Osler's small book on the subject had therefore the amplified title: *Lectures on Angina pectoris and Allied States* (1897). In a later publication (1910) Osler introduced a small chapter with a caption 'Pipes and Pump'. Though used by him in another context, this chapter shows an increased interest in the 'pump' (myocardium), *versus* the 'pipes' (coronaries), the latter having been already fully discussed during the later part of the eighteenth century. In fact, the notion of an impairment in the 'very substance of the heart' is of ancient Galenic origin. Much of the newer knowledge about myocardial infarction was brought together in the nineteenth century. Herrick, one of the modern scholars to substantiate this knowledge, wrote (1942, p. 229) of it in his modesty: 'these facts had been written about before. They had to be rediscovered'. This is obviously going somewhat too far, but it was probably dictated by Herrick's historical awareness.

From the facts already presented and discussed it becomes clear that long before Obrastzow and Straschesko (1910) and Herrick (1912) published their papers, a vast amount of material had been accumulated. On the other hand, they deserve the credit given to them for having initiated the definitive understanding of cardiac infarction as a clinically recognizable morbid entity, which was later acknowledged to be a very common condition and of paramount statistical importance. These papers no longer call the condition 'angina pectoris', but 'thrombosis and obstruction of the coronaries'. The clinical features they described are decidedly incomplete, but the general aim at the recognition of coronary thrombosis with induced damage to the myocardium is explicit. This was a decisive step towards the terminological differentiation of myocardial infarction from the old notion of angina pectoris, a disease which might or might not precede the myocardial event.

Indeed, the best clinicians about the year 1900 did not usually separate these two entities. Osler in his informative and beautiful book on the subject (1897) could not avoid reference to numerous cases of coronary thrombosis (p. 12); he includes most of his cases of 'angina vera' and a full reproduction (pp. 34–36) of Latham's case 1846 (*vide supra*). He quoted previous authors to the effect that there are attacks without pain (pp. 68, 74) and quoted a passage: 'These which have lost the title to the name angina have an equally serious significance'. Indeed Osler was aware of the significance of the myocardial lesion in coronary diseases, yet he was reluctant to place the infarction of the heart into a separate section of his system. His Lumleian Lectures (1910), in which he returned to the subject of angina pectoris, is again a very learned, warm and clever exposition, but the clinical picture of coronary thrombosis is not too clear, though he does mention very briefly that 'blocking of a [coronary] branch with a fresh thrombus is very common in cases of sudden death in angina'.

Huchard's section on 'Maladies des coronaires' (*vide supra*) is very detailed (259 pages in the third edition, 1899) and is also full of important facts pointing to muscular damage in the heart. Not inclined to create a nosological entity for this kind of disease, he is more precise in his brief conclusions (pp. 132–34). There he discusses only two of the eighty [*sic*] theories of angina pectoris: (1) arterial coronary disease with myocardial ischaemia; (2) 'Cardiodynie' with anginal pain only.

This was the last rank, next in time to Obrastzow (for brevity named alone as senior author) and Herrick, on the long march of the researchers into the essence of coronary thrombosis and myocardial infarction. In fact it is thrilling to learn how much had been already brought to light. Neither Obrastzow nor Herrick are 'discoverers' of the clinical picture of acute coronary thrombosis and they did not make such claims. The former listed quite extensively his predecessors, and so too did Herrick, who quoted many of them, including Obrastzow. What distinguishes them from their immediate forerunners is their way of approach: explicit, definitive and unreserved in expression, and free from obscurity of meaning. In contrast, most of the best clinicians immediately preceding them only implied the diagnosis of coronary thrombosis, the notion being contained in the mind, without being clearly formulated. We now read both these papers as classics, but they evoked no response for years. Much later, Herrick, referring to his paper of 1912, commented: 'When it was presented it was discussed by only one person, there was no repercussion for six years. It had fallen like a dud'. We may add that even later the repercussion was limited to a small group of researchers while the general acceptance in medical practice came only in the 1930s. In spite of this late recognition, many excellent papers continued to appear and the leaders of the profession were cognizant of the diagnosis. This was the situation, e.g. in the case of the medical appraisal of James Mackenzie's disease and death from myocardial infarction in January 1925, when Sir Thomas Lewis' comment was given in terms quite up-to-date and with full consideration of the myocardial damage.

It took some time not only for the clinical diagnosis to be largely accepted, but also for the more favourable prognostication. Thrombosis of the coronary arteries was no longer only a concern of the pathologists, or a problem of clinical diagnosis in immediately fatal cases

(Osler, Krehl's 'Sekunden-Tod'). It is appropriate to quote D. Evan Bedford, who himself largely contributed to this knowledge. Writing in 1933 he stated:

> 'The knowledge that coronary thrombosis is often compatible with life and even health, and that it can be recognized during life with certainty in many cases, has only come to us during the last twenty years'.

It might be added that the knowledge became more widespread at the very end of this time-span (P. D. White). In fact the estimation of a more recent author is that only one of four or five people with acute myocardial infarction dies immediately (W. B. Bean, 1962).

It can be accepted that before the early 1920s the knowledge of coronary artery disease including myocardial infarction became firmly established. However, only a few particularly interested physicians were able to venture on diagnosis and properly evaluate their cases. The situation changed with the advent of electro-cardiographic studies.

While the first period of clinical electrocardiography was chiefly covered by studies of disorders of the heartbeat, already in 1919 a tracing from a patient with myocardial infarction was published by Herrick. These years between the second and third decade were very fruitful: 1918, Bousfield's first electrocardiographic record, obtained before and after an episode of angina pectoris in a man, and Fred Smith's tracings after ligation of the coronary arteries in dogs; 1919, Herrick's quoted case; 1920, Pardee's classical demonstration with the coved RS-T segment. This was the beginning of further progress, to the point where not only the presence of infarction, but also its magnitude and localization could be assessed. Owing to accumulated knowledge and experience, the medical profession became aware of the high incidence of the disease. Its manifestations were studied until finally it could be diagnosed or at least suggested even before taking an electrocardiogram. The instruments became gradually simplified, easier to handle and smaller, though the original tracings by Einthoven are even now unsurpassed. The first commercially-produced Einthoven string electrocardiograph was released in 1908. According to a recent authority its weight in 1914 was 188 pounds, which was reduced to only 7 pounds in 1938. The ubiquity, relatively low price, and portability (since 1928) of the instrument resulted in its indiscriminate use, a fact that became rightly disquieting for the specialist who is often called upon to give a competent interpretation of the tracings for the benefit and often for the reassurance of the patient. Moreover, it became apparent that the method is only one of the ways to a correct diagnosis and cannot be a substitute for a balanced clinical judgement.

Additional diagnostic help came from the laboratory. The blood-count in cases of myocardial infarction is useful since the number of the white cells in the peripheral blood is often increased, mostly very soon after the event. It seems that Libman was the first to draw attention to this laboratory aid (1916). This phenomenon was even more obvious in one of the early cases communicated by S. A. Levine (1918), where the leucocytes reached the unusual figure of 33,500.

In the same manner a raised erythrocyte sedimentation rate of the blood, beginning later after the attack than the leucocytosis but persisting much longer, can be of importance as an adjunct to diagnosis. It may serve as well as an aid to prognosis, a subsequent fall in the rapidity of the sedimentation often indicating improvement or recovery. This test was first applied to the evaluation of myocardial infarction in 1933 by G. Scherk. In general medicine this quick and simple test had long been extensively used in continental Europe, but was adopted only later in England and the United States of America.

Again, since 1954 the determination of the transaminase in a blood specimen, introduced by La Due and Wroblewski, became an important diagnostic criterion. The serum glutamic oxalo-acetic transaminase increases after acute transmural myocardial infarction, often twelve hours after the event, and returns to normal after some days.

The tendency to strengthen the diagnosis by quantitative data led physicians to pay attention to the often raised body temperature and to the fall of blood pressure. Fever, usually moderate, in acute coronary thrombosis was noted in 1916 (Libman), though Kernig had described it in 1905 in cases of so-called 'status anginosus'. The lowered arterial tension in cardiac infarcts seems to have been known since 1895 (quoted by R. Marie), though it was not always referred to in the earlier classic descriptions. Both fever and lower blood pressure may be absent in some cases of myocardial infarction, but generally they do occur, thus supporting the diagnosis.

Our task will now be to describe in detail the evolution of medical knowledge with regard to coronary heart disease from antiquity to modern times. Much of the information obtained from old sources will necessarily be fragmentary: often merely a symptom, a reference to an anatomical structure, or an example of sound reasoning. On the other hand, striking evidence of signs and symptoms of ischaemic heart disease will be found at remote periods when few facts, methods, and concepts had yet made their appearance.

CHAPTER II

Antiquity and the Middle Ages

1. ANCIENT EGYPT

(a) Pathological evidence

THIS phase of medical civilization is singled out for the wealth of non-literary material preserved in the mummies. Accordingly, palaeopathology[1] has been able to delineate some of the diseases of Ancient Egypt with a good deal of accuracy. It has used inspection, histology, chemistry, X-rays, and, more recently, stain technology and electron microscopy (Leeson, 1959). Only the morbid changes of the heart and the vessels will be here mentioned and, as far as possible, the findings will be critically evaluated.

The first author to describe calcification of the aorta in a mummy was J. N. Czermak (1852), who was at the time a young assistant at the Physiological Institute in Prague. His paper is constantly referred to in historical surveys; in 42 pages he gives a description and a microscopical examination of two Egyptian mummies. It is worth reading, for the author conveys his emotional reaction to his handling a pathological specimen of such great antiquity. The first mummy was of a boy 15 years of age; the other of an elderly woman. Her heart and lungs had been taken out (p. 443). The aortic arch was in its place, the aorta having been cut near the heart (p. 444). The more detailed description by Czermak comprises: skin, nails, hair, fibrous and elastic tissues, cartilage, bones, teeth and muscles. The vessels are treated rather sketchily and the only relevant phrases bearing on our topic are:

> 'The anterior wall of the descending part of the aortic arch contained several, not inconspicuous, calcareous deposits. These pathological products, along with the other characteristics of the body, testify to the advanced age of this female' (p. 463).

The paper contains a table (No. 36 of the volume) with 13 illustrations, but unfortunately none of them depicts the vessels. A more detailed investigation into vascular pathology was not undertaken by Czermak,

---

[1] See also S. Jarcho, ed., *Human Paleopathology* (1966).

3

nor was the time ripe for such an attempt, despite promising beginnings which were not yet generally accepted by physicians.

After this publication, anatomical research into vascular changes in mummies suffered quite a long intermission. The more easily performed examination of the bones, greatly helped by X-rays, and the spectacular findings of communicable disease (bilharzia, 1910) came more to the fore. Then, in 1909, came a more detailed paper by S. G. Shattock, which was also abstracted in the weekly journals. It bore upon the pathological condition of the aorta of King Merneptah, a famous Pharaoh. His mummy had been unwrapped in 1907 by G. Elliot Smith, whose contributions to Egyptian palaeopathology are well known (1912, 1924). Smith mentioned that 'the aorta was affected with severe atheromatous disease, large calcified patches being distinctly visible'. He sent a specimen for histological examination to London, and this came into the hands of S. G. Shattock, then President of the Pathological Section of the Royal Society of Medicine.

His report, summarized, is: The piece of aorta examined is 3 cm in length. Gross anatomy: a slightly curved calcareous plate 6 mm in diameter, which lies in the deeper part of the internal and muscular coat. Microscopically (p. 126): extensive groups of particles of calcium phosphate are deposited in the intralamellar substance. The illustration of the microscopical appearance in the mummy (Fig. 1) has been placed opposite a modern section of the aorta of a man aged 79 (in Fig. 2) in order to stress the similarity of both findings. Shattock's methods of examination were: (1) unstained; (2) treatment with hydrochloric acid; (3) with Ehrlich's Haematoxylin and Eosin; and (4) with Carbol Thionine.

The pathology and nomenclature of arterial sclerosis underwent some changes during the period 1909–31, but the fact of its existence in Egyptian mummies, and also in those from Peru, is established without doubt. Sir Marc Ruffer (1911) was able to bring much additional evidence. His *Studies in the Palaeopathology of Egypt*, posthumously collected and edited in 1921, contain an observation which is worth quoting (p. 27):

> 'In one subclavian artery of the 18th–20th dynasties the lumen of the artery near its origin was almost blocked by a ragged calcareous excrescence, depicted in Plate III, Fig. 5. There can be no doubt that this person narrowly escaped embolism (calcified atheromatous ulcer).'

Ruffer's paper 'On arterial lesions found in Egyptian mummies' (1911) is very informative. Most of the preparations came from a number of arms and legs from broken-up mummies which were of no possible use as museum specimens. They were mutilated by the embalmer, but the posterior peroneal artery, owing to its deep situation, often escaped the embalmer's knife. After fully describing his technique for restoring the dry and brittle material, Ruffer reported twenty-four dissections of arteries. The findings were: complete and incomplete calcification (after decalcification and staining one sees shreds of endothelium), degeneration of the muscular coats, the above-mentioned atheroma of the left subclavian artery, and numerous patches non-calcified. According to recent information (Pickering, 1964), the pathogenesis of arteriosclerosis is basically connected with intimal changes in the arteries, and these alone lead to thrombus formation. The rigid 'bony' tubes which Ruffer mentioned with regard to the appearance of the pelvic arteries do not indicate a possibility of a thrombotic outcome. It is not the place here to enlarge upon details of thrombotic disease, this being deferred to a later chapter, where due credit will be given to a fact, hitherto unmentioned, that the stress on the significance of the inner coat (the intima) in the pathogenesis of degenerative arterial disease must be credited to Scarpa (1804) in his work on aneurysms. Keeping in mind the crucial importance of the degeneration of the intima in particular, which is the anatomical basis of 'atheroma', it seems that in Ruffer's classic paper atheroma was not fully proved and depicted, and his repeated emphasis on the similarity to the lesions 'of the present time' was not fully substantiated.

Calcification of the leg arteries was also demonstrated and depicted by Ruffer; later, in 1931, R. L. Moodie was able to visualize these calcified arteries by X-rays of unwrapped mummies. Tortuous, calcareous temporal artieries were also mentioned (G. Elliot Smith in his *Royal Mummies*, 1912). Degenerative arterial changes were observed also in a Peruvian mummy; the thickening of the intima, together with a calcified thrombus, was described by H. U. Williams in 1927.

However, changes of the coronary arteries proper in a mummy were recorded only once, when A. R. Long (1931) 'was fortunate enough to examine the coronaries in one case,' as A. T. Sandison (1962) put it. This was indeed a very fortunate occasion not met with by earlier or later pathologists, who worked on the aorta and peripheral arteries of mummies but never succeeded in examining a coronary vessel or found a myocardium with even slight signs of coronary heart disease. It seems worth while to summarize Long's concise and well-illustrated paper.

The organs of seven Egyptian mummies were offered by the Metropolitan Museum of Art, New York, to the laboratory of the Department of Pathology of the University of Buffalo School of Medicine. A disease of a female mummy, about fifty years old, of the 21st dynasty (about 1000 B.C.) is here described. The heart was reduced to about the size of a hen's egg, not much thicker than an eggshell and much more fragile. The mitral valve showed a small calcified mass on one leaflet indicating old endocarditis. The coronary arteries showed well marked fibrous thickening, chiefly of the intima, with calcification. There were areas of fibrous tissue in the cardiac muscle, like small scars. The aorta showed moderate nodular arteriosclerosis. Other findings were: pneumokoniosis, few areas of caseation, many glomeruli of the kidney, fibrous, thick capsule and sclerosis of the medium-sized arteries.

The importance of Long's paper rests upon the fact that for the first time in the pathological examination of mummified material the degenerative process was demonstrated in a coronary artery (see photograph in Long's paper). Likewise, the fibrous areas in the myocardium point to an older stage of small coronary obstruction with replacement of parts of the heart muscle by fibrous tissue. This histological finding, so often described by pathologists of the late nineteenth century, led clinicians of the time to the wrong diagnosis of 'chronic myocarditis', later to be known as a manifestation of ischaemic heart disease. The concomitant occurrence, in Long's mummy, of lung and kidney pathology together with coronary findings does not detract from the historical significance of the latter.

One may wonder why coronary pathology in mummies was not recorded earlier. A tentative explanation may be found in the lack of interest in coronary disease prevailing around the year 1910. If an interest in it had existed, the early investigators (especially Ruffer) with their good connections would probably have succeeded in procuring specimens for a pathological examination of the coronaries. Nowadays this is not easy to achieve, though many mummies are lying in the cellars of the great museums (Sandison, 1962).

The pathological studies in mummies after 1931 suffered again a longer interruption, on which H. E. Sigerist (1951) made some comments. They were, however, revived when Sandison, after 1951, took up these studies vigorously. He has utilized modern technical methods and shown good preservation of certain tissues. His own examinations of arteries (1955, 1957, 1959, and 1962) describe and beautifully depict atheroma with lipid deposits, reduplication of the internal elastic lamina, and medial calcification. His paper (1962) on degenerative vascular disease in the Egyptian mummy serves best the needs of a critical evaluation from a pathological point of view.

As to the future of these researches, much will depend upon the pathologists' interest and the availability of material. Dried bodies without embalming were often also well preserved, like those found in Peru. For some time assertions were made that in Egyptian mummies the heart was taken out by the embalmer and often preserved in a special jar (e.g. E. A. Wallis Budge, 1899). However, most of the authorities are quite certain that the heart remained *in situ* (G. E. Smith and others). Sometimes the heart was removed in error, since it is no easy matter to remove the right lung through a left abdominal incision (J. Thompson Rowling, 1961). Accordingly, hearts and coronaries can, theoretically, be examined in the future. The mummies should be screened in advance for presence of degenerative disease, and those which yield some prospect could be searched for evidence of coronary disease.

(b) Literary Sources

The medical historian in trying to trace some allusion to ischaemic heart disease in ancient Egyptian writings must overcome difficulties of a linguistic, formal and methodological nature. The fascinating story of the deciphering of the hieroglyphs (sacred carvings) begins with Young's early attempts, followed in 1822 by Champollion's discovery of the key to Egyptian writing and has often been told.

Our task here is a presentation of those facts and ideas as found in the ancient Egyptian writings which have some bearing on coronary heart disease. Not only symptoms and signs which may point specifically to precordial pain or an eventual fatal outcome of the disease will be taken into account; even more interesting is the idea of some kind of obstruction, though not as a finding of morbid anatomy, which did not exist as such in this ancient civilization. The idea of obstruction will later on be one of the leading points in the appraisal of Greek, medieval and Renaissance medicine in relation to our topic. In ancient Egypt, and also in some later periods, this idea of obstruction emerges in the form of reasoning and hypothesis and was not necessarily based on actual inspection of dead bodies. Perhaps one exception in an ancient civilization can be conceded, and this is to Talmudic medicine, where obstruction (e.g. atum ba-rëah = imperviousness to the passage of air in the lung) was actually observed at the ritual inspection and autopsy of slaughtered animals.

Before embarking on an analysis of the texts, a word should be said about the different editions. The historian of medicine when himself not an Egyptologist would not dare to discuss controversial points of translation. However, we feel ourselves on the safe side if we refer only to those passages which, in the available translations, show but minor variations.

The most important source of information is of course the famous Ebers papyrus. During the winter of 1872–73, G. Ebers spent several months with L. Stern in Thebes and was fortunate enough to buy the manuscript. Stern remained in Cairo where he served as librarian to the Khedive, but participated in the edition (1875) by composing the second volume, which is a hieroglyphic glossary in Latin. The papyrus was later given by Ebers to the Leipzig University Library. It is the most substantial Egyptian medical papyrus found so far, being 30 cm high and 20.23 metres long; the text is divided into pages, numbered at the top. The pagination totals 110, but numbers 28 and 29 are missing without interruption of the text's continuity. In his preface Ebers assumes, on circumstantial evidence, that it had been written in the year 1552 B.C. However the text must be older, being a therapeutical compendium from an earlier manuscript, as is evident from the occasional remark by the scribe: 'found damaged'. The splendid edition contains a facsimile reproduction of the original in hieratic script, which is a cursive form of the hieroglyphic. The text has been translated into German; however, this version is not a continuous one, as Ebers finds it necessary to stress on page iii of the preface. The concise introduction by Ebers does not fail to emphasize the difficulties. For our purpose the remark that the same word may mean at one point the stomach, and at another the heart, as it also does in Coptic, is of some importance. This double meaning occurs also in ancient Greek texts, as already briefly mentioned in our introduction.

In 1890 H. Joachim translated the Ebers papyrus into German, this time producing a full, consecutive version. Joachim was a practising physician and was prepared to venture upon a medical interpretation. It is remarkable that he was able to teach himself the Egyptian language, so far as the early stage of Egyptology made it possible. Though censured by later specialists, Joachim's more handy volume gives a convenient access to the text, always with the need to check the translation against more modern renderings. Joachim was bold enough to use the word 'heart' whenever it seemed to him appropriate, while some later and more competent scholars adhere always to the word 'cardia', even when they admit in the commentary that the significance of the symptoms is connected with the heart.

From this German version C. P. Bryan produced, in 1930, his volume, *The Papyrus Ebers*, the first version in English. It is not consecutive, but arranged in chapters, among them one on the heart. The quotations do not refer to the pagination of the original Ebers edition. The volume is prefaced by an important introduction by G. Elliot Smith, who speaks of Bryan's book as belonging to 'works of popularization'.

J. H. Breasted's great and scholarly edition, in 1930, of the Edwin Smith Surgical Papyrus does not, strictly speaking, belong to our survey. It should, however, be mentioned here, since the only passage which has some bearing on our topic is repeated in the Ebers papyrus almost word for word. It is a passage suggestive of some kind of counting the pulse (Breasted, p. 430, a parallel to Ebers, page or column 99 of the original papyrus). In this edition Breasted incorporated a very long commentary (pp. 104–14) on this passage, not avoiding exaggeration as to a presumed knowledge of the circulation of the blood; these have been recently commented upon, with all due respect, in a paper by the Egyptologist John A. Wilson (1962). As this important passage does not bear on symptoms of disease and is not to be discussed later, it will be reproduced here, using Wilson's (ibid., p. 120) recent English translation. For the sake of brevity the quotation is shortened:

> 'When any physician . . . puts his hands or fingers upon the head . . . upon the hands . . . upon the seat of the heart . . . he is examining for the heart . . . it speaks throughout the vessels of every part of the body.'

In 1937 B. Ebbell, a provincial physician in Norway, produced the only consecutive translation of the Ebers Papyrus in English. It is arranged in a scholarly manner and the beginnings of the pages of the original text are marked by large Roman numerals in the margins. This arrangement facilitates the checking of the translation against the later editions, especially that by the Grapow school. The translation has been rightly censured by O. Temkin (1938) for many errors. H. Grapow's criticism has been expressed quite often, e.g. in the 'Grundriss', 1955, pp. 89, 92. Fortunately, those passages suggesting coronary disease have been free from later criticism and the translation of this source material has been approved. The attempts at diagnoses in Ebbell's edition are incorporated in short footnotes rather than in plethoric commentaries; they can be accepted or rejected by critical students of the ancient text.

The most recent, competent and critical arrangement of the source material has been given by H. Grapow and his school. The publication began in 1954 under the title *Grundriss der Medizin der alten Aegypter* (Outline of Medicine of the Ancient Egyptians), of which eight volumes or parts have now been issued. The Papyrus Ebers has not been consecutively translated, as the *Grundriss* covers the whole of ancient Egyptian medicine and does not contain editions of single manuscripts. The pertinent material can be looked up under the headings Heart and Vessels, and more specifically, under Stomach-Heart, in Volume IV (1958), 1 (texts) and 2 (explanations), both parts being a joint publication by H. V. Deines, H. Grapow and W. Westendorf.

Our first quotation is from the Papyrus Ebers (p. 37, and repeated on p. 38) which is highly suggestive of the precordial pain syndrome. As early as 1875 Ebers, on page v of his introduction, proposed his interpretation. Ebbell was sure of the diagnosis Angina pectoris, and even the very cautious editors (1958) of the Grapow school (vol. IV 2, p. 84) supported this diagnosis. This is the text:

> 'When you examine a man for illness in his cardia, he has pains in his arm, in his breast, on the side of his cardia; it is said thereof: this is the w3d-illness. Then you shall say thereof: it is something which entered his mouth; it is death which approaches him. Then you shall prepare for him stimulating herbal remedies: fruits of pea, bryony [and other vegetable remedies]; let them be boiled in fat [Ebers 38: in beer] and be drunk by the man.
>
> Put then your bended hand on him, until the arm gets well and free of pains. Then you shall say: this illness has descended to the rectum, to the anus.
>
> The remedy shall not thence be repeated.'

It seems not unreasonable to find in this text features and elements of Heberden's 'angina'. As already mentioned several times, cardia or stomach stands for heart, as in the other medical sources of bygone civilizations. Pains (*Grundriss*: 'suffers') in the arm and sensations in the left side of the breast, and the death threatening the patient are clearly outlined. The disease has the character of an attack: 'until the arm gets well'. The remedies are difficult to explain on pharmacological grounds; the beer prescribed as a vehicle for the herbs only remotely recalls the wine prescribed in Heberden's classical account. The supposed connection between a cardiac condition and the rectum is typical of Egyptian medicine; 'the illness [which entered his mouth] has descended to the rectum, to the anus' is a notion of elimination of noxious substances. F. Jonckheere also refers to the 'coexistence of an anal happening with cardiac disturbances' (1947, p. 54) in his edition of the Chester Beatty Papyrus on the diseases of the anus. The last phrase that 'the remedy shall not be repeated' is probably intended to stress its efficacy; this would be in conformity with other concluding formulas as: 'so he will be soon healed' (e.g. Ebers 37, 4; 38, 10 and many more).

The Ebers Papyrus, besides containing incantations, is basically a compilation of remedies, made by a professional scribe, not a physician (cf. *Grundriss*, Vol. II, p. 95); more or less coherent descriptions of disease as in the quoted passage are very rare. We have, therefore, to proceed as with a mosaic: small pieces of sentences and expressions may then reveal the amassed information. Most of the data on the heart and the vessels are to be found in the glosses, beginning on page 99 of the Ebers Papyrus. They are very brief, additional remarks to diagnosis, or explanations of words:

> 'As to: his heart is darkened, he tastes his heart; this means that his heart is constricted and there is darkness in his belly . . .; he produces states of faintness' (Eb. 102, 9–11).
>
> '. . . the heart is hot from burning as a man who is tormented by a biting insect' (Eb. 101–102).
>
> 'As to: the kneeling position of the heart; this means that his heart is tied up (101); that the heart assumes the kneeling position because of pain-producing-matter.'
>
> '. . . the heart is inundated' (Eb. 99).
>
> 'As to: the heart is tired; this means that the heart does not speak or the vessels of the heart are mute. Nor are their statements apparent under both your hands, which are due to air [pneuma] which fills them' (Eb. 100).
>
> 'As to: his heart is widened; this means that the vessels of the heart contain faeces' (Eb. 100).
>
> 'Forgetfulness of the heart' [Adams-Stokes?] (Eb. 102).
>
> 'As to: A round mass has fallen on his heart; this means that a ball of tȝw-heat has fallen on his heart. This is a frequent weakness. This means that he faints. The filling of his heart with blood, this is what does it' (Eb. 102).

So the individual elements of this mosaic, such as precordial pain, oppression, and heaviness; and also some indication of collapse or fainting, which is connected with a diseased state of the heart or the vessels, are denoted in this ancient Egyptian source.

When we turn to one of the underlying medical theories in these ancient texts some notion of impediment and occlusion becomes apparent. The word šn< has indeed this meaning. The dictionary (*Grundriss*, VII 2, 1962) lists this word beginning with page 859. To quote one of the entries:

> p. 860, 2, 'all mentioned parts of the body in which ob-
> struction may occur, possess channels for drainage; the word
> always refers to a stoppage in the canalisation system of the body;
> i.e. the draining of faeces, of blood or of other matter is impeded.'

Since faeces were regarded as a paradigm of obstruction, it is possible that the 'descending' of the suffering in Eb. 37 to the anus was an expression also for an improvement in the vascular system.

Another word whdw, which is translated in the dictionary (VII, 1, pp. 207–217) as 'Schmerzstoffe', has often been commented upon, especially by R. O. Steuer (1948, 1959) and J. B. de C. M. Saunders (1963, p. 27). It has been explained as the noxious agent entering the vascular system, leading to putrefaction or to coagulation of the blood. This is a difficult problem, but reduced to a few more easily-under-standable examples, the assumption of some vascular occlusion is a part of the theoretical substructure which can be perceived in ancient Egyptian medical writings.

Actual observations are also of some interest: the vessels become hardened, and there are remedies against the condition (e.g. Eb. 81, 7–10). Or: local swelling, a vascular tumour ('due to wounding the vessel'), probably aneurysm, with the advice of 'knife-treatment' (surgery) (Eb. 108, 3–9); or varices (Eb. 108). At the same time there exist, as we have just mentioned, concepts and ideas not based on observation but on reasoning, as for instance that vessels contain faeces, a substance which, when not eliminated from the body, causes disease. Along with our previous discussion, this shows again that the concept of obstruction in the blood vessels is found in ancient Egyptian medicine.

As to possible pictorial representations of coronary death in ancient Egyptian art, an interesting example has been discussed by W. L. Bruetsch.[2] His subject is the relief of a tomb from the Sixth Dynasty (2625–2475 B.C.) illustrated with a balanced and detailed explanation by von Bissing.[3] There seems to be no proof of the supposition that the relief can be interpreted as a representation of death due to coronary occlusion, since any other cause of sudden death might likewise be implied. Nor did von Bissing suggest any connection with heart disease.

---

[2] 'The earliest record of sudden death possibly due to atherosclerotic coronary occlusion', *Circulation*, 1959, **20**, 438–41.

[3] F. W. von Bissing, *Denkmäler ägyptischer Sculptur*, Munich, 1914 (Plate No. 18B).

2. ANCIENT GREECE AND ROME

This period of about one thousand years abounds in literary medical sources which have been scrutinized by generations of medical historians and philologists. The extensive medical literature of the classical period offers an opportunity to approach the question whether in fact signs and symptoms of coronary artery disease have been recorded. While a full-fledged picture of the disease is certainly not to be found, there are, however, many references to its constituents. In particular, descriptions of attacks resembling cardiac syncope and also of precordial pain are mentioned, as will be seen in the following discussion.

The problem which faces the historian is first to uncover the often-hidden sources of information and then to provide a critical evaluation of this material The difficulties which have to be overcome are those of obscure terminology, and of descriptions often accompanied by theoretical reasoning which is very different from modern biological concepts. It is small wonder that conflicting opinions have been held as to the very core of the question. Some more recent authors have been inclined to deny almost any evidence of the existence of this disease in classical medicine; others feel that the disease has been present from time immemorial.

A conclusion would best be reached by presenting the facts and ideas pertaining to this disease in verbal quotations, and by offering a critical analysis of the sources. For the sake of convenience a chronological order will be kept, bearing in mind the clinical symptomatology, the prognosis and the localization as reported by the ancient authors, starting with Hippocrates.

Hippocrates

The information derived from the Hippocratic writings is arranged in two groups: first, clinical descriptions (symptoms, prognosis and localization) having some bearing on, or at least allusions to, coronary artery disease; second, biological ideas concerning every kind of impediment in the blood flow, not really understood by the ancient author through lack of physiological and pathological knowledge, but leading ultimately to the newer concepts of thrombosis prevailing in more modern medicine.

(a) The clinical data are often presented in very brief terms:

1. *Coan Prenotions* (Littré V, 601, § 70).

> 'Sharp pains, irradiating soon towards the clavicle and towards the back, are fatal.'[4]

[4] Compare the Akkadian prognostication: 'Si le malade, sa poitrine lui fait mal, main de son dieu' (meaning a catastrophe). See R. Labat (1951), I, p. 101.

The *Coan Prenotions* consist of very short sentences bearing mostly on fevers, 'phrenesis' (§ 69), fatal prognosis (§§ 71, 72, etc.), and delirium (§§ 83, 84, etc.) The context of the paragraph quoted above, i.e. its position between phrenesis and fatal prognosis, makes it uncertain to which organ the disease is thought to belong. However, this is an acute disease producing in a very short time deferred pain[5] (from the heart?) to the clavicle, and is fatal. The localization of the disease is not specified, and one could think even of acute pancreatitis being involved. Nevertheless, this brief description may fit exactly into the frame of an acute coronary event.

2. *The Aphorisms, II, 41* (Littré IV, 483; English translation by W. H. S. Jones, *Hippocrates*, vol. 4, p. 119).

> 'Those who suffer from a frequent and extreme prostration without any manifest cause die suddenly.'

This aphorism has often been quoted and commented upon in the historical literature. Again, the heart as the seat of disease is not mentioned, but the aphorism appears to be compatible with a special form of repeated coronary attack and implies also the grave prognosis. Parenthetically it may be added that two aphorisms preceding No. 41 bear on diseases of old age, and it is possible that the type of coronary lesion found in the aged provided the subject of this observation.

3. *Aphorisms II, 44* (Littré IV, 483; Jones, l.c. p. 119).

> 'Those who are constitutionally very fat are more apt to die quickly than those who are thin.'

This aphorism, not specifically mentioning the organ involved, adds to the better knowledge of prognosis which in modern times has been established on statistical evidence. It is indicative of the sure prognostication to which the Hippocratic writings adhere, often to the detriment of diagnosis.

4. *Coan Prenotions* (Littré V, 647, § 280).

> 'Frequent recurrence of cardialgia, in an elderly person, announces sudden death.'

Here the meaning depends on the interpretation of the word 'cardialgia', which was used for pain in the heart as well as in the stomach, more specifically at its orifice. The precise meaning and interpretation of the word was a puzzle even in classical times, and

---

[5] See also A. Souques (1937) on the subject of pain in the Hippocratic writings, pp. 209 ff.

Galen in his Commentary on the sixty-fifth Aphorism, Book IV, is indecisive about the real significance of the term. Galen concludes, after a lengthy discussion, that cardialgia or 'cardiogmos' may describe a disorder of the heart 'which is a most grave evil, surpassing all others since this signifies the burning down of life's base'.

5. *Aphorisms II, 48* (Littré IV, p. 485; Jones l.c. p. 121).

> 'In every movement of the body, to rest at once when pain begins relieves the suffering.'

While many kinds of pain react favourably to rest, this is most pronounced in precordial pain.

6. *Aphorisms III, 17.* (Littré IV, p. 495; Jones, l.c. p. 127).

> 'Of daily constitutions, such as are northerly brace the body, giving it tone and agility, and improving the complexion and the sense of hearing, drying up the bowels and make the eyes tingle, besides aggravating any pre-existing pain in the chest; southerly constitutions relax and moisten the body, bring on heaviness of the head, hardness of hearing and giddiness, make the eyes and the whole body slow to move, and the bowels watery.'

This rather lengthy passage has been quoted for the sake of the few words which are relevant to our topic. The aphorism denotes its Mediterranean origin and praises the salutary influence of a bracing northerly wind, so welcome in a hot country. However, in pointing to the less agreeable consequences of this cold spell the author stresses its provocative and noxious influence on preexisting pain localized in the chest. This is a rather common clinical observation and fits again into the frame of precordial pain which is often provoked by walking against a cold wind.

7. *Regimen in acute diseases, chapter 7* (Littré II, 273; Francis Adams' translation (1849), I, p. 290).

> 'but if the pain point to the clavicle, or if there be a heaviness in the arm, or about the breast, or above the diaphragm, one should open the inner vein at the elbow . . .'

Though the chapter covers other chest diseases as well, and probably pleurisy, this passage may be regarded as fitting into the symptomatology of anginal pain.[6]

---

[6] I am indebted to Dr K. D. Keele for drawing my attention to the above passage.

This collection of scattered pieces of information is compatible with signs and symptoms of anginal manifestations as understood in recent times. One weakness lies in the author's not mentioning the heart as the seat of the disease. Hippocratic medicine was never too keen on diagnostic and topographic endeavour. Its main object was always prognosis based on knowledge of syndromes. Even the classical publication by Heberden in 1772 failed to locate precisely the seat of the disease. Incidentally, those writers who have tried to trace the evolution of the medical knowledge of coronary artery disease have not for some reason used the information found in the Hippocratic works.[7] However, some less comprehensive papers not dealing exclusively with coronary artery disease do contain some information on Hippocratic views. For instance, some of our material has been discussed in a paper by H. M. and Ph. B. Katz (1962). This is duly acknowledged, even when their statement that Hippocrates 'may have been describing myocardial infarction' (*Prognostics*, Chapter 23; Littré II, p. 177), where Hippocrates is referring to a very severe throat infection, does not seem to be substantiated.

(b) The following discussion of biological ideas concerning impediment in the blood flow will present a more intricate analysis based on lesser-known material gathered from the Hippocratic sources. These ideas concern disturbed physiology arrived at by theoretical reasoning about supposed morbid conditions in the blood vessels. They have a bearing on blood-coagulation[8] and on so-called obstruction in the vessels. Ideas which were ultimately to lead to the now-accepted doctrines are represented in some texts which do not directly refer to the coronaries or to the myocardium, but they do reflect the theoretical concepts of the ancient Greek authors regarding impediment of the blood flow.

The most striking text which will be reproduced in part is found in Hippocrates' *Regimen in Acute Diseases*, Appendix; Littré II, 407. These theoretical concepts appear in a most striking form in the following text, as also do their clinical implications, and the enumeration of symptoms and signs to which the impediment gives rise. Without the kind of material evidence revealed in later times by pathology and dissection, and purely on theoretical grounds, a correlation is reached between the supposed clotting of the blood leading to obstruction, and the ensuing clinical results of this stoppage.

---

[7] Those who have written on this topic are: Herrick, 1942, Willius, 1945-6, East, 1958 and Klemperer, 1960.

[8] That coagulation of the blood was at least considered by Aristotle also is shown by the following quotation from his *Historia Animalium*, 520b, 20: 'Blood, if it corrupts in the body, has a tendency to turn into pus, and pus may turn into a solid concretion'.

8. *Regimen in Acute Diseases, Appendix,* chapter 5 (Littré II, 407; Adams I, 316).

> 'With this alteration in the blood, air [*spiritus vitalis, pneuma*] cannot pervade the natural passages. This stasis produces a cooling down, obscuring of the sight, loss of speech, heaviness of the head, and convulsions as soon as the stasis reaches the heart or the liver or the great vein; such occurrences as epilepsy or palsy follow when the fluxions or swellings occur in those organs through the adjoining vessels; and when, owing to desiccation, [9] the air cannot follow its course.'

This passage requires some explanation in the light of more modern concepts, while remaining faithful to the old terminology and notions of morbid processes. First the alteration of the blood apparently means a kind of deterioration if its normal state which leads to an obstruction of the blood vessel. The notion of air pervading the natural passages is in conformity with the so-called pneuma which according to the ancient biological theories provides the organs with the necessary substance for survival. This is not very far from the modern concept of oxygenation.

The stasis is freely acknowledged as a pathological condition which is the basis of the morbid states mentioned in these texts. These conditions are chosen at random and not systematically, just as they come to the ancient observer's mind. First, the 'cooling down', which is easily observed in peripheral obstruction affecting a limb, gangrene, which is preceded by a fall in the skin temperature, having been known to the ancients. The 'obscuring of the sight' in the present context again implies a vascular disturbance, for its cause is now known to be the clotting of a retinal vessel. The symptom 'loss of speech' foretells aphasia, more precisely described in the nineteenth century; and that of 'heaviness of the head and convulsions' would indicate a vascular brain disorder which was more extensively studied in later periods of medical history. The same refers to epilepsy or palsy, with a statement that these morbid states occur in the organs through a lesion in the adjoining vessels. Even the etiology of all the named signs and symptoms has been tentatively described by the ancient author, who assumed that all these morbid conditions came about 'owing to dessication'. This last word must be more fully explained. The older commentators on Hippocrates interpreted the term as being identical with coagulation, since the latter process is accompanied by loss of the liquid state of the blood. This interpretation has been given by Vassaeus

---

[9] The term 'desiccation' was used for obstructive processes in the vessels as late as the end of the sixteenth century (see this page and also page 58).

(Vassé), a French author of the Renaissance period, already quoted by Littré, and known by his work *In anatomen corporis humani tabulae quatuor* (1540).

It may be presumed that this remarkable and relatively unknown passage in the Hippocratic corpus is a description of what was later known as thrombosis. According to the classical definition by Virchow of thrombo-embolic processes, the factors involved are: (1) hyper-coagulability of the blood; (2) retardation of the blood flow; (3) lesion located in the coat of the vessel. Of these, two factors are indeed referred to in this passage: (a) 'the alteration in the blood'; (b) the 'air (the pneuma in the blood vessels) cannot pervade the natural passages'; while the third factor is not mentioned. Again let us stress that all these deliberations and biological conjectures have been set down by the ancient author without any actual inspection in autopsies. It is indeed an example of sagacity and penetrating analysis at a remote time, when no facilities for anatomical investigation were available.

In order to round off this chapter on the biological views of Hippoc-rates, only one further item shall be touched upon. This refers to the Hippocratic views on the myocardium, and deals with the significance of the heart as a muscle, an item long neglected in the clinical evaluation of heart diseases. The quotation runs as follows:

9. *On the Heart* (Littré, IX, p. 82).

'The heart is a very vigorous muscle, vigorous not through its tendinous tissue, but owing to its interlacing fibres.'

The great importance of the conception of the heart as a muscle has an immediate bearing on the history of myocardial infarction. His-torical literature places the emergence of this notion in a later period and connects it with the name of Nicholaus Steno in the seventeenth century. I have drawn attention elsewhere (1965b) to earlier statements of the heart's muscular nature, more specifically in the later Renais-sance literature. It is of some importance to find the idea of the heart fibres as an essential structure already expressed in the Hippocratic writings.

Aretaeus

This Greek author of the second century appeals to the medical re-searcher for his basically clinical descriptions. He is well known as probably the first to describe diabetes and diphtheria. His work is relatively concise and well organized. In studying his views and statements, it is important to compare the descriptions of diseases given in each part of his work, i.e. in *Causes and Symptoms in Acute Diseases*, and in his *Therapeutics*. This method of arrangement of his material is almost unique insofar as everything belonging to signs and symptoms is concentrated in the first section, while the management of disease and its cure is relegated to the second part.

In the case of our topic the description of the disease is contained in chapter III, 'On Syncope' (p. 270 in the Francis Adams edition[10]). Here, pain in the heart is not mentioned, but is indeed reported in his *Therapeutics* (p. 430).

The chapter contains a most impressive description of syncope with clear indication of its cardiac origin. This is implied in his rhetorical question: 'What other organ more important than the heart for life or for death? Neither is it to be doubted that syncope is a disease of the heart'.[11] In this respect the cardiac origin of collapse as an etiological factor is more clearly stressed than in the description by Caelius Aurelianus, to be mentioned later, where many other causes of collapse and shock are by far predominant.

Aretaeus pays much attention to the state of the heart which is responsible for the syncope. Since the terms for heart and stomach in Greek are confusing, he tries to prove in a lengthy discussion that the heart and not the stomach is involved.

The cardiac collapse is described in its most intense, acute and fatal form:

> 'those dying in such cases have symptoms of heart affections, namely, pulse small and feeble, bruit of the heart, with violent palpitation, vertigo, fainting, torpor, loss of tone in the limbs, sweating copious and unrestrainable, coldness of the whole body etc.'.

As distinct from other forms of collapse, the cardiac syncope, according to Aretaeus, is different from others inasmuch as the patient remains undisturbed in his mental faculties until his death. The author even ventures a statement that the patients in cardiac affections are more acute in their senses and are more clear in mind. This observation does not appear in other descriptions of cardiac syncope. In the clinical symptomatology a prominent place is given to excessive sweating and coldness of the limbs.

[10] All quotations are taken from the Francis Adams translation.
[11] The term 'syncope' in historical literature does not imply loss of consciousness, but rather sudden weakness of the heart muscle. This definition has been provided by D. Evan Bedford (1968) with reference to the work of C. H. Parry.

On the whole, Aretaeus is very precise in describing syncope as a disease of the heart, distinguishing it from 'ardent fevers' as another cause of death.

The gloomy picture of the chapter just discussed is much mitigated when we look up its fellow chapter in the *Therapeutics*, where the author considers also a happy outcome. Of this, two types are described: (1) complete recovery of the patient, who 'calls to his memory the circumstances of the disease like a dream'; (2) a conversion to 'marasmus' with some morbid signs left. Here supportive measures are required, 'and by these means the patient is to be brought back to convalescence and his accustomed habits'. Again a happy end is promised and the conclusion drawn that the disease is not always fatal. Indeed, this conclusion was reached comparatively late in medical history, and after long years of experience in the natural course of the disease.

In the discussion of therapeutic measures, Aretaeus advises bleeding if the syncope arises from 'redundancy'. He gives wine, advises cataplasms to procure a flow of blood, silence and cheerfulness. Food may be supped rather than masticated. The requirement for wine is indicated when there is much sweating and the pulse is coming to a stop. The patient must be stouthearted and courageous, and the physician must encourage him with words 'to be of good cheer'. After a long enumeration of supportive measures the author concludes:

> 'From these things there is hope that the patient may thus escape. If everything turns out properly, sweat is nowhere, but restoration of the heat everywhere, even at the extremities of the feet and the nose; but the face is of good colour; pulse enlarged in magnitude, not tremulous, strong; he recovers his senses, and sprouts out into a new nature'.

We could not abstain from the above quotation so beautifully supporting therapeutical optimism, at least in some cases. The author seems to have grasped the full significance of cardiac syncope in its fatal but also reparable forms, while the anginal form has been at least briefly mentioned, and the heart clearly conceived as the seat of the disease.

Galen

The amount of information on coronary disease increases spectacularly when we turn to the numerous works of Galen. This Greek physician was privileged to display his immense knowledge owing to the fact that he lived in the great Roman metropolis with many facilities and a large audience to listen to his lectures and to encourage his endeavours.

Not only clinical material and some concepts, but also actual anatomical descriptions can be extracted from his works.

Let us begin with the text referring to the anatomy as well as to the physiological significance of the coronary vessels. This is remarkable enough to be quoted almost in its entirety.

On Anatomical Procedures. Book VII, Chapter 10 (translated by Charles Singer, 1956).

> 'The veins that nourish the heart spring in all animals from its cavity. People speak of them as "enwreathing" the heart, since two of them do so surround it, just as two arteries come down from the left part into the substance of the heart [coronary arteries]. . . . It is easier to see them in large hearts' (p. 186).
>
> 'You can observe the vessels that wreathe the heart in a mani-fold series of branches passing over the surface in various ways, all from the junction of the cavities' (p. 188).

These brief passages show Galen's acquaintance with the anatomy of the coronary vessels largely derived from animal dissections, since we have no proof that Galen practised dissection on human bodies. In this case, his findings readily yield valid information, applicable to human anatomy as well. When Galen mentions the veins first in his discussion, he is following his system of the blood flow, supposing that blood originates in the liver and is distributed through the veins. He knows that the veins and the arteries are often parallel structures running close together. What is remarkable in his description is his knowledge of a special supply to the heart muscle, to which effect he returns again in the sixth book of his *De Usu Partium*.[12] That the coronary vessels were already known to anatomists before Galen can be derived from his words, 'people speak of them'. The name 'coronary', based on a similarity to a crown or a wreath, was not coined by him, but the knowledge of this structure became widely spread through his extensively studied works. He is very precise in allotting to the coronaries the function of blood supply to the heart muscle, based on his observation that these vessels 'come down from the left part into the substance of the heart'. The small interpolation 'from the left part' clearly denotes their origin from the aorta. Galen was also conscious of the muscular nature of the heart[13] since he discusses this topic at

[12] This work has recently been translated into English for the first time by M. T. May and published with the title *Galen on the Usefulness of the Parts of the Body* (2 vols., 1968).

[13] In his *De motu musculorum*, lib. I (Kühn IV, 377 ff. and Daremberg II, 327) Galen notes, however, that the heart differs from other muscles in its denseness, configuration, texture, hardness, and its involuntary action. He makes a similar comment in another treatise, *De probis pravisque alimentorum succis* (Kühn VI, 771).

considerable length (see pp. 181–84 in Singer's edition). As yet ignorant of the very nature of the circulation of the blood, he nonetheless
allots a central position to the heart muscle in the blood transit: 'the
power of pulsation has its origin in the heart itself'.

The whole passage is refreshingly short and not encumbered, as is
often the case, with theoretical speculation. It is included in the relatively concise volume *De Anatomicis Administrationibus*, a title which
Daremberg very aptly translated as 'Manual of Dissections', conforming to the purpose of the book as a short guide to the practice of
anatomy.

To this item Galen returns in his *De Usu Partium*, Book VI, Chapter
14 (Kühn III, 497; Daremberg I, 431.)

> 'The vein which "enwreathes" the heart, and this is why it is
> called [the coronary vein], has [its] origin outside the part from
> which the valves emerge'.

In another part of this work (VI, 17, Kühn III, 499; and Daremberg
I, 446) we find a variation of the same theme.[14]

> 'The heart is not nourished by its own blood; but before the
> vena cava penetrates the right ventricle, a rather thick branch
> [the coronary vein] leads off for the nourishment of the heart,
> and spreading over the base of this viscus it reaches all its parts.
> Together with this vein an artery entwines and branches off,
> this branch originating in the great artery and being considerable
> enough to refresh this vein and to maintain in the exterior parts
> of the heart [walls] an exact balance of inner heat.'

Here Galen differentiates between arterial and venous function.
However, though perceiving the aeration of the blood by the artery
he has not grasped the true function of the veins, believing that it is they
which nourish the organs.

In accordance with his teleological views he stresses the need for an
adequate and special system of blood supply [coronary vessels] for the
heart, the latter being a dense and compact organ. Parenthetically it
may be recalled that already Hippocrates had spoken of the heart as
'a solid and dense structure which is less affected by pain' (*On Diseases*,
Book IV; Littré VII, 555). Galen is very explicit in bringing out the
fact of a self-sufficient blood supply for the heart, describing the branch
which leaves the great vessel for this purpose. One can consider this
idea as an ancient parallel to Harvey's 'third circulation', when Harvey
refers to the coronaries.

[14] See translation of the complete passage in M. T. May (1968), p. 325.

As to the diseases of the heart, insofar as they concern our topic, another passage in Galen must be considered. He concentrated his pathological findings and explanations in his work *De Locis Affectis*. In Book V, Chapter 2 (Kühn II, p. 623, Chapter 2; Daremberg II, p. 627, as Chapter 3) he deals exclusively with heart diseases. While pericardial effusions are described in a more detailed and specific way, diseases of the heart muscle proper are mentioned less explicitly. For a better understanding[15] of the rather difficult arrangement of this chapter, the data can be divided into three parts, each presenting a different type of heart lesion. Their description will be given as far as possible in Galen's own words. First he described 'slight dyscrasias', which make the pulse vary (pulse anomalies), each dyscrasia being different according to its nature. Secondly, he speaks of 'serious dyscrasias', but still affecting only the homoïomeric parts, a term taken from Aristotle and translated by medieval authors as *partes similares*. This means that only parts are damaged, but not the heart as a functional entity. Consequently these diseases are not followed by rapid death. Finally, he speaks of 'organic dyscrasias',[16] where death is instantaneous and is preceded by initial signs as found in Hippocrates' Aphorism II, 41:

> 'Persons subjected to frequent and serious faintings occurring without any apparent reason, die suddenly'.

This passage shows that Aphorism II, 41, was understood by Galen as related to the heart, which makes its inclusion in a history of coronary heart disease more acceptable.

Let us again return to Galen's definition of organic dyscrasia, to which apparently, in his terminology, a coronary thrombosis would have belonged. He would not have called it a homoïomeric dyscrasia, which would be more applicable, for example, to a disease of the type of myocarditis, while a coronary thrombosis would not fit into a homoïomeric disorder since it would seem to follow an obstruction from outside. In Galen's pathological system homoïomeric lesions are chronic while a coronary thrombosis could be a sudden event.

To proceed with Galen's theoretical views as expressed in the same chapter, it is worthwhile to quote the following phrase: 'When the heart is deprived of respiration it dies instantaneously' (Kühn V, 299;

[15] I am indebted to Dr. O. Temkin for his kind assistance in the interpretation of this chapter.
[16] The chapter is of a more speculative nature and does not refer to specific heart affections, with the exception of pericarditis. However, it may be assumed that myocardial damage is hidden under the term 'organic dyscrasias'. It may be added that among heart symptoms Galen, in his *Praesagium de pulsibus* (Kühn IX, 403) mentions pain in the heart, explaining the pain by 'copius humours'.

Daremberg II, 626). Translated into more modern terms this gives an insight into the role of oxygenation. Some heart diseases have been termed by Galen as palpitations. Then he mentions patients who died after frequent cardiac syncope, often between the ages of 40 and 50. These types of disease have been included in the same chapter in which he speaks of the different dyscrasias of the heart.

The physiology of the coronaries always aroused Galen's curiosity, as is evident in Bk. III, ch. 15 of his *Natural Faculties*. This work contains Galen's system of physiology, just as his *Anatomical Procedures* reflect his views of anatomy, and the *Affected Parts* those of pathology. Chapter 15 refers briefly to the physiology of the coronaries.[17] Galen speculates about the quantity of the blood supplied to the heart and its ultimate distribution. He then asks whether 'a fraction of the blood is used up in the nutrition of the substance of the heart itself': and adds immediately,

> 'In fact, there is another vein branching into the substance [muscle] of the heart, and which does not originate in, or take its share of blood from the heart itself.'

Admittedly the short sentence just quoted is only a slight reference to the coronaries, and perhaps based on rather crude physiology. Besides, it is embedded in a lengthy theory of 'attraction' in order to explain the blood transit in the vessels. It is a wonder that Galen paid any attention at all to such a specialized question as the blood flow in the coronaries. Most striking is his attempt at quantitative reasoning, when he is considering the amount of blood which is used in the nutriment of the heart itself.

Though not directly belonging to our topic, we may stress Galen's deliberations about quantitative questions regarding the blood transit. They take the form of a mechanical exercise, taking into account the width of the channels and the vascular orifices.[18] The smaller calibre of the pulmonary artery compared to the greater width of the vena cava led Galen to his erroneous hypothesis of blood passage through the septum. Thus the ideas about coronary physiology are linked closely to those of the general flow of the blood as expressed in Galen's physiological system.[19]

[17] The same passage can be found in Kühn II, p. 209, in Daremberg II, 317, and also in A. J. Brock's translation into English, Loeb Classical Library, p. 323.

[18] L. G. Wilson, 'Erasistratus, Galen and the pneuma', *Bull. Hist. Med.*, 1959, **33**, 293–314, especially p. 309. J. Prendergast, 'Galen's view of the vascular system', *Proc. roy. Soc. Med., Section Hist. Med.*, 1928, **21**, 79–88. A. Fishman (ed.), *Circulation of the Blood, Men and Ideas* (1964); pp. 15 (A. Cournand), 645 (S. E. Bradley).

[19] For further discussion of these points see R. E. Siegel, *Galen's System of Physiology and Medicine* (1968); pp. 41 (coronary vessels); 272 (thrombus); 337 (narrowed or obstructed vascular connections); 344–7 (angina pectoris); 347–52 (syncope).

Caelius Aurelianus

A much later author, Caelius Aurelianus, lived in the fifth century A.D. and wrote not in Greek, but in Latin. Most of his writing is based on and translated from Soranus, the Greek physician of the early second century. He is in fact the greatest Latin medical writer after Celsus. When we examine closely the long chapter on 'The Cardiac Passion', we meet with a multitude of signs and symptoms, among which a few allusions to coronary artery disease may be discerned. However, we would not venture to claim that a clear and consistent description of what was later called coronary thrombosis can be attributed to this author. What is characteristic of the description is the full coverage of a morbid state (now termed as 'shock'), which may accompany a coronary event, but which can also be provoked by other etiological factors. The points suggesting a possible relation to coronary artery disease were assembled and commented upon by R. E. Siegel (1961). The shock symptomatology in Caelius recalls the description by Aretaeus. However, Aretaeus is less ambiguous in stressing the heart as the origin of this morbid state. Caelius writes more in the form of a medical compendium, not always naming his sources, and he assembles many etiological factors not related to heart pathology.

The edition of the Latin text with an English translation by Drabkin (1950) will be used in the following references. A general remark concerning the theoretical assumption of 'obstruction' has already been mentioned in the section on Hippocrates. The parallel in Caelius is:

> 'The followers of Asclepiades say that it [cardiac disease] is an inflammation in the region of the heart due to a heaping-up or stoppage of the corpuscles' (p. 243).

Circulatory collapse is characterized by a weak and rapid pulse, and sometimes, 'because of its rapidity the beats become confused and it lacks regularity' (p. 245). The author sometimes observed this morbid state after excessive blood loss and severe diarrhoea (p. 245). Like Aretaeus he refers also to coldness of the skin and sweating. He mentions heaviness of the chest on the left side near the nipple (p. 257). As to the pain, he states:

> 'There is also a disease called by some Cardimona (in Greek cardiogmos). In this disease there is always pain at the mouth of the stomach, a condition which many laymen call "pain of the heart"' (p. 263).

While collapse has been classically described, a few anginal symptoms are mentioned.

In Caelius' own words, the etiology does not even include an affection of the heart. He states on p. 245:

> 'The usual causes are continual indigestion, excessive drinking of wine, bathing after taking food, vomiting after dinner, and grief or fright in which the body is sympathetically affected and dissolved in sweat.'

This is rather far from a clear cardiac etiology and is more vaguely connected with heart disease than the description by Aretaeus.

On the other hand, a quite unusual conception was brought to light by this author when he extended the term 'paralysis' to be applied also to the heart (p. 575):

> 'Thus Herophilus tells us that, when death comes suddenly without any apparent cause, it is the result of paralysis of the heart. Erasistrates terms *paradoxos* [strange, paradoxical] a type of paralysis in which a person walking along suddenly stops and cannot go on, but after a while can walk again.'

This quotation from Caelius was used as a footnote by Heberden in the final version of his paper 'Pectoris dolor', as it appears in his *Commentaries*. In this context Caelius was apparently referring to a condition of the heart rather than to intermittent claudication, and this was also the interpretation given to it by Heberden.

Cassius Felix

This minor Latin author, close in time and origin (Africa) to Caelius Aurelianus, uses the same term 'cardiac disease', which is not too clear and certainly does not correspond to modern usage. The term, also styled 'kardiakos'[20] is the title of a chapter. Cassius's small book, entitled *De Medicina*, is a therapeutic guide which he had written for his son and which was edited rather late by V. Rose, in 1879. The small chapter 'Ad Cardiacos' (pp. 156–57) does not add materially to the clinical picture of what would now be termed 'shock', apart from the author's supposition that it can be brought about by a pericardial distension:

> 'When the heart membrane is swollen a slight fever may occur, and the pulse is weak. Some physicians call this disease syncope, and the patient loses his life through a mortifying sweat.'

[20] Francis Adams reviews this subject in *The Seven Books of Paulus Aegineta* (London, 1844–7), I, pp. 292–96.

As therapy Cassius proposed:

> 'cataplasma of woollen cloths soaked in oil of myrtle mixed with sharp wine, etc. This drives away sweat and revives strength.'

Some recent writers, as for instance W. D. Sharpe (1964), felt that the description could be compatible with acute myocardial failure. Even if the clinical picture is not adequate and convincing, Cassius may be mentioned here for a further contribution to syncope.

3. BIBLE AND TALMUD

Although no clear-cut clinical descriptions pertaining to coronary artery disease are to be found in the Bible, a few data alluding to it may be briefly reported. The word heart[21] is mentioned eighty-five times in the Old Testament, mostly in a figurative, non-medical sense. Occasionally a cardiological meaning is attached to the word, for example, in Genesis 45:26, 'And Jacob's heart fainted'; according to Hebrew scholarship the word 'fainted' can be replaced by 'stopped'. On the other hand we cannot fail to be impressed by the number of figurative predications in connection with the word 'heart'. Some authors stress the frequent occurrence of these expressions referring to heart pains in the Bible: 'My heart is aching' (Jer. 8:18); 'I am pained at my very heart' (Jer. 4:19); 'My heart within me is broken' (Jer. 23:9), and so on. The frequent mention of the heart in a context of sorrow leads us to suppose that heart pains were considered in Biblical times, though they were far from actually depicting angina pectoris.[22]

One controversial and relevant 'case history' was repeatedly discussed in the historical literature.[23] The case is that of Nabal in the 25th chapter of the first book of Samuel. This man was described as a heavy eater and drinker, with a harsh temper which brought him into conflict with King David at the time when the latter was persecuted by King Saul. Nabal's wife Abigail learned of David's intention to assail their house, and only through her personal charm and diplomacy was she able to avert the disaster. We proceed with the story in quoting the King James' translation, 1 Samuel 25:36-38.

> 36. And Abigail came to Nabal; and behold, he held a feast in his house, like the feast of a king; and Nabal's heart was merry within him, for he was very drunken: wherefore she told him nothing, less or more, until the morning light.

[21] Cf. F. H. van Meyenfeldt (1950), see Bibliography.
[22] Any reference suggestive of precordial pain in the Bible aud the Talmud is denied by I. van Esso (1954).
[23] See for example, D. C. Peete (1955).

37. But it came to pass in the morning, when the wine was gone out of Nabal, and his wife had told him these things, that his heart died within him, and it[24] became as a stone.
38. And it came to pass about ten days after, that the Lord smote Nabal, that he died.

In commenting upon these verses it must be admitted that an expression like 'stony heart' in Ezekiel 36:26 is sometimes used metaphorically for obstinacy and an unrelenting nature. However, the context of the quoted verses precludes this interpretation. Some authors took it quite literally even to the extent of interpreting stone as calcification. In a medical thesis written under our guidance J. Danon was reluctant to see in the story a coronary event, an opinion we also held at that time (1960). We should like to revise that view, and are now more inclined to find an allusion to a cardiac infarction in this Biblical narration on the following grounds. Nabal was perhaps prone to it owing to his nutritional habits; which, coupled with the great fear and anxiety of a man harbouring guilt feelings because of his ingratitude towards King David, may have been responsible for his cardiac death. In this case death overcame him after ten days of great tension, perhaps as the result of a second, and fatal, heart attack.[25]

The Babylonian Talmud is a huge compilation of Hebrew knowledge, law, and philosophy in which some items belonging to medicine and natural sciences have been interspersed. The final revised text was completed in the fifth century A.D., but it contains much older matter, for instance, the Mishnah, assembled by Rabbi Judah ha-Nassi, a contemporary of Galen. As remarked in the introduction to this study (p. 19), the diseases mentioned were often verified by ritual inspection and autopsy of slaughtered animals. The data pertaining to pulmonary lesions are much more detailed than those relating to the heart, since slaughtered animals present more pulmonary than heart pathology. Indeed, coronary lesions in animals used for food are extraordinarily rare;[26] only traumatic cardiac lesions are more common,

[24] In most translations this is given as 'he became'; however, the Hebrew word used is compatible with our translation 'it became'.

[25] Some Hebrew commentators of the fourteenth to sixteenth century have stressed the psychogenic factor in Nabal's death. Don Isaac Abravanel (1437–1508) suggests that Nabal lived these ten days in a constant state of fear, which led to his death in a fit of 'melancholic disease'. The case was also commented upon by Dr. John Smith in his book *Portraiture of Old Age* (1666, p. 229) where we are given a cardiological interpretation of Ecclesiastes 12:2–6 (cf. J. O. Leibowitz, *J. Hist. Med.*, 1963, **18**, 283; and Sir Geoffrey Keynes, *The Life of William Harvey* (1966) pp. 166–8).

[26] See, however, H. L. Ratcliffe (1963) who reports from the Philadelphia Zoo that the frequency of coronary arteriosclerosis, including myocardial infarction, in the animals increased tenfold in a 14-year period up to 1961.

and such cases are reported in the Talmud since it is forbidden to eat the affected animals. As for human patients, however, a short aphorism, not devoid of a humorous touch, shows that pains in the heart were quite common and well known. The quotation runs as follows:

> 'Rather any disease, but not a disease of the bowels; any pain, *but not heart pain*; any ache, but not head ache; any evil, but not an evil wife' (Babylonian Talmud, Tractate Sabbath, fol. 11 recto).

So anginal pain and its implication might be seen in a Talmudic saying.

It is worth noting that the sages of the Talmud knew that an organ could become obstructed. In the Tractate Hulin, 47, an 'obstruction in the lung' (*atum ba-rëah*) is incidentally referred to as consolidation and hardening in the tissues; air is unable to enter an obstructed lung and therefore inflation cannot take place. There are even methods mentioned in the Talmud of examining these hardenings and of making a differential diagnosis between them and other pathological findings, as for instance lung abscesses. It seems that though vascular obstructions are not reported in the Talmud, obstructions in other organs have been described. A possible interpretation of the word *atum* as pertaining to thrombosis can also be deduced on linguistic grounds, since the verb derived from it means 'to block', not unlike the Greek derivation of the term 'thrombosis'.

4. THE MIDDLE AGES

The Greek medical literature of the fourth to the seventh centuries, including Byzantine medicine, is more or less a compilation and new arrangement of the ancient Greek authors. It is a rich field for historical investigation, often clarifying such topics as surgical procedures. However, in a search for allusions or facts pertaining to coronary artery disease, no new vistas are revealed. This was a period of copious, all-embracing medical writing, often systematically arranged, and setting the pattern for the works of later medieval medicine as represented by Avicenna. In Oribasius (fourth century), Aetius and Alexander of Tralles (sixth century), and Paul of Aegina (seventh century) we may find the Galenic references to possible manifestations of coronary disease without many additions or alterations. It may be that this over-systematized and very detailed way of writing, which aimed at covering the whole of medicine, precluded special research of limited scope, which might have shed some light on our topic.

An item like precordial pain tended to be buried in these huge compilations. The time was not ripe to make a real discovery in this field, not only because of the lack of adequate knowledge and concepts, but also since the literary convention was directed towards this compilative form of writing. Only with the advent of short papers in more recent times could an author draw attention to a hitherto unnoticed or not specifically labelled morbid condition. Even in medieval times, occasional smaller treatises, such as the concise tract on smallpox and measles by Rhazes, were instrumental in furthering medical knowledge. Indeed, the most striking advances in our subject were incorporated into relatively brief papers, such as those by Heberden (1772) or Herrick (1912). Besides, the whole period was authority-bound and leaned heavily on the ancients, which made any individual investigations, or the desire to innovate, practically impossible. These remarks have been inserted here as a general introduction to the more important medical writings of the Middle Ages.

With these limitations in mind, we shall turn to some literary sources of the Middle Ages, where indeed distinct references to pain of the heart are to be found.[27] More rewarding sources are often not the formal medical works of the type already described, but shorter collections of recipes, in which our attention is drawn not to the alleged therapeutical measures but to the fact that they were prescribed for coronary manifestations.

We begin with Anglo-Saxon magic and medicine as compiled by J. H. G. Grattan and Charles Singer (1952), taking into account the ailments themselves rather than the details of the remedies which do not belong directly to our purpose. Let us quote a few of them:

> 'For pain at the heart: A handful of rue (Ruta). Seethe in oil, and add one ounce of aloes. Smear with that; it stills the pain' (p. 197).
> 'For ache at the heart: If he have within him a severe pain at the heart, then wind groweth in his heart, and thirst consumeth him, and he is without strength. Prepare for him then a "stone" bath [form of vapour bath], and in it let him eat southern radish with salt. By that can the hurt be healed.'

[27] A definition of cardiac disease with pain in the heart was given by Isidore of Seville (died A.D. 636). In his *Etymologiae*, lib. IV, 'De medicina', chapter 6, he writes: 'The word *cardiaca*, from the Greek *kardian*, is used for the heart, because it is affected by any fear or pain. For it is a pain of the cardia accompanied by formidable apprehension'. See also the monograph on Isidore by W. D. Sharpe (1964), p. 56.

'For ache at the heart again: Take cockle; seethe in milk; give to drink six days.'

'For tightness of the chest. Thus must the medicine be wrought,' etc. (p. 199).

Apparently pain at the heart, tightness of the chest, and similar conditions were not unknown to the anonymous writers of the ninth century and were already a medical problem at that time.[28]

There is an even older source, discussed by J. Stannard, providing references to pain of the heart. We quote the English translation by this writer from his paper 'Benedictus Crispus, an Eighth Century Poet':

'When furious pain strikes the diaphragm in the side,
And bitter anguish greatly torments the heart
Strong fluids are a help, joined by the power of coral:
Next pipinella is mixed with a broth of fennel;
Zedoary then is taken, also potent tansy
Which calms fevers and repels poisons of the heart.'

The same mention of tightness and anguish in the heart can be traced to the Basle recipes of the eighth to ninth centuries, as reported by K. Sudhoff in 1910.[29] Sudhoff was able to adduce a recipe from a ninth-century Latin MS. supposed to cure certain ailments, among them constriction of the heart. The heading reads: 'A powder against all fevers and against all venoms and the bite of all snakes, and against all kind of constriction in the heart, etc.' In another recipe from a MS. of the twelfth century ingredients are recommended 'against pains in the heart'.

We have been able to detect the same diagnosis, termed pain or anguish or constriction in the heart, in two as yet unedited MSS. by an Arabic and a Hebrew author respectively: Abd al Rahman ibn Haitam (tenth century), and Abraham Ibn Ezra (eleventh century).[30] The symptoms put under different headings such as 'sadness about the heart', 'pain in the heart', 'anguish' or 'constriction', were quite often described in the medieval literature. The remedies proposed by Abraham Ibn Ezra were opium and rue, the same rue as was used in Anglo-Saxon magic as mentioned above. The particular association of pain in the heart with a feeling of fear and sorrow leads us to think that

[28] Wellcome MS. 46 (early eleventh century) is a collection of prescriptions in Anglo-Saxon, the first being a remedy for 'heartache'.

[29] 'Die gedruckten mittelalterlichen medizinischen Texte in germanischen Sprachen.'

[30] See J. O. Leibowitz (1953) where the Hebrew manuscript of Ibn Ezra's *Book of Medical Experience* is fully described. A scholarly edition of this MS. and of the Hebrew version of Ibn Haitam's work, is now being prepared by J. O. Leibowitz and S. Marcus.

some form of coronary disease was implied by the medieval authors. In the same way, the herbal by Rufinus of the thirteenth century recommends a remedy 'contra cardiacam et sincopim', as well as 'contra melancholiacam passionem'. The many unpretentious tracts about plants and their medical properties in the Middle Ages thus testify to the fact that some form of anginal pain was known to the medieval doctors and was the subject of their therapeutical endeavours.[31]

Avicenna (980–1037)

The information given in the last few paragraphs has been derived from therapeutic guides and lists of drugs. It is these less elaborate pieces of literature which are of great value to us because they faithfully depict the current practice of medicine of the time. In examining the greatest work of systematic medicine produced in the Middle Ages, the *Canon* of Avicenna, we find the material pertaining to the heart neatly arranged in the Third Book, more especially in the eleventh section or 'Fen'. On the other hand we encounter difficulties in sorting out information on what would now be termed coronary artery disease, since no paragraph deals specifically with this disease, which had not been clearly distinguished in the period when this author lived. Indeed, heart disorders are treated more *en bloc*. In order to trace the material relevant to coronary disease, we begin by giving a few quotations from this extensive work, taken from the eleventh Fen, which is subdivided into three parts. The material contained in paragraphs 1, 2, 5 and 6 of the first part are relevant to our topic.

Paragraph 5 is entitled 'Signs of heart diseases' and contains the following remark:

> 'One of the physicians said: If a wound (or abscess) is formed in the heart, blood issues from the left nostril, and the patient dies. In this disease pain occurs in the region of the left nipple.'

Though bleeding from the left nostril does not form an acceptable symptom of coronary disease, the localization of the pain and its occurrence in heart disease are to be noted.

> Paragraph 6: 'Among the causes of heart disease are those connected with emotional disturbance.'

Even though the author speaks in more general terms, the remark is noteworthy and applicable to our topic.

---

[31] See J. O. Leibowitz, 'Early attempts at therapy in coronary disease', *Proceedings of the 19th International Congress of the History of Medicine* (Basle, 1966), p. 325.

With regard to pains in the heart, Avicenna echoes the ancient belief that this pain is incompatible with life and kills the victim immediately, as is evident from the following quotation from Paragraph 1:

> 'The heart cannot sustain pain nor tumour; therefore diseases which are usually found in other organs, will not be found in the hearts of slaughtered animals.'

The rarity of coronary pathology in domestic animals has been mentioned already in the discussion of Talmudic medicine.

In paragraph 2 mention is made of swelling and obstruction occurring in the heart, which brings about the death of the patient.

Also included are notions of cardiac collapse, recalling the classic description by Aretaeus, which Avicenna explains as 'suffocation of the innate heat'.

Paragraph 6 is very detailed as to the kinds of collapse or fainting. Some points referring to the heart or the vessels may here be reproduced. For instance,

> 'Collapse is an abolition of the moving force of the heart.'
> 'Elderly people cannot bear collapse; it occurs more often in cold than in warm weather.'
> 'The deficiency of coction leads to the filling-up of the arteries.'
> 'The dyscrasia is the cause of the filling of the arteries anywhere in the body, thus blocking the pathways of the pneuma, and resulting in an accumulation of humours which lead to death.'

These are Avicenna's views on possible vascular obstruction, and also on signs and symptoms which bear on our theme. Like those of Hippocrates and Galen discussed above, they are milestones on the long way to the recognition of coronary disease. We have been impelled to quote at least some of them, for the obvious reason that the *Canon* was the most influential book in world medicine for six hundred years, extensively studied in East and West alike. This work was printed fifteen times in the last part of the fifteenth century in the Latin translation by Gerard of Cremona. It was fully translated into Hebrew in 1279 and printed in 1491/2 in Naples, being the only Hebrew medical incunable. There are different opinions as to the intrinsic value of the *Canon*, and Garrison[32] was not too lenient in his criticism. Besides, the parts belonging to cardiology are difficult to

---

[32] *Introduction to the History of Medicine*, 4th ed. (1929), p. 130.

study, with the exception of the description of pericardial effusion. In some respects these difficulties are due to its model, the Galenic writings. It shares the merits and shortcomings which were referred to in our discussion of Galen's views on heart diseases.

Maimonides (1135–1204)

A description of Maimonides' views about signs and symptoms of what we now understand as coronary artery disease is facilitated by the smaller bulk of his work, the *Aphorisms*, and the more restrained form of presentation.

The *Aphorisms* of Maimonides, written in Arabic and very soon translated into Latin and Hebrew, represent a concise system of medicine divided into 25 sections, called in Latin 'particulae'. The relevant material is contained mostly in the third section, and does not differ very much from the views of Galen and Avicenna. They are reminiscent even of some old notions we referred to in the section on Hippocrates. Though some of these aphorisms could refer to other heart conditions as well, they contain allusions to states and symptoms definitely belonging to our topic. Some relevant passages will now be given in English translation.

> Section 3: 'Great dyscrasia, when established in the heart, be it primary or derived from another organ in the vicinity, weakens the vital force and destroys it. This is analogous to brain dyscrasia, which suffocates the brain and leads to obstruction.'

The analogy between an obstruction in the brain and in the heart later became an important factor in the understanding of thrombotic processes.[33]

> Section 3: 'The blood not only nourishes the organs, but also preserves the natural heat. Therefore, when blood undergoes changes such as excessive accumulation or diminution or change in quality,[34] then the natural heat suffers damage. When this takes place in the heart, the whole body will suffer.'

In the same section Maimonides refers to 'humours located in swellings of arteries undergoing obstruction'. He distinguishes smaller obstructions which can be healed by 'coction'; when, however, the

---

[33] In the nineteenth century terms used in brain pathology were applied to the cardiac condition which is now known as infarction. Thus, Cruveilhier wrote of 'heart apoplexy' (see below, p. 111) and Ziegler of 'myomalacia cordis', after the term encephalomalacy (see below, p. 138).

[34] In severe anaemia, anginal attacks do not respond to the usual therapy of coronary disease, but to blood transfusions, as long as they are able to control the anaemia.

transforming faculty is weak then 'putrefaction' [necrosis] is irreversible.

In the 24th section Maimonides refers to morbid states in the heart in which the blood becomes thick and the spirits [pneuma] in the arteries are diminished to such a degree that life ceases. A special form of sudden death is referred to in another part of the third section which the author explains as due to the so-called heart dyscrasia. In this special case the sudden death had been preceded by severe and repeated faintings. This recalls the Hippocratic aphorism which we quoted earlier, but here Maimonides attributes the syndrome to cardiac etiology. Later commentators on the Hippocratic aphorism, II, 41, stressed the relation between the symptoms mentioned therein and heart disease.

Mundinus (1275–1326)

From the beginning of the fourteenth century dissections of human bodies were occasionally performed. In Bologna the opening of corpses was permitted by the authorities, though on a very small and restricted scale. The first existing record is that of a post-mortem performed there by Bartolomeo Varignana in 1302, by order of the Court, as a legal autopsy. Only in 1316 were two bodies of deceased persons permitted to be examined for the sake of anatomical studies proper. This gave occasion to the appearance of probably the first text on human anatomy in medieval Europe, by Mondino de'Liucci or Luzzi. We have used the Paduan edition of 1484 of his *Anothomia*, being a reprint of the first edition published six years earlier, as well as the Italian translation, a fifteenth-century manuscript, published in 1930. Mondino's work is admittedly not an original contribution to anatomy, and is not based on extensive observations arrived at during the autopsy. It leans too heavily on the Galenic writings, translated into Latin from the Arabic versions. Mondino gives a short description of the anatomy of the heart in a special chapter, in which some information on the coronaries is to be found on ff. 13r–15v in the Latin, and on p. 120 in the Italian editions. He stresses the fact that the heart draws the appropriate portion of blood from the vessel for its nutriment, and even speculates on a quantitative problem. He admits that sometimes during disease the quantity of blood drawn through the vessels is too small; in Mondino's words, 'offered with avarice'. This, however, belongs to a general discussion on blood supplied either profusely or sparingly to every part of the body. The anatomical description of the coronary vessels can be rendered into English as follows:

5

> 'From this vessel [aorta], before it enters the cavity of the heart, rises a vessel which surrounds the base of the heart. Branches project from it into the substance of the heart. By this vessel the heart is nourished, that is, by the blood from this vessel.'

The unusual choice of the word 'avarice' quoted earlier, anticipates the later notion of coronary insufficiency, a fact which brings Mondino's contribution near to an inquiry into disturbed physiology, irrespective of his adherence to Avicenna and to scholasticism at large.

Even lesser authorities who were not professionally engaged in medical or anatomical problems paid attention to the small structure of the coronary vessels. The popular encyclopaedia *Shevileh Emuna* (*The Paths of Faith*), by Meïr Aldabi (1360) can be quoted as an example from the Hebrew literature. It was published rather late, the first edition being printed in Italy, Riva di Trento, in 1559. When the author describes the aorta he adds:

> 'From the aorta two vessels branch off. One of them is directed to the cavity of the right heart, and the other surrounds the heart and then enters it and divides into two branches.'

The quotation is remarkable for its being included in a general encyclopaedia, and also for the fact that the left coronary is more fully described with regard to its ramification (ramus circumflexus and left descendens).

CHAPTER III

The Renaissance and the Seventeenth Century

1. THE RENAISSANCE

THE transition from Middle Ages to the Renaissance is smooth rather than sudden in medical science and practice. In fact Renaissance physicians tended to purify the Greek sources and improve the translations into Latin. Often their chief motives seem to have been philological rather than medical. Only in anatomy and medical botany did they add materially to basic medical knowledge.

Yet the clinical picture, and still more the anatomical facts and ideas pertaining to coronary artery disease, became during this period more explicitly defined. The prominent place given to art in the Renaissance influenced also the pictorial aid to literary production, though this trend became apparent only later, through Vesalius, who made illustrations an important part of medical literature.

The number of books available in Renaissance medicine steadily increased. With the development of the universities, far more people were engaged in research and book-writing. For this period it would not be advisable to arrange our material under headings referring to the individual authors. However, medicine in the sixteenth century lost much of the anonymity and even modesty which had characterized it in the Middle Ages, when authors had felt themselves to be the apostles of a medical tradition and were reluctant to stress their own achievements. The Renaissance writers were often not far from vanity and self-publicity and sometimes engaged in the struggle for priority. This corresponded with the frame of mind in a period which sought to cultivate a new individualism. In spite of these features we have from now on to abstain from arranging our material under individual names, simply because they became too numerous each to be treated under a separate heading.

The intimate connection between medicine and art is best represented by Leonardo da Vinci (1452–1519). Since we cannot do justice to his almost universal interests and activities, we will limit ourselves to discussing what he contributed to knowledge in our subject. From about 750[1] of his separate anatomical drawings, nearly all preserved in Windsor Castle, we can use only very few pertaining to our study. Historically they had no influence on the development of medicine, being kept in private collections. In 1796,[2] a few of them were published, mainly on the initiative of William Hunter (1718–1783), who himself had 'hoped to engrave and publish the designs'.[3] In the meantime all the drawings, together with Leonardo's notes on them in mirror writing, have been published.

In his anatomical studies of the coronary vessels, Leonardo developed an admirable attention to detail, and an appropriate technique. Thus he mentions a difficulty in anatomizing the coronaries since 'they are surrounded by waxy (*sevoso*) fat'; cf. Keele (1952), p. 96. This was one of the reasons why these vessels were liable to be overlooked by the early anatomists. Edward Jenner (see below, p. 94) came to a similar conclusion in 1778. Referring to a dissection of a patient who died from angina pectoris, he stated in his letter to W. Heberden: '. . . as these vessels lie quite concealed in that substance [fat], is it possible this appearance may have been overlooked?'

Quite remarkable is the fact that Leonardo was able to demonstrate and depict for the first time the origins of the coronary vessels from the coronary sinus. He used the technique of a transverse section; cf. McMurrich (1930); Keele (1952), Fig. 29; O'Malley and Saunders (1952), facing p. 262. The figure is found in Q II, 9 v and was drawn about 1513.[4]

Leonardo was very much interested in the blood vessels and the changes produced by the ageing processes; in fact his drawings are probably the first to give a pictorial representation of sclerotic vessels. He depicts the tortuous vessels in his striking print of the 'Anatomy of the old man'. He says: 'Vessels in the elderly, through the thickening

---

[1] According to L. Choulant, *History and Bibliography of Anatomical Illustration*, English translation by M. Frank, New York, 1945 (p. 105). According to E. Belt (1966) 'there were 779 drawings, of which today only 600 remain at Windsor Castle; the fate of the others is not known'.

[2] John Chamberlaine, *Imitations of Original Designs by Leonardo da Vinci*, fol. London, 1796, cf. p. 10. 'I was encouraged by the favourable opinions of the late Dr. William Hunter, the physician, and John Hunter, the surgeon, as well by the ablest anatomists of the present day, with regard to the utility of such a publication.'

[3] R. H. Fox, *William Hunter* (1901), p. 50.

[4] Vesalius was likewise interested in the origin of the coronaries. In his *Tabulae anatomicae sex* (1538), plate III, the ramifications on the heart-surface are depicted. The explanatory text (translated by Ch. Singer (1946)), runs: 'The origin of the coronal arteries cannot be depicted in this plate for they are hidden beneath the valves.' In the *Fabrica* (1543) the description is found in Lib. III, cap. XII, and the references are mainly to fig. 10 of the 6th book.

However, no illustration is given portraying the origin from the aorta, as shown by Leonardo.

of their tunics, restrict the transit of the blood.' Leonardo did not mention these sclerotic changes expressly in the coronary vessels, but often refers to them in other parts of the body; for instance:

> 'The artery and the vein in the aged which extend between the spleen and the liver, acquire so thick a covering that it contracts the passage of the blood which comes from the mesenteric-portal vessels.'

As to the anatomy of the coronary vessels, Leonardo's drawings are the most beautiful specimens to be found among old illustrations, surpassing in precision and detail those included in Vesalius' work. In fact the illustrations of the coronaries in the *Fabrica* are too small and technically inadequate and do not reveal the details of the coronary branches. That Leonardo had in mind the blood supply to the heart can be deduced from his 'Anatomy of the old man' where he speaks of 'debility through lack of blood and deficiency of the artery which nourishes the heart and the other lower members'. This quotation, in all its beauty, is not indicative of Leonardo's pointing to impaired coronary blood-flow, and leads us to think that it refers to the aorta, since he states that the artery provides blood also to the lower members.[5]

A slightly older contemporary of Leonardo was the Florentine physician Antonio Benivieni, whose small book *De abditis nonnulis ac mirandis morborum et sanationum causis* was published in 1507, five years after his death. The volume is available in a facsimile edition (1954) with a translation by C. Singer, and prefaced by E. R. Long. Benivieni is sometimes regarded as a precursor of pathological anatomy. In fact, among the hundred and eleven cases he describes, some twenty are accompanied by post-mortem findings, which, however, are rather sketchy. Case 35 belongs to our topic. The author mentions a woman who

> 'was sometimes troubled with pain at her heart. At last the pain began to attack her more frequently and at length she was carried off. The corpse being cut open, there was found a small piece of dark flesh shaped like a medlar in the left ventricle of the heart, above the artery'.

The post-mortem report closes with the words that this tubercle had been the cause of her death. The case is noteworthy for the confrontation of the clinical course with the results of the autopsy. The

[5] On Leonardo and the Heart see the volumes by K. D. Keele (1952) and by E. Belt (1955).

word 'tubercle' is not used in the modern sense, but implies any protuberance or excrescence. The description is compatible with thrombosis, while the words 'above the artery' lack precision as to topography, but are still meaningful as a link between the arterial system and the pathological structure.

Another case presented under number 89 concerns a male criminal. Unfortunately the clinical data are not given. The report is called simply: 'Things of interest found in an opened body'. The pathological finding was 'an abscess in the left ventricle of the heart, the abscess being overflown by phlegm'. The interpretation is questionable,[6] but we are benefited by many later descriptions of so-called heart abscesses which can probably be identified as softening of the myocardium by an infarction. Benivieni's book is an early specimen of the collections of case histories popular in the Renaissance period, which provides a mine of actual observations from which we have been able to quote at least two pertinent narrations.[7]

In searching the older medical literature for sources prior to the time of definitive diagnosis of myocardial infarction, we came across a significant passage which was added by Vesalius to the second edition of his *Fabrica* (1555). We have discussed this passage at some length in our paper on 'Thrombo-embolic disease and heart-block in Vesalius' (1963) and we may be permitted to quote it in our translation into English and also reproduce part of our discussion and interpretation. As the passage has been interpolated by Vesalius in a section which deals not with the heart and its vessels but with the anatomy of the cranium (Lib. I, cap. 5, p. 24), it readily escaped the attention of the historians of coronary artery disease. The references to heart block, which do not strictly belong to our topic, will likewise be reproduced, as this condition is not infrequently met with in cases of coronary disease. The patient was 'the most noble and learned Dominus de Imersel', a member of the court of Charles V, whom Vesalius accompanied on his travels until 1555.

> 'Almost at the same time, our astonishment was roused by the [anatomized] heart of a most noble and also learned man; in the left ventricle of his heart we found almost two pounds of glandulous (though somewhat dark) flesh, whereby the heart was

[6] Pyaemic abscess in the heart may have been more common in the past.

[7] Another Renaissance author, Berengario da Carpi (d. 1530), appears to have been acute enough to differentiate between the function of the coronary arteries and veins. He even hints at the existence of an actual circulation between the arterial and venous systems of the coronary blood-flow (*Isagoge breves* (1522) in the English translation by L. R. Lind, p. 95). Colombo (1559) referred in almost the same words to the functions of the coronary arteries, but suggested that their blood was 'vivified' in the lungs (see p. 55).

distended like a belly around this flesh and similar to the brain of the above-mentioned girl. This man was, before his death, in a persistent melancholic and somewhat wakeful state, his pulse being really astonishingly unequal and changeable, manifestly demonstrating the contraction of the artery. For, during many months before death (though he walked about generally as a fit person), it was observed that the pulse—or more accurately the artery—was contracted, and remained constricted during the interval of three or four pulsations, or beats, as if labouring upon the expulsion of the blood. Indeed, during the last weeks of his life it was sometimes possible to palpate out of a [time-] interval of nine beats only three or two dilations of the artery. Then, to the very time of his death, he possessed enough of animal faculties as to the principal functions of the soul, death being not so nearly related to a fault of the heart as to the gangrene of the left leg; the gangrene, naturally, was provoked by the impediment of the arterial pulsations, as if these beats, intermittent through the fault of the heart, were insufficient in providing the natural heat for the legs; even more so as some years ago the artery leading to the fibula had been contused by a bullet.'

We may draw from this account the following deductions:

1. Vesalius assumed that 'a sad feeling and pain in the heart' is associated with some form of heart disease. He reported that the patient, de Imersel, died before some sad feeling at the heart became manifest, and, had not the irregularity of the pulse indicated heart disease, nobody would have thought of it. Apparently Vesalius inferred that precordial pain does denote some disease, this narration having preceded Heberden's description by more than two hundred years. The narration in the *Fabrica* stressed the fact that the patient was able to walk about ('ambulare') like a healthy person. This detail, of the general report, seems to imply that Vesalius knew that a person afflicted with a diseased heart of the type of 'tristi in corde sense doloreve' would not have been capable of free ambulation. The precordial pain without dyspnoea was one of the constituents of the diagnosis stressed in the early descriptions of ischaemic heart disease.

2. The striking post-mortem finding of a big fleshy mass in the left ventricle of the heart is obviously an intra-cardiac parietal or lateral thrombus, possibly embedded in a partial aneurysm of the heart. The details make this very probable and they preclude taking the finding for a 'heart-polyp'. The 'polypi cordis' were described many times in the older medical literature, but they proved to be agonal artefacts of

no pathological significance, whereas Vesalius' fleshy mass or mole
has features of a real thrombus. Since the description is so brief, there is
no possibility of more precise pathology.

A similar case with an autopsy was included in Vesalius' last work,
Anatomicarum Gabrielis Falloppii Observationum Examen.[8] Once again
a thrombo-embolic disease of both the legs and the heart is described.[9]
This is indicative of the interest Vesalius took in the problem.

In surveys of the history of coronary artery disease we failed to
find any discussion of Vesalius' contribution to this field. M. Roth in
his *Andreas Vesalius Bruxellensis* (1892, p. 223) gave a brief paraphrase
of the Imersel case, and lately it has been included in C. D. O'Malley's
definitive biography of Vesalius, 1964 (p. 252; see also p. 460, note
114). As to the earlier medical literature, however, it was repeatedly
referred to by authors of the seventeenth and eighteenth centuries.
It was mentioned by Caspar Bauhin in his *Theatrum anatomicum*
(1605, marginal note 1, p. 412) and by William Harvey in his manuscript *Prelectiones*, 73v. Hercules Saxonia, whom we will mention
later, discusses the case in his *Prognoseon practicarum lib. II* (1620, pp.
131–32) and significantly enough he alludes to the often-quoted
Aphorism II, 41 of Hippocrates. Bonet reproduced it in his *Sepulchretum*
(Vol. I, 1679, p. 672; 1700, p. 845) and came nearer to modern
terminology, using a derivation from the verb *infarcire* in the title he
gave to the case history: 'Pulsus inaequalitas ob cordis sinistrum
ventriculum subnigricante carne infarctum'. Finally, Morgagni (Epistle
24, par. 22) also paid due attention to Vesalius' remarkable case.

It is astonishing, however, to read in Vesalius' report that 'death
was not so nearly related to a fault of the heart as to the gangrene of the
left leg'. Vesalius' remark shows that the time was not yet ripe to
evaluate the case and the cause of death. Needless to say, the coronaries
were not mentioned in the case-report, although this structure was an
object of his studies in that part of the *Fabrica* where he described the
heart and its vessels.[10]

This is not Vesalius' only contribution to cardiovascular pathology;
in his letter to Achilles Gasser of 1557, he refers to his diagnosis of an
aortic aneurysm which had subsequently been verified by autopsy.
Here Vesalius stresses the coagulation process in the sac, and so anticipates the later, more elaborate, studies on thrombosis.[11]

---

[8] Venice (1564) p. 154; Hanau (1609) p. 236. In his *Observationes Anatomicae* (1562) fol.
124 ff. Falloppio describes the nerves of the heart and refers to cardiac pain.

[9] An interesting historical parallel is found in Dupuytren (1839); see our paper on this
case (1963, p. 261).

[10] *Fabrica* (1543), Lib. III, cap. 12.

[11] See J. O. Leibowitz, *Med. Hist.*, 1964, 8, 377.

Vesalius' successor to the Paduan chair, Realdus Columbus (?–1559) was able to add his share to a more precise understanding of coronary physiology. In his book *De re anatomica* (Venice, 1559, p. 177) he says that the coronary artery vivifies the heart substance by the vital heat thereby conveyed to it. However, the vital spirits are not engendered in the heart [as Galen put it] but in the lungs. He argued that if the heart vivified the blood, then there would be no need for the coronary arteries to supply vital spirits to the heart substance. This is an important contribution to the physiological significance of the coronaries, coming closer to the modern notion of oxygenation.*

Another Renaissance physician, almost contemporary with Vesalius, Amatus Lusitanus (1511–68), gave a purely clinical case-report which is one of the earliest to depict sudden death due to myocardial infarction. No post-mortem examination is described. Since death was attributed by Amatus to 'obstruction in the heart', an unusual diagnosis at that time, we understand why he insisted on the fact that death had not occurred from apoplexy, which was then commonly and easily diagnosed. Although too much space is allotted to measures for ascertaining death[12] as they were taken in the Renaissance period, the case history may be reproduced for better understanding of the attached scholia. The report, being one of the earliest in medical literature, is reproduced from the sixth 'Centuria', a name coined for a collection of one hundred cases. An English translation from the *Curationum medicinalium centuria sexta* (Venice, 1560) follows:

> 'The sixty-second case treating of sudden death from syncope and not from apoplexy.
>
> A reverend abbot from the Isle of Croma, one or two miles distant from Ragusa, when he was in good health and talking to several persons, said that he suddenly felt pain in his heart and with his hand moved rapidly toward the region of the heart, he fell, though slowly, to the earth and rapidly lost all his animal faculties. When called in I said he was dead. Not only was the pulse at the metacarpium and the temples missing, but even no motion upon the heart could be perceived. In order to satisfy the assistants I brought to the nostrils a burning candle whose flame did not move at all. Also a bright mirror was advanced near the mouth and nothing of respiratory contraction was seen on it. We then applied a glass vessel filled with water upon the

---

* I am indebted to Dr. J. J. Bylebyl for having drawn my attention to the passage.
[12] For methods of ascertaining death see also Antoine Louis, *Lettres sur la certitude des signes de la mort*, Paris, 1752 (376 pp.). This problem has lately become of the utmost importance in quite a different setting, namely with regard to the donor in heart transplantations.

thorax but the water was unmoved. Thereupon I ordered to keep him unburied until the next day; and if nothing happened, I advised them to dismiss him till the third day, since, as you know, the humours complete their motion within seventy-two hours which denotes three days.'

Scholia

'Some people contended that this abbot met his death from apoplexy, but verily not without error, since this [man] ended his days due to syncope, his heart lancinated, and his spirits dissolved, either through some venomous humor or, to be more precise, through some obstruction engendered in the heart which is attested by the following signs. First, because he had pain in the heart and as you know from Hippocrates: where the pain is, say there is the disease. Secondly, since no froth was brought to the mouth, nor was there any distortion of the mouth or retraction of the limbs. The mouth even remained almost opened, so that he had his teeth not tightly closed. Therefore it may be rightly and with greater probability asserted that, his nerves being without lesion, he died not from apoplexy, but suddenly and unexpectedly from a primarily affected heart. If somebody contends this comes from the nerves and he supposes that in a vehement apoplexy some kind of dissolution of the limbs may occur without retraction (an assertion which we contest) then he may be aware that an apoplexy cannot supervene without lesion of the brain and the nerves, which in this violent and sudden death did not appear. Therefore, since this [man] suffered from pain in the heart, and no damage of the nerves became visible, it seems to me more plausible that he died from a badly damaged heart than from apoplexy.'

The Scholia appended to the case-report contains a few points to be commented upon: (1) 'his heart lancinated' (lancinato corde), or lacerated, could have a figurative as well as an anatomical meaning; (2) 'through some obstruction engendered in the heart' (in corde obstructione aliqua parta), a very significant expression, calling to mind the term of occlusion, but derived no doubt from the Hippocratic-Galenical terminology; (3) 'primarily affected heart' (ex corde primario affecto), a successful and well-reasoned attempt at nosological classification. The wording of the case-history is self-explanatory. The last words about the humours completing their motions within three days is an Hippocratic notion. (Cf. the Littré edition, Vol. VII, p. 567, par. 44).

Though we have mentioned repeatedly that the word 'obstruction' in old medical literature does not always mean vascular obstruction, in the case quoted both the clinical history and the emphasis laid on the heart as the affected part do in fact refer to a vascular disease.

Looking for relevant material in the works of other Renaissance authorities led us to Paracelsus (1493–1541). We did not find much of precise clinical evidence. However, Paracelsus' notion of 'tartaric diseases', which signifies the formation of deposits, implies obstructive processes in the cardio-vascular system as well. In his work 'Tartarus cordis' (Vol. 9, p. 154 of the Sudhoff edition) Paracelsus ridicules the doctors who foolishly explain the diseases which they call 'cardiaca, tremor cordis', etc., on the grounds of disturbances in the humours. He asserts that 'tartar' is formed in some parts of the heart, especially in the pericardium, and is responsible for the aforementioned heart troubles. This is a kind of solidism as against the prevailing humoral pathology.[13] In Volume 4, p. 618, Paracelsus speaks of a pulsus tartareus: 'pulsus sine tactu, est ex sanguine coagulato, qui impedit essentiam' (pulse that cannot be felt, caused by coagulated blood which impedes the essence). The meaning of 'essence' is not explained in this context. Paracelsus may be alluding to the absence of the pulse in peripheral artery disease. The word 'dura' inserted in the margin of the text would thus refer not to the pulse but to hardening of the vessel itself.

The great work on surgery by Ambroise Paré (1510–90) contains some interesting references. He describes a person suffering from repeated swoons, in whom he found, in the autopsy, a bony constitution of the internal coat of the arteries. The post-mortem also showed a haemorrhage in the thorax probably due to a ruptured vessel. This case is not easy to interpret, since it is not evident whether the ruptured aneurysm is that of the aorta, or of the heart (Book VI, ch. 28). Though the coronary pathology is not expressly referred to in Paré's works, this surgeon records some cases of probable arteriosclerotic disease as well as post-mortem findings of sclerotic plaques, and a corresponding history of disease, as for example, in the 1579 edition (pp. 280–281). The same reference contains a passage which shows his ideas of blood coagulation as causing death.

> 'The blood solidifies into a thrombus,[14] which then rots, as the parts are not fanned and not sustained by the natural heat of the

---

[13] W. Pagel, in his book *Paracelsus* (p. 170), refers to the doctrine of 'tartar' as an early attempt at the localization of disease.

[14] The French original has the word 'thrombus'.

heart; violent grief ensues, then gangrene and mortification of the part, and finally death'.

Paré, who was in no way a classical scholar, significantly refers in this passage to the last chapter of the 4th Book of the *De praesagitione ex pulsibus* by Galen.[15] It seems that at the end of the sixteenth century the notion of 'obstruction' in the heart and the vessels became fairly well known and was referred to occasionally in the non-medical literature of the period. This is exemplified by quotations from two learned authors of that time, differing in background and in the subject of their works. Both authors use medical items only as examples for their views on the mind and soul, but they reflect current medical opinions.

Francis Bacon[16] (1561–1626), philosopher and fighter for scientific methods of research, in his essay on 'Friendship', writes:

> 'A principal fruit of friendship is the ease and discharge of the fulness and swellings in the heart, which passions of all kind do cause and induce. We know diseases of stoppings and suffoca-tions are the most dangerous in the body; and it is not much otherwise in the mind.'

Rabbi Hayim Vital (Safed 1543—Damascus 1620), Hebrew philoso-pher and leading kabbalist, in his *Shaare Kedushah* (*Gates of Holiness*, Aleppo, 1866, fol. 1a and 2b), writes:

> 'God created the body, which is the garment of the soul, of 248 organs, to which He gave 356 vessels uniting them and supplying them with blood and vitality. If the channel concerned should become occluded, the organ will desiccate'.

An author not commonly known among historians of Renaissance medicine is Petrus Salius Diversus (second half of the sixteenth century). The study of his principal work *De Affectibus particularibus*, published in his *De febre pestilenti tractatus, etc.* (1586), is very instructive as to his descriptions and theories of pain in the heart and sudden death. Under the influence of Galen, Diversus wrongly pays too much attention to pulse irregularity as an absolute requirement for the diagnosis of circulatory collapse. But for that he could in fact have ep icted myocardial infarction in its fatal form.

---

[15] Kühn IX, 421–30.
[16] Cf. G. W. Steeves, 'Medical allusions in the writings of Francis Bacon', *Proc. roy. Soc. Med., Section Hist. Med.*, (1912–13), **6**, 76–96; see p. 91.

The fourth chapter (p. 215) 'De syncope cardiaca'[17] did not escape the attention of those writers who were primarily interested in arrhythmias. It was quoted by Scherf and Schott in 1953, as follows:

'Two signs indicate impending cardiac syncope and sudden death: first, a sensation of sudden constriction of the heart associated with collapse, pallor and perspiration, and the second, that in those [patients] an intermittent pulse sometimes occurs; if the intermission extends beyond one pulse great danger threatens and it signifies that such syncope is imminent; which intermission, as well as the feeling of suffocation, originates nowhere else but from that amount of thickened blood which obstructs and impairs those vessels and internal parts'.

This translation is an almost verbal rendering into English of the Latin original on page 216 of Diversus' tract, with omission of certain phrases which are not significant. The crucial point in our investigation concerns the words, 'amount of thickened blood which obstructs and impairs those vessels and internal parts'.[18] The Latin original uses the expression 'sanguinis coalescentis copia'; the meaning of this 'coalescence' is very suggestive of clotting, which would correspond to the modern conception of the cause of myocardial infarction. The Dictionary of Classical Latin translates 'coalesco' as 'to unite, agree together, be consolidated'. It is significant that the sub-headings in the margins of Diversus' book are consistently stressing the role of the blood which coagulates, or in a slightly-changed nomenclature they refer to a so-called concretion of the blood.

Though Diversus repeats the older views underlining the role of extinction of natural heat as a factor responsible for syncope, in his insistence on the clotting process in the vessels he does not lack originality. As to the coincidence of pulse irregularity and syncope, which Diversus emphasizes, we might add that this has been repeatedly mentioned in modern publications. For instance, the occurrence of ventricular fibrillation in cases of myocardial infarction at the moment of circulatory collapse has been reported in the Lancet, 1962, i, 1306.[19]

[17] An earlier author, Bartholomaeus Montagnana (d. 1470), in his Consilia Medica (1476), mentioned 'copious matter in the heart leading to lipothymia and syncope'. See the chapter 'De egritudinibus cordis', ff. 185a–193a in the Lyons edition of 1525.
[18] See also Sebastianus Pissinus (1609), who refers to 'thickness of the blood which obstructs the little cavities of the arteries in the vicinity of the heart'. Incidentally, John Freind, in his History of Physick (1725–26; 2nd ed., London, 1727, Part II, p. 82) gives full credit to Diversus' ideas on this matter. And see also E. Rudius (1602), fol. 153: 'ex crudis humoribus syncopes periculum imminent'.
[19] G. H. Hall, G. Neale and D. M. Young, Letter to the Editor on Ventricular Fibrillation, with successful resuscitation of one patient.

Heart rhythm disorders figure prominently as a cause of sudden death in patients with myocardial infarction. We will later return to this item in commenting upon Heberden's patient 'Dr. Anonymus'.

In view of the restricted knowledge of coronary pathology in his period, and as yet unaided by Harvey's theory of the circulation of the blood, Diversus' statements are bound not to be very precise. Thus he refers to coagulation occurring not only in arteries but also in veins, as the cause of syncope. Stating rightly that coagulation takes place during life (thrombus formation) he postulates that the blood in the corpse remains liquid, which according to modern knowledge holds only in some cases of cardiogenic shock.[20] In spite of these and other smaller inadequacies, the ideas expressed by Diversus seem to be nearest to the present-day conception of the pathology of a coronary event, notwithstanding the total lack of indication as to where the clotting process takes place.

The Renaissance authors we have just mentioned were thus instrumental in providing observations and ideas which suggest coronary artery disease. However, their knowledge of heart diseases and their subdivision into well-defined clinical and pathological entities remained only rudimentary, a state of affairs which persisted until the end of the eighteenth century. Very few heart diseases had been clearly described, as for instance those of the pericardium, known already since classical antiquity. Works devoted exclusively to cardiovascular diseases began to make their appearance rather late, the most complete one being that of Sénac, in 1749. When we examine older books for information on the heart, we find that symptoms are described rather than the diseases themselves. The chapters are given such headings as 'Syncope', 'Palpitation', 'Tremor of the heart', 'Intermittent pulse', and so on, whereas these manifestations are in fact common to several heart diseases.

Other organs were given a more thorough representation. Though the descriptions may not always be in conformity with recent knowledge, historical study is facilitated by appropriate headings and fuller accounts. In his paper of 1928, Max Neuburger deplored the low state of older cardiology as compared with the history of other fields of medicine. The great delay in the inquiry into cardio-vascular diseases is partly explained by the old classical doctrine that the heart cannot survive any damage. This preconception held back the earlier physicians from investigating more thoroughly heart diseases at large. However, even in classical times authors were not too consistent.

[20] See our discussion of blood-fluidity in the chapter on Heberden.

Hippocrates and Galen, though teaching that the heart cannot be diseased without sudden death intervening, described, nevertheless, quite a number of cardiac symptoms and morbid states.

2. THE SEVENTEENTH CENTURY

Keeping in mind these limitations we proceed to the seventeenth century in further search of material pertaining to our topic. The first two authors to be mentioned belong chronologically more to the preceding one, but their works were published early in the seventeenth century. They lived before the scientific revolution which characterized this epoch, though it did not immediately influence medical practice.

We refer first to the physician of Padua, Hercules Saxonia (Ercole Sassonia, 1551–1607), and to his work, *De Pulsibus*, published in Frankfurt in 1604. We became interested in this author while investigating the early history of heart block,[21] and found that this condition was mentioned by him long before the generally accepted 'first descriptions'. Saxonia discusses in detail the question whether this condition, which he calls 'rarity of the pulse', is or is not a sign of impending death. In chapter 100 of his volume he pays attention not only to this symptom, but also to the condition of the heart. 'When the rarity stems from an essential disorder of the heart itself', he writes, 'it is the most lethal of all'. In a further elaboration of this proposition he speaks also of 'significant damage to the solid substance of the heart' (solidae cordis substantiae insigni laesione).[22] He supposes, further, that 'the acute attack arises from a heart which is essentially affected in its substance'. We should like to draw attention to this not so well-known author and his work for the following reason. Besides clinical descriptions suggesting coronary artery disease, every reference to damage in the heart muscle in older literature should be carefully recorded. Saxonia did not speak of real pathology and probably did not participate in autopsies. His remarkable statement just mentioned must have come to his mind through reasoning, as was the case in the examples referred to in earlier chapters. His younger contemporary, Amatus, as already mentioned, also spoke of a 'primarily affected heart' as an etiological basis for sudden death.

The second author to be considered is Felix Platter of Basle (1536–1614), whose extensive work, *Observationes* (abridged title), was published in Latin in Basle in 1614. Platter was a renowned physician,

[21] See J. O. Leibowitz and D. T. Ullmann (1965).
[22] Almost the same wording was used by Duretus (1527–86) in Jac. Hollerius (1611): Syncope . . . a dissolutione solidae substantiae cordis'.

a clinician who also had a great interest in investigating mental and
nervous diseases. This fact is not irrelevant to the case we are about to
discuss, which appears (pp. 174–75) with the caption, 'A lethal suffocation of the uterus' (Uteri suffocatio lethalis). This obsolete term was
used extensively in medieval and Renaissance medicine, in a way more
or less conforming to the word 'hysteria' of later periods. That this
diagnosis was far from being precise is manifested by the gloomy
adjective 'lethal'. Incidentally, the case is included in the section,
'Reduced action of breath'. It should be noted that heart diseases in
Galen to which we referred earlier were also incorporated under the
general heading of 'Respiration', in De locis affectis. A heart case
similarly classified by Platter will not, therefore, take us by surprise.
We shall quote our translation of the case-history with some omissions:

> 'A maid, about thirty-six years old, a virgin, robust, dark-
> haired and healthy, who was employed in my house, left on the
> 4th June 1613, in order to go to the market. Quite suddenly she
> fainted and fell on the ground, and when we picked her up she
> began to speak. She told us that she had never before suffered
> from anything similar. At the same time she complained of a
> very sharp pain in her heart, saying something was gnawing
> inside her. . . . A short time afterwards she again lost conscious-
> ness, and neither moved nor breathed. Her pulse failed com-
> pletely. The woman's face was yellowish and covered with a
> cold sweat. She did not regain consciousness, though we had
> hoped the attack would subside, since the case appeared to me
> to be a "suffocatio uteri", which through constriction of the
> heart causes a grave syncope. However, she did not recover,
> and within half an hour she expired'.[23]

In this case, myocardial infarction is very probable, though age and
sex would not favour the diagnosis, since women of this age are not so
prone to this disease. Other possible diagnoses, such as acute pneumo-
thorax or some form of pulmonary embolism are not very likely.
Details which support our diagnosis are: the patient's constitution,
described as robust, which may indicate obesity; her possibly hurrying
to the market; localization of the pain in the heart; and recovery after a
while, followed as is so often the case by a second and this time fatal
event. A diagnosis 'suffocation of the uterus' is also incidentally
mentioned by Saxonia in his De pulsibus with an additional comment:
'few of them die'. The fact that the patient was regarded before this

---

[23] See also the German translation of Platter, edited by H. Buess (1963), pp. 134–35,
and note 37, p. 170.

event as healthy does not speak against our diagnosis. In people not yet advanced in years, myocardial infarction can often occur without previous complaints or symptoms.

With regard to the first half of the seventeenth century, we refer to Harvey's work which throws light also on our subject. His theory of the circulation of the blood did not exert as yet a direct influence on the medical profession or on its awareness of coronary artery disease. On the other hand, Harvey was not only physiologist and experimentalist. His close contact with the practice of medicine led him to make observations and in two of them he described cases highly suggestive of coronary manifestations. We shall quote his first observation contained in his 'Second Disquisition to John Riolan' (1649), which has been inserted in the apology for his theory, a matter of physiology rather than of clinical medicine, exemplifying his general concept of circulation. To our mind this case is the most remarkable reference of the pre-Heberden period. We wonder whether Heberden knew of this passage when he wrote in his classic paper of 1772: '. . . a distemper hitherto so unnoticed that it has not yet, as far as I know, found a place or a name in the history of diseases'.

> 'I add another observation. A noble knight, Sir Robert Darcy, when he had reached to about the middle period of life, made frequent complaint of a certain distressing pain in the chest, especially in the night season; so that dreading at one time syncope, at another suffocation in his attacks he led an unquiet and anxious life. He tried many remedies in vain, having had the advice of almost every medical man. The disease going on from bad to worse, he by-and-by became cachectic and dropsical, and finally grievously distressed, he died in one of his paroxysms. In the body of this gentleman, we found the wall of the left ventricle of the heart ruptured, having a rent in it of size sufficient to admit any of my fingers, although the wall itself appeared sufficiently thick and strong. This laceration had apparently been caused by an impediment to the passage of the blood from the left ventricle into the arteries.'

This passage is taken from the translation by Robert Willis, published in 1847, which in spite of some archaisms is generally satisfactory and is preferred by some readers as retaining the flavour of the original Latin. A more modern and very scholarly rendering into English was produced by Kenneth J. Franklin in 1958.

Comment: clinically, anginal syndrome with a protracted course of disease leading in the later stage to heart insufficiency ('dropsical').

This precedes similar descriptions by Parry (1799) and Leyden (1884). Pathological findings reveal rupture of the left ventricle; the hypertrophy is probably based on a concomitant disease, e.g., hypertension or severe aortic valvular disease; while a transmural infarct, the probable cause of the rupture ('rent'), was at Harvey's time beyond the range of diagnostic possibilities.

A modern pathologist[24] found spontaneous rupture of the heart in 5–10 per cent of deaths from coronary artery disease or myocardial infarction. In the history of disease, the most striking and dramatic forms were the first to be described. For instance, peptic ulcer, in its chronic form, characterized by hunger pain, was noted as late as 1832. By contrast, the first case with an autopsy described by Marcello Donato in 1586 was that of a stenosis due to pylotic ulcer. So was the diagnosis of myocardial infarction, described but not named as such by Malmsten and Düben in 1859 (the first report with a histological finding of myocardial necrosis), also occasioned by the dramatic event of a ruptured heart ventricle.

In the same letter to Riolan, another case of what will now be termed coronary artery disease immediately follows. Here Harvey uses the words: 'the patient fell upon a strange kind of disease and was miserably tormented with very great oppression and with pain in the heart and chest'. (Franklin's translation.) This second case is very interesting as to Harvey's concept of the etiological factors.

> 'The man, having received an injury and affront from one more powerful than himself and upon whom he could not have his revenge, was so overcome with anger and indignation, which he yet communicated to no-one, that at last he fell into a strange distemper.'

This conjecture seems to favour a psychogenic theory of the disease. The opening of the body in this second case did not show a cardiac rupture but only an enormous hypertrophy and an enlargement which Harvey called a 'bovine heart';[25] this term remained in use until the present day. It is noteworthy to record that Harvey occasionally used the word 'infarcted' in the meaning of impeded (*De motu cordis*, end of the third chapter).

So far the clinical and some pathological features as found in Harvey's *Disquisition* have been dealt with. No less interesting is a short passage on a purely physiological matter which is inserted in the first letter to

---

[24] A. Levene, 1962; see Bibliography.
[25] Cor bovinum. Also a plant, Bullock's Heart, the fruit of Anona reticulata, was known in old medical botany; see Gerard's *Herbal*, 1597.

Riolan, and refers to the 'third circulation'.[26] Harvey states that besides the first circulation of the blood through the whole body, and the second through the lungs, there is a third, which he describes[27] as 'a very short circulation; namely, from the left ventricle of the heart to the right one, driving a portion of the blood round through the coronary arteries and veins, which are distributed with their small branches through the body, walls, and septum of the heart' (translation by Franklin), p. 23 in English and p. 117 in Latin.[28]

In the next paragraph Harvey adds 'that a valve is very commonly found in the opening of the coronary vein (sinus) preventing entry into it, but favouring egress from it. So a third circulation must certainly be admitted'.

The details of this so-called third circulation have in fact only been elucidated in quite recent times, when the blood flow in the coronary vessels could be quantitatively measured by means of catheterization and complicated laboratory procedures.

An early case description of angina pectoris, this time not given by a physician, has been found in the autobiography of Edward, Earl of Clarendon (1609–74), Lord High Chancellor, and concerns the case-history of his father who died in 1632. The report is purely clinical and does not provide anatomical data. However, the lively description by a layman is a fine specimen of the author's powers of observation. In medical literature we found a reference to the case in John Blackall's book *Observations on the Nature and Cure of Dropsies*, etc., 1813, pp. 378–79. It first came to the attention of medical historians in a paper published in 1922.[29] A few lines from the Memoirs may be quoted:

'He was seized by so sharp a pain in the left arm . . . that the torment made him pale as he were dead; and he used to say that

[26] Since the completion of this manuscript, we have had the pleasure of reading the paper (*Brit. med. J.*, 1968, **4**, 273) by D. Evan Bedford, in which he stresses the importance of Harvey's concept of 'a third circulation' which has been neglected by other writers on Harvey.

[27] The Latin original begins with the words: 'Poterat hic addere doctissimus vir tertiam circulationem brevissiman . . . per arterias et venas coronales, etc.', on page 34, 1st line, of the 1st edition: *Exercitationes duae anatomicae de Circulatione Sanguinis. Ad Joannem Riolanum filium*, etc. Roterdami, Ex Officina Arnoldi Leers, 1649.

[28] In this connection, Galen's views of the coronaries as a separate system for supplying blood to the heart are interesting enough to be recalled here. See our discussion above, on pages 33–36; especially the quotation on page 34: 'The heart is not nourished by its own blood; but . . . a rather thick branch [the coronary] leads off for the nourishment of the heart,' etc. Harvey was an assiduous student of Galen, whom he mentions very often. From the inception of our work, we have been captivated by Galen's concept of coronary physiology and were induced to regard it as an ancient parallel, *mutatis mutandis*, to Harvey's Third Circulation (see above p. 34).

[29] J. Rosenbloom, see Bibliography.

he had passed the pangs of death, and he should die in one of those fits; as soon as it was over, which was quickly, he was the cheerfullest man living . . . . But he had the image of death so constantly before him in those continual torments, that for many years before his death he always parted with his son, as to see him no more. Death came quite suddenly, after one of his usual attacks, and the writer stresses that it could not be apoplexy, "nor could the physicians make any reasonable guess from whence that mortal blow proceeded".'

The exclusion of a possible apoplexy recalls the case earlier quoted from Amatus Lusitanus who used almost the same words, finally concluding that death had been due to 'obstruction in the heart'.

Clarendon's case is one of the few descriptions of the disease to be found in the early non-medical literature. It recalls a still earlier account of this kind as given in Froissart's *Chronicles* concerning the sudden death of the Count de Foix (1331–91). Froissart (1333?–after 1400), a contemporary of the Count, was an able chronicler, writing with grace and naivety. From his account we extract a few features relevant to the case-history. The Count was a patron of literature and the arts and himself wrote a Treatise on Hunting.

'The day he died, he had all the forenoon been hunting a bear. The weather was marvellously hot, even for the month of August. In the evening [at the inn] he called for water to wash and stretched out his hands; but no sooner had his fingers . . . touched the cold water, than he changed colour, from an oppression at his heart, and, his legs failing him, fell back on his seat, exclaiming, "I am a dead man: Lord God, have mercy on me!" He never spoke after this, though he did not immediately die, but suffered great pain . . . In less than half an hour he was dead, having surrendered his soul very quietly.'

The case is suggestive of a coronary event, though the description is not detailed enough to warrant a definitive diagnosis. The clinical features include: sudden onset, collapse-like phenomena with loss of tone in the limbs, oppression at the heart, and great pain. Predisposing factors were: the long strain of a full day's hunting; very hot weather, and possible reflex spasm from the cold water.

An illustration entitled 'The sudden death of the Count de Foix' is to be found in MS Harl. 4379, fol. 126 in the British Museum (Plate iv). It does not, however, show the typical movement of the hand towards the heart, due perhaps to the loss of muscular tone which is clearly depicted as part of the state of collapse.[30]

The second half of the seventeenth century was characterized by the steadily progressive integration of scientific methods into medical inquiry. Medicine again adopted experimental methods inaugurated by Galen but almost forgotten during the long intervening period. Medical scholarship made fuller use of the advances in natural sciences than was the case during the Renaissance period. More precise instruments were invented and used. A physiological approach to problems of health and disease became more widely adopted, as exemplified not only by the work of Harvey but also that of Malpighi. Since technical methods were not so well developed as they later became, scholars experimented on lower species, and also on the hen's egg. In this endeavour the Royal Society of London, established in 1660, played an important rôle, since the meetings were combined with practical experiments—biological, chemical and mechanical. In comparison with other branches of learning, our subject played, quite understandably, only a minor part in the activities of the Royal Society.

One of the scholars inspired by these trends and aspirations, Richard Lower (1631–91), turned to investigations of the heart and the blood flow. In 1669 he published his *Tractatus de Corde*, in which some information on the coronaries is to be found, the main content of the book being the anatomy and physiology of the heart at large. Lower also described transfusion from one dog to another in 1665, and in man, two years later. Bearing directly on our subject and of high import are the details about coronary anastomoses, which he proved by a technique of injecting fluid into the vessels. The question of anastomoses became momentous in coronary research only in the 1880s, when the possibility of collateral circulation was denied by the experimental pathologist Cohnheim, but proved by other investigators. Here is what Lower has to say about the coronary vessels and their anastomoses:

> '. . . they come together again, and here and there communicate by anastomoses. As a result, fluid injected into one of them spreads at one and the same time through both. There is everywhere an equally great need of vital heat and nourishment, so deficiency of these is very fully guarded against by such anastomoses.'[31]

[30] I am indebted to Dr. M. H. Armstrong Davison of Newcastle-upon-Tyne for drawing my attention to both the case and the illustration.
[31] Quoted from K. J. Franklin's English translation of Lower's treatise (1932), p. 13.

With the exception of this quotation, no clinical data about coronary disease can be found in this work. However, on page 207, Lower mentions mechanisms 'to prevent resistance or obstruction of any kind'. This phrase indicates that pathological findings were at least considered, even if not elaborated upon, the book being, as already mentioned, devoted solely to anatomy and physiology of the heart. In some respects his observation on the absorption of air by the blood belongs to our topic since coronary disturbances have much to do with inadequate oxygenation of the tissues.

It is tempting to associate the name of Marcello Malpighi (1628–1694) with our topic for his treatise *De Polypo Cordis*.[32]

As to the term 'heart polyp', it was used very often in the sixteenth and seventeenth centuries when the early anatomists described dissections in heart patients. Very seldom did this finding correspond to a thrombus in the modern sense, and the so-called cardiac polypi were artefacts arising after the death of the patient and due to stagnation and postagonal coagulation of the blood in the heart chambers. This was convincingly demonstrated by Th. Kerckring (1640–93). However, the great merit of this brief tract lies in Malpighi's lucid presentation of blood clotting and the role of fibrin in this process.

Although cardiac polypi, a term used at the time when Malpighi wrote his treatise, are not always identical with thrombi, there is a possibility that the author included the latter in his considerations. This is suggested by his statement, 'In cardiac syncope, which closely resembles apoplexy in its symptoms, they readily appear in profusion in the heart and lungs' (p. 129), which could perhaps refer to thrombo-embolic phenomena. Incidentally, not all authors of the sixteenth and seventeenth centuries use the word 'polyp', as is evident from our previous discussion of Vesalius, who spoke of a 'fleshy mass'. At any rate, Malpighi holds a place of honour in connection with our topic, since he discusses in detail the fluidity and coagulation of blood. That he also treated a case of what is now known as coronary artery disease is evident from a note by Morgagni (Epistle 35, par. 16 and 17) in which he mentions a patient,

> 'the Commander of the city fortress, who was frequently seized with a pain at the region of the heart. Being under the

---

[32] First published in 1666. Carlo Frati (1897) in his *Bibliografia Malpighiana* (photolithograph, Dawsons, 1960) lists 14 editions of *De Polypo Cordis*. It is included in many editions of his *De Viscerum Structura*, as well as in his *Opera Omnia* (pp. 123–32). This treatise has also been commented upon by the assiduous Bonet (*Sepulchretum*, ed. of 1700, vol. III, 574). There is also a modern edition (1956) with an English translation by J. M. Forrester. Also Luigi Belloni's scholarly Italian edition of Malpighi's *Opera scelte* (1967). See especially pp. 33–34 of the introduction, and the translations, pp. 193–216, preceded by three pages on the history of the treatise.

cautious and diligent care of Malpighi he seemed likely to have recovered, when at length, being seized with an acute fever, he died. In the heart were found both polypi and an ulcer.' (Translation by Alexander.)

The 'ulcer in the heart', in view of the case history, may correspond to a softening due to infarction.

As to the clinical picture reflected in medical writings of this period, coronary artery diseases occasionally seem to be disguised by descriptions in which the respiratory distress comes more to the fore. Some writers[33] have suggested that F. Bartoletti (1576–1630) may have had in mind coronary attacks when he described distress on exertion. He speaks of the impediment of blood flow through the lungs, calling it 'obstructio laevium arteriarum pulmonum', the same words Galen had used in the case of Antipater (*De locis affectis*, IV, 8). We have studied Bartoletti's *Methodus in dyspnoeam* (1633), containing the text of his lectures given in 1628, but we have failed to find there any record of severe pain. However, Bartoletti did refer to a 'characteristic dyspnoea from which sudden death can be predicted, where the patients had suffered for a long time from respiratory difficulties when walking and they are forced to stop because they experience a sort of suffocation, accompanied by a certain irritating sensation around the sternum which is indescribable and gradually ascends toward the throat'. (Lib. III, Par. IV, cap. 3, pp. 383–84). The dyspnoea was probably a result of left heart insufficiency complicating coronary heart disease.

Thomas Willis (1621–72), a medical authority of that period, paid attention to several manifestations of the disease with which we are concerned, and he described heaviness and great oppression in the heart. However, according to his tendency to attribute diseases to the nervous system, he assigned this disease to an influence of the nerves on the aorta[34] rather than to coronary pathology. Using the English translation of his *Pharmaceutice Rationalis* (1679) we find in Chapter 3, entitled 'Palpitation of the Heart', a few relevant observations which are worth while noting. Here the author refers to a patient who 'began to be afflicted with palpitation continually, night and day, with grievous pursiness [perhaps congestion]'; when he died, the post-mortem revealed that 'the heart appeared tumid with concreted blood' (p. 125). Willis goes on to describe what he terms 'convulsive passion':

'The arteries belonging to the heart have been in fault. This

---

[33] Erik J. Warburg (1930); P. Klemperer (1960).
[34] Cf. the aortic theory of Allbutt (p. 143).

affection does sometimes proceed from the blood clotting within the bosom of the heart and the adjoining vessels, and being concreted as it were into a fleshy crust' (p. 126).

There is also a remark to the effect that

'arteries being suddenly constrained stop the sanguineous flood; blood heaped up and stagnating, there is presently felt a mighty burden and a great oppression' (p. 127).

Though the pathological findings are not described in terms conforming with present-day usage, the recognition of blood-clotting as an etiological factor is quite pronounced. As to the clinical side, the wording 'mighty burden and a great oppression' would readily fit into the picture of coronary artery disease.

The question of anatomical lesions in the coronary vessels was only occasionally approached by the seventeenth-century investigators. Particular attention to findings of calcification in these vessels in autopsies was delayed until the end of the eighteenth century, when the clinical picture of angina pectoris became known. Occasional descriptions do, however, emerge before this period. There is, for instance, some evidence that Carolus Drelincourt (1633–97) found ossification of the coronary artery, a fact reported by Théophile Bonet (1620–89) in his three-volume work *Sepulchretum*. We have not been able to trace this particular piece of information to its original source, though other cases collected by Bonet can be verified, often after considerable effort. Incidentally, this comprehensive work, especially pages 863–901 in the first volume of the 1700 edition, as well as the fourth book in Volume III, abounds in observations which are relevant to our topic and which the compiler took from books which have since become rare.

One of the observations by J. Fantoni appended to the last volume of Bonet's work (1700) is worth quoting:

'From 1680, the patient was under observation for two years, and suffered from great oppression in the heart, and substernal pain. Before his death cold sweat and imperceptible pulse were reported. In the post-mortem a huge thrombus ('polypus') and small ulcers on the surface of the heart were observed' (Lib. IV, Sect. XII, Obs. 22).

In spite of the abundance of information on our subject offered by Bonet, there are not too many quite typical and convincing cases of coronary artery disease confirmed by post-mortem. The *Sepulchretum* represents a collection of source material aiming at the correlation of diseases and anatomical findings, a real precursor of Morgagni's work, so that the perusal of its volumes is rewarding. It seems to us that in present-day historical research into the history of disease this book is almost neglected.

Several forms of heart disease, especially of the syncopal type, were reported by Lorenzo Bellini (1643–1704) in his book *De urinis et pulsibus* (1683). Bellini discusses the state of the coronary arteries and admits that the condition which he calls 'pressio' is dangerous and may cause the contraction of the heart to be abolished (p. 541). He also has in mind external pressure by tumours, fat and so on. However, an intra-arterial coronary impediment of blood-flow by calcification was clearly described by this author. Bellini reported of a patient who died of a condition similar to the clinical picture of coronary disease as we now understand it, in whose coronary arteries he found a 'stone'. It seems quite reasonable to deduce that Bellini saw in the post-mortem a coronary occlusion. This case was later quoted by Morgagni (Epistle 24, par. 17) as follows: 'I have seen a stone growing to the larger branches of the coronary artery, where they divide the right from the left ventricle.' Thus, the localization of the occlusion in the ramus descendens has been mentioned.

A special position must be allocated to the French physician Pierre Chirac (1650–1732) for having performed the first experimental ligation of a coronary artery in a dog. His book *De Motu Cordis Adversaria Analytica* (1698) is an early attempt at experimental pathology with regard to the coronary vessels. Likewise there is much information on the fibres of the heart; some ideas are also expressed as to measuring the heart's power: 'Quocirca aestimandas nobis ac mensurandae potentiae metrices hinc inde agendes'; the blood volume too was estimated (p. 305). The main purpose of the book was to describe the heart's mechanism; the experimental ligation of the coronaries is referred to in order to explain the contraction of the auricles and ventricles. In fact, Chirac does not say that he himself made the experiment (p. 234), but since he later refers to a ligation of the pulmonary artery apparently made by him (p. 302), it may be assumed that his is the first experimental ligation of a coronary vessel.

Since the description of the effects of coronary ligation was quite a novum in medical literature it is appropriate to reproduce Chirac's account in a slightly abridged form. In the case of

'interrupted entrance of blood into the coronary artery, the heart once contracted cannot afterwards perform the movement of dilation. When the coronary artery is tied up, then [at first] the movements of contraction and dilation are exercised in the usual way, whilst in a heart excised completely [from the body] the coronary arteries, almost empty of blood, at that time, cannot impel the humours contained within, into the usual channels.'

To examine the excised heart of an animal was an accepted practice in Galenic anatomy, as evidenced by Galen's *De anatomicis administrationibus* (Lib. VII, cap. 8):

'But the fact that the heart, removed from the thorax, can be seen to move for a considerable time is a definite indication that it does not need the nerves to perform its own function' (p. 184, Charles Singer's translation).

It is not unlikely that Chirac's experiments were performed in emulation of Galen's experimental approach, forgotten for many centuries.

CHAPTER IV

The Eighteenth Century

THE most significant feature of this period in connection with our topic is Heberden's introduction of the name and notion of 'angina pectoris', which occurred in the last third of the century. Before going into details of this turning-point in the history of our subject, a survey covering the previous decades of the century will be given. They were rich in individual observations, experiments and techniques and paved the way for a better understanding of coronary artery disease. Greater and lesser authorities concurred in assembling an increasing volume of knowledge, and we shall refer to them in the following paragraphs.

Notable among the merits of the Dutch physician Fredrik Ruysch (1638–1731) are his anatomical preparations which show the arborization of the vessels. Ruysch applied the so-called corrosion method, by injecting metallic salts into the blood-vessels, with the result of their representation as a metallic tree. By this study he furthered the knowledge of the coronary arteries.[1]

Raymond Vieussens (1641–1716) is best known for his classical studies of valvular disease, and especially for giving us what is probably the first description of mitral stenosis. However, he also promoted the idea that the coronary vessels have direct communication with the chambers of the heart. In his book, *Novum vasorum corporis humani systema* (1705),[2] he describes his experiments on the structure of the coronary vessels, using both the corrosion method and microscopic examination. He found ducts [capillaries] which he later called 'fleshy ducts' or 'conduits charneux'. So two modes of venous drainage of the heart were considered by him: a superficial system (anterior cardiac veins of the coronary sinus), and a deeper system of veins which communicate directly with the heart chambers (p. 108).

Almost at the same time a small book by Adam Christian Thebesius (1686–1732) was published, including two illustrations which are

---

[1] Ruysch's anatomical museum at Leyden was purchased by Peter the Great in 1717 for the Imperial Academy of Sciences. Quite recently it was found in Leningrad in a still fair state of preservation. Cf. G. Mann, *Sudhoff's Arch.*, 1961, **45**, 176–78, and the same, *Bull. Cleveland med. Libr.*, 1964, **11**, 10–13.

[2] See also his *Nouvelles Découverts sur le Coeur* (1706); and for further information see F. H. Pratt (1898, 1932) and C. E. Kellett (1959).

both beautiful and exact. The book is entitled *Dissertatio medica de circulo sanguinis in corde* (1708). In some respects the ideas it contains are similar to those of Vieussens, but experimentally it is sounder and more precise. Thebesius injected materials into the coronary veins of cadavers and observed the passage into the chambers of the heart through small orifices in the endocardium. His name is still remembered by the term Thebesian valves, or valvulae sinus coronarii cordis (Thebesii). These are the openings of the Thebesian veins on the inner surface of the right atrium of the heart, which provide a drainage bed known as the Thebesian system. This discovery is of importance for the understanding of some reparative mechanisms after arterial thrombosis.

Besides the study of the above-mentioned structure bearing his name, which corresponds to that of Vieussens ('fleshy ducts'), Thebesius gave accurate descriptions of ossification in the coronary arteries. This process, as far as it occurs in other vessels of the body, had been mentioned of course much earlier, for instance by Leonardo da Vinci, who also provided drawings of tortuous vessels in the aged. Thebesius in fact quotes quite a large number of authors who had described degenerative processes in the arterial walls before him—Ruysch, Willis, Platter, Forestus, Realdus Columbus, and Lower. His own merit consists in having dealt specifically with ossification in the coronaries, not unlike Bellini's earlier and more inclusive observation. This important finding corresponds to the later notion of coronary sclerosis, and the author also stresses its dangerous nature. Thebesius' observation was regarded as significant enough to be quoted by Morgagni (Epistle 24, par. 17): 'The larger branches of the arteries . . . which run down upon the convex surface of the heart, quite to the apex, partly ossified in several places' (Alexander's translation, p. 729).[3] It is amazing to find so much in so small a book as Thebesius', numbering only 31 pages. (We have used the second edition of 1716.)

Among the early authors of the eighteenth century G. M. Lancisi (1655–1720), a papal physician in Rome, is to be noted. His famous and quite concise book *De subitaneis mortibus* (On sudden deaths) (1707) was occasioned when the Pope became aware of a large number of sudden deaths in the metropolis; he summoned his court physician, Lancisi, to investigate the matter by opening the bodies of the deceased persons.[4] Lancisi began his book with a historical survey, in which he

---

[3] See F. H. Pratt's paper, 'The nutrition of the heart through the vessels of Thebesius' (1898), and also his paper, 'Swedenborg on the Thebesian blood flow of the heart' (1932).

[4] The initiative of the Pope in commissioning this study is quite remarkable. This must be the first epidemiological study of a non-communicable condition.

quotes Hippocrates in his 'Coan Presagia' and proceeds to define the Greek word 'cardiogmos' to which we referred earlier. It is significant that he stresses the conjunction of pain with dyspnoea (chapter 18, 9), an item to which we referred in the discussion of Bartoletti and which will also be touched upon in later chapters.

A reference to precordial pain is made in Chapter 19, 7–8, in which it is regarded as a forewarning symptom, especially when the pain occurs in elderly persons and recurs frequently. This is of course a repetition of the famous Aphorism II, 41 of Hippocrates. Lancisi also repeats the Hippocratic notion that obese people are more prone to fall victim to sudden death.[5]

In his book, *De Aneurysmatibus*, published posthumously in 1728 and which is available in a more recent edition with an English translation by W. C. Wright, Lancisi often speaks of obstructions in the heart and vessels. However, he mainly considers dilated cavities of the heart, and obstructed blood-flow through aortic anomalies, for instance, but not coronary obstruction as such. He does not omit mentioning polyps, a term which was used for coagulation of the stagnant blood in the cadavers, and he also refers to a clotted substance which encrusts the membrane of the artery as found in the aneurysmatic sac (p. 325 in Wright's edition).

In the first more comprehensive manual of heart diseases by J. B. de Sénac (1693–1770), quite a number of items pertaining to our topic are to be found. His two-volume work, *Traité sur la structure du coeur, de son action et de ses maladies*, was published in Paris in 1749.[6] In the preface he stresses the difficulties in the diagnosis and treatment of heart diseases, which, in the author's words, are 'commonly a stumbling block to so many patients and so many doctors'. He is very precise as to the anatomy of the coronaries, in the second volume, and quotes many authors. In the chapter on syncope (p. 542) he quotes Salius Diversus, whom we mentioned earlier (pp. 58–59), duly recognizing the importance of the coagulation of the blood. Again, the signs of suffocation are recorded along with oppression felt in the region of the heart.

Sénac later supplemented this work with two volumes entitled *Traité des Maladies du Coeur* (1781). We have used the second edition (Paris, 1783). Several of the descriptions it contains suggest to us some kind of myocardial infarction or at least a softening of the heart

---

[5] Papers dealing *inter alia* with Lancisi's views on our topic include J. J. Philipp (1847–1848), M. Hoffman (1935), and M. Calabresi (1944).

[6] This work contains the beautiful plates drawn by Jacques Pottier (spelt 'Potier' on the figures) and engraved by J. Robert (see Vol. I, p. 504). For general information on the author see Degris, *Etude sur Sénac* (1901).

substance. In one observation he stresses the fact that the disease must have been quite a sudden one, since the patient had been playing cards three or four days before (I, 197). The substance of the lesion was 'soft as butter'; 'one could easily put one's finger into it'. In another case (I, 208), 'half of the heart was entirely decayed'. Previous to his death the patient had suffered for a long time from frequent swooning. In the chapter headed 'Concrétions osseuses du coeur' Sénac asserts: 'The great Harvey[7] had seen a piece transformed into a round bone' (p. 268). As to the ossifications in the coronary vessels, he quotes observations by Drelincourt, Bellini, Thebesius and also Crell (1740), the latter stating that the coronary artery was as hard as bone. In the same connection he mentions the names of Bonet and Morgagni. Finally he introduces his own observation, where the coronary arteries had been ossified to such an extent that they were like branches of coral, while the heart ventricles were covered with a dense crust; the walls of the heart could be stretched or compressed only after considerable force had been applied (I, 279). It is possible that Sénac described in this observation a case of coronary sclerosis combined with pericarditis, as later demonstrated by Kernig (1892, 1905) and by Sternberg (1910).

Johann Friedrich Crell (1701–47) has to be credited with a quite early observation of coronary sclerosis (1740). It seems that his dissertation[8] described not only the induration, but also a thrombus in the coronary artery. The autopsy of a patient who died in his 70th year revealed not only a left descendent coronary artery 'hardened like bone', but also a solid wormlike cylinder of atheromatous matter which the dissector had squeezed out from the lumen.

> 'It was apparent that the exterior tunic had not changed at all from its natural condition, but that it contained, within, a harder body. When the channel was dissected lengthwise, its interior tunic, which is called the nervea, had remained whole and through it there appeared likewise a body of a different character, of a yellowish-white colour, of which I observed a greater density near the point where the branches emerge, particularly from the trunk. As I desired to ascertain the nature of this hard body and the reason for its appearance, I turned the artery in every way and, happening to press lightly on the inner tunic, I observed that there came out through its pores a substance

---

[7] This remark refers to ossification in the aorta and not in the heart in spite of the misleading title of the chapter!

[8] *Dissertatio de Arteria coronaria instar ossis indurata*, in A. von Haller, *Disputationes* (1757–60), 7 vols; Vol. II, 566.

similar to that found in an atheroma or a meliceris; this was squeezed out in a wormlike shape and the majority of it, which was more solid but of the same colour, remained inside, so that there was no doubt that it was caused by the hardening of this and would coagulate if it remained there longer and the thinner part of it continued to be expelled in the same way.'[9]

When discussing pathological descriptions of coronary disease during the eighteenth century, one is naturally led to seek for detailed information in the classic work by Morgagni (1682–1771). It is not necessary to enlarge on the importance of this great work, published in 1761 and translated into English by B. Alexander in 1769, *The Seats and Causes of Diseases investigated by Anatomy*.

Covering the facets of pathology in all parts of the body, Morgagni did not overlook the diseases which are the topic of our investigation. We will pay due credit to his achievements and quote some of the more pertinent passages.[10] However, that the Epistle (24, par. 16) acts as a testimony that 'Morgagni included an early description of the anginal syndrome', as Willius (1945, 1946) put it, is to be questioned. In this epistle, a clinical description of anginal pain is missing though calcification of the coronaries is mentioned. On the other hand some cases which clinically suggest to us coronary artery disease lack information on the state of the coronary vessels. With this limitation in mind we will try to present Morgagni's knowledge of what we now call coronary artery disease.

In Epistle 44 (par. 15) a physician aged fifty-eight is described, who, twelve months before the fatal catastrophe, began to suffer from a sensation of pain ascending from the abdomen to the thorax, accompanied by convulsive and anxious respiration. He was carried off in a very short time. The dissection showed: 'Pericardium contained a considerable quantity of blood which had effused from the left ventricle by three foramina. The cavity of this ventricle was dilated to three times its usual extent'. This case appears to be a partial aneuryism with rupture of the wall. The symptoms are those of coronary disease, but the coronary vessels are not referred to.

In examining Epistle 17 (par. 6) we find a description of a man of about fifty-five who suffered from pain in the thorax especially in the left side, on which he was prevented from leaning. He coughed frequently, bringing up phlegm. Likewise, he suffered from oppression

[9] We are indebted to Mr. H. J. M. Symons, B.A., the Wellcome Institute of the History of Medicine, for this translation from the original Latin.
[10] See also the paper by Ch. Laubry and M. Mouquin on Morgagni's cases of angina pectoris (1950; see Bibliography).

in the breast, with difficulty in breathing, and anxiety in the heart region. Post-mortem: 'Serous fluid in the thorax, heart very much enlarged'. In commenting upon this case, there is a full clinical description of coronary disease and left heart failure. However, the state of the coronaries is not mentioned at all.

The case in Epistle 17 (par. 17) is complicated by different disorders but the sudden death and the circumstances which brought it about are compatible with a final acute coronary event. A man of fifty-five suffered for about ten years from many diseases; first fever, then splenic disorders, cachexia, then hydrops; afterwards jaundice, dyspnoea, throbbing of the jugular vessels, hard pulse, cough; in the last days, swelling of the face. When put to bed he died suddenly. The dissection showed: pleural adhesions, bronchial stasis; aorta hard, osseous and dilated, aortic aneurysm with a polypous concretion, ruptured.

Epistle 26 (par. 31) provides the most apt instance of angina, the opening paragraph not dissimilar to Heberden's description. It is worth recalling that the observation was made as early as 1707, and the clinical signs are clearly delineated. However, again the pathological findings are less spectacular. The patient was a woman, forty-two years old. We reproduce the case report in Alexander's translation, slightly abridged.

> 'On using pretty quick exercises of the body, a kind of violent uneasiness came on, within the upper part of the thorax, on the left side, join'd with a difficulty of breathing, and a stupor of the left arm: all which symptoms soon remitted when these motions ceas'd. This woman then, having set out about the middle of October, in the year 1707, from Venice, to go up the Continent in a wheel carriage, and being cheerful in her mind, behold the same paroxysm return'd: with which being seiz'd, and saying that she should die, she actually died on the spot.... The body ... was examined by me on the following day.'

Morgagni found 'the heart large, very hard, aorta not without bony scales,[11] marks of ossification; other great arteries partly ossified. Blood in the heart ventricles altogether fluid'.

In epistle 24 (par. 22) some historical considerations about the formation of polyps are recalled. Morgagni quotes from Galen, to show that the ancient author, quite unexpectedly, had already some notion of these pathological formations. Galen's findings did not refer to the cavity of the heart or vessels but to the pericardium. In *De Locis Affectis*

---

[11] 'from the very origin behind the semilunar valves' (Alexander's translation, p. 820, line 2) recalls Allbutt's aortic theory of anginal pain.

(Book V, Ch. 2; Ch. 3 in Daremberg's translation), Galen writes: 'We found in the pericardium of a cock a scirrhous tumour just as if many thick membranes had been wrapped up one over the other. It is thus likely that in man similar processes occur' (cf. M. Neuburger p. 81).

In the same Epistle (par. 23) Morgagni shows his interest in thrombotic processes and recalls the correspondence (see above p. 54) between Gasser and Vesalius in the year 1557, in which Vesalius refers to an aortic aneurysm as 'a flesh-like substance', or as a formation 'which resembled melted hog's lard'. In the same context Morgagni quotes Coiter, the Dutch anatomist of the sixteenth century.

As to the changes in the myocardium as described by Morgagni, the best references are found in letter 27, paragraphs 15–17,[12] in which hardening of the fleshy fibres is repeatedly reported.

Pathological changes in the myocardium to which Morgagni refers under different descriptive terms such as cartilage, bony scale, or tendinous hardness, are, historically, of great documentary interest. In the light of modern knowledge they indicate those areas in the myocardium which can be observed in a late stage subsequent to occlusion of coronary arteries, more often of their smaller branches. Incidentally, Sénac also refers to the opposite consistency in the heart substance, that of softening or 'heart abscess'. In the nineteenth century, when there was as yet little understanding of the underlying etiology, the indurations were incorrectly named 'chronic myocarditis';[13] the term myocarditis is now reserved for an inflammatory process.

Letter 27 is important enough to be quoted in parts, even though Morgagni's own observations did not refer specifically to scars located deep in the heart muscle, but to those on the inner surface of the heart. However, he also quoted intramuscular induration as reported by other authors. In paragraph 15 (p. 844 of the English translation) is noted:

> 'The heart had a bony scale (squamum osseum), of no inconsiderable size, and another in the right auricle. Both scales were close to the fleshy fibres, without laceration of which they could not be separated.'

These scars, which he calls 'scales', correspond to fibrosis resulting from older infarcts. The patient had died suddenly, so that the fresh lesions could not be anatomically ascertained. The pathological report adds that the aorta was marked by whitish spots. In paragraph 17 of

---

[12] We are indebted to Dr. Saul Jarcho of New York for his information contained in a personal letter of 3rd September 1959.

[13] The term 'myocarditis' was first used by J. F. Sobernheim, who in fact applied it to conditions which appear to have been of coronary origin.

7

this epistle Morgagni uses the terms cartilaginous or tendinous and describes indurations in the following references:

> 'Our Columbus[14] saw the septum of the heart, in some bodies really cartilaginous; and in like manner, our Veslingus[15] saw the left ventricle internally surrounded with a cartilaginous crust.'
>
> '... those cartilages in the fleshy fibres, must by their hardness also be injurious to the motions of the heart and the auricle.'
>
> '... It is certain that the fleshy fibres of the heart themselves sometimes degenerate into a tendinous hardness.'

In the following discussion (p. 846) Morgagni refers to autopsies made by himself in the years 1707, 1717, and 1719, all pertaining to hardenings in the fleshy fibres of the heart:

> 'In my opinion the indurations consisted of fleshy fibres, previously changed into tendon, by force [as a consequence] of the disease.'

He also quotes Boerhaave to the effect 'that the septum of the heart, and its cavities, had put on a bony nature.' He goes on to mention (p. 847) a French author of 1726 who found a 'bone' lying internally in the fleshy fibres, and again Sénac (1749) who found 'the left ventricle and the carneae columnae also changed into a bony substance.'

Our discussion shows Morgagni's insight into myocardial patho-physiology based on a degenerative process. This concept is, as we have already noted in the introduction (p. 4), Morgagni's most precious contribution to our problem. With this in mind, we add one quotation more to illustrate his broader view of this matter:

> 'The "bone" must so much the more have diminished the force of the heart, as this always decreases in proportion to the decrease of the fleshy fibres (tante magis imminuere debuit cordis vires, ut quae, decrescente ejus carneae substantia), and have been so much prejudicial to both the motions of the heart, by its inflexible hardness' (p. 847).

In other words, the force of the heart decreases so much more in proportion as the greater number of its parts become tendinous instead of being fleshy. This dictum is the culminating point in Morgagni's patho-physiological approach to the problem of myocardial damage.

[14] Realdus Columbus (1515?–1559). Morgagni writes 'our' since both Columbus and Vesling were former members of his university (Padua).
[15] Johann Vesling (1598–1649).

On reviewing our studies on Morgagni's contribution to our subject, we increasingly felt that the case histories with coronary pathology proved not to be his main achievement. More interesting seemed to us his pathological findings in the myocardium, which in the light of modern knowledge are sequelae of coronary occlusion. Thus he developed his own view and philosophy which ultimately led to the recognition of myocardial ischaemia.

Earlier in our study we referred to the importance of papers published in periodicals, as against the material found in books. We felt that the shorter papers are more likely to shed light on our topic, being devoted exclusively to one cardiological item. In fact the last reference from Morgagni's great book was based on a paper by Garengeot, published in the *Histoire de l'Académie Royale des Sciences* (1726). From this Morgagni deduced his remarkable patho-physiological concept mentioned above.

In the course of our search in the literary sources we came across another paper in the Academy *Mémoires* (1732, pp. 428–34). The author was S. F. Morand (1697–1773). His main publications deal largely with surgical problems; however, the paper under consideration bears on a cardiological topic and is entitled: 'Sur quelques accidents remarquables dans les organes de la circulation du sang.' It is a scholarly piece of writing and makes ample use of the cardiological literature then available. His two cases were accompanied by a detailed report of the following post-mortem findings: in the case of the Duchess of Brunswick a rupture of the right ventricle; and in that of 'a gentleman of distinction . . . a red mass in the left ventricle, formed by a clot of congealed blood, and a blackish narrow spot conforming to the tear of the myocardium'.

The rupture has been reported in some detail. In the case of the lady an erosion of the muscle fibres was described, which seemed to have been ulcerated and hollowed out gradually until the ventricle was torn. In the second case, the muscle of the heart had softened to such an extent that when the affected part was touched by the tip of a metal probe without applying any force, the very weight of the instrument, which was not considerable, caused it to enter and traverse the heart.

In conclusion, Morand's finding of a 'concrétion polypeuse' may be interpreted as a parietal thrombus; while in the case of the gentleman, the softening of the muscle substance may be due to a transmural necrosis, extending to the surface of the ventricle where the rupture was visible as a narrow blackish spot, 'long d'environ huit lignes' (old French unit of measure). By putting the probe into the tear the author was able to enter freely the left ventricle, which is a testimony to the transmural nature of the lesion.[16]

It is appropriate to mention briefly the clinician Friedrich Hoffmann (1660–1742), the first Professor of Medicine at the newly-founded University of Halle. In his *Medicina rationalis Systematica*, 1738 (Vol. III, ch. 12, par. 12, p. 274), Hoffmann expressly declared the impaired passage of blood in the coronary vessels to be the cause of the disease. In this respect he is quite exceptional and comes nearest to our modern concept. However, it is not the clinical picture of precordial pain that he has in mind here, but rather the unequal pulsation in the arteries. What is so important in his discussion is the statement that this 'may occur when the free passage of the blood through the coronary arteries ... is impaired by some obstacle, or the tenacious, thickened blood adheres in the coronary vessels.' Later, he paid due attention also to the clinical manifestation of precordial pain, with a sense of oppression radiating in all directions and especially to the arm.[17] Hoffmann seems to have imparted his great interest in cardiology even to his theological colleagues, as is suggested by G. H. Michaelis' unusual and detailed medical comment in his *Biblia Hebraica*, 1720, on Ecclesiastes XII, 6.[18]

A report submitted to the Royal Society by Frank Nicholls[19] (1699–1778), on the post-mortem findings in the autopsy of King George II (1683–1760), contains some material pertaining to our subject. The case was that of a rupture of the right ventricle of the heart showing an effusion of blood into the pericardium and an aneurysm of the aorta. The King had complained for some years of frequent distress about the region of the heart. His death[20] was due to a tamponade by the extravasated blood from a tear in the myocardium, probably caused by a coronary occlusion. Descriptions of ruptured hearts were not uncommon in medical literature, William Harvey's case having been published already in 1649. Though complicated by a 'transverse fissure in the trunk of the aorta, one and a half inches long,' Nicholls' report may be regarded as a contribution to the history of myocardial infarction.

This case was mentioned by Morgagni (27.10)[21] as that of 'a most

---

[16] Morand's case was mentioned by several subsequent authors: Morgagni (1761), 27.5; James Johnstone (1792), *Mem. Med. Soc. London*, I, 376–88; Testa (1831) 2nd ed., II, 294; Huchard (1899) 3rd ed. II, p. 228.

[17] See F. Hoffmann, *Operum omnium supplementum secundum*, Genevae, 1753, p. 243.

[18] See J. O. Leibowitz (1963).

[19] *Phil. Trans.*, 1761, vol. 52, pt. 1, pp. 265–75.

[20] See Horace Walpole, *Memoirs of the Reign of King George the Second*, 1846, vol. III, 302. 'In falling, he [the king] had cut his face against the corner of a bureau. He was laid on a bed and blooded, but not a drop followed' [shock!].

[21] Cf. English abridged translation by William Cooke, London, 1822, I, 426–27; A. Scarpa, English translation, 1819, p. 91. For comments see: H. B. Burchell and Th. E. Keys (1942), and J. O. Leibowitz (1960).

powerful monarch,' but he has erroneously reported an oblong fissure in the left ventricle (instead of right). It was referred to by Hebb, the translator of Corvisart into English, and also by Scarpa in his book on aneurysms. The coronary arteries were not regarded by the anatomists of that time as significant, and were not mentioned in Nicholls' report of the autopsy.

Proceeding in chronological order, we move on to the work of William Heberden (1710–1801), who quite understandably occupies a central position in our study. We cannot confine ourselves to a mere narration of his achievements pertaining to our subject. These have been laid down in an astonishingly brief form. The very concise texts call for a deeper probing and for a textual criticism in order to understand better Heberden's contribution to our topic as well as to draw attention to some words and details which later led to the much broader concept of ischaemic heart disease.

Although it is not our practice to bring in biographical material, however interesting it may be historically, one brief digression might be appropriate. Throughout his long life Heberden was highly esteemed for his integrity and scholarship, an esteem out of proportion to his purely literary work. During his lifetime he was revered like a figure from Antiquity, and Samuel Johnson called him 'ultimus romanorum.' His integrity and self-constraint in writing may throw some light on the fact that, despite the rich content of his work, he restricted himself to a purely observational presentation. It is known that he was never connected with a hospital and that he recorded his observations, made over more than forty years, 'in the chambers of the sick', as he puts it. This would explain the striking fact that Heberden does not even attempt an anatomical localization of the angina pectoris which immortalized his name. His disposition prevented him from making statements and theoretical deliberations for which he could not provide sound verification. He read his paper, 'Some account of a disorder of the breast' at the College of Physicians on 21st July, 1768, and had it published in 1772.[22] He took a long time to publish another of his observations: his paper on Dr. Anonymous (see below, p. 88) was read on 17th November, 1772, but was not printed until 1785.[23]

We may dwell awhile on the caption and its formulation. Heberden was a regular contributor to the *Transactions*. It is tempting to compare the unusual styling which begins with the words 'Some account' with, for instance, his paper on p. 216 of the same volume, which is called simply 'An account of the noxious effects of some fungae.'

[22] *Med. Trans. Coll. of Physns Lond.*, 1772, vol. II, pp. 59–67.
[23] *Med. Trans.*, 1785, vol. III, pp. 1–11.

The cautious wording of the caption seems to imply that Heberden was aware that only the future could provide more information on the disease and arrive at an explanation. He even states explicitly at the end of the paper that 'time and attention will undoubtedly discover more', etc. Instead of inscribing this paper, his main donation to medicine, with the words 'Angina pectoris', we find only the vague and modest title '. . . a disorder of the breast.'

To continue with the investigation into the minor question of captions, we looked these up in the *Commentaries*, which is quite a substantial volume of 483 pages in the 1802 edition, and provides indexes both in English and in Latin. The names of the chapters are given in Latin throughout the English edition, where chapter 70, pp. 362–69, has been entitled 'Pectoris Dolor', a much bolder form of inscription compared with that of 1772. The English index goes even farther when it lists the chapter as 'Pains of the Breast, and Angina Pectoris.'

The history of the composition of the *Commentaries* is not irrelevant to our study. In this we have been helped by the Preface, which is a useful tool for every student of Heberden's work.

It seems reasonably certain that the *Commentaries* were composed in 1782, and the preface reveals that the author read over his notes every month and 'such facts, as tended to throw any light upon the history of a distemper . . . were entered under the title of the distemper in another book, from which were extracted all the particulars here given.' Another unusual feature is provided by the absence of references throughout. Heberden states that his *Commentaries* are taken exclusively from his original notes and that he did not 'borrow any thing from other writers.'[24] These notes 'were written in Latin, the distempers being ranged alphabetically.' Heberden bequeathed the manuscript 'to any of my sons, who may choose the profession of physic.' It was published by William Heberden, Jr., both in the Latin original and in the English translation. In order to show that Heberden was quite conscious of some shortcomings in his method of investigation, we quote in full the last sentence of the preface.

'An useful addition might have been made to these papers by

---

[24] The only exception is one note referring to both Erasistratus, as quoted by Caelius Aurelianus (see above p. 38), and Saussure (Horace Benedict de Saussure (1740–99) of Geneva) which is found in the *Commentaries* (1802) but not in the original version of 1772. The reason for Heberden's deviation from his stated policy of not mentioning other authors was his impression that these authors had in mind angina of effort as described by himself. In fact, de Saussure seems to have been describing the 'effort sickness' of high altitudes, a condition which, incidentally, will be considered in a forthcoming series entitled 'Medicine and Sports', edited by E. and P. Jokl. (S. Karger, Basel.)

comparing them with the current doctrine of diseases and remedies, as also with what is laid down in practical writers, and with
the accounts of those who treat of the dissections of morbid
bodies, but at my advanced age it would be to no purpose to
think of such an undertaking.'

Before discussing all the details and implications derived from the
original texts it is worth while to evaluate Heberden's view on the
history of the disease which he described. It seems that in 1772 he had
no knowledge of previous descriptions either by ancient authors or
even by his great compatriot Harvey, who might have had the same
disease in mind, for Heberden writes, '. . . a distemper hitherto so
unnoticed,[25] that it has not yet, as far as I know, found a place or a
name in the history of diseases.' This statement is slightly mitigated in
the revised version as given in the *Commentaries*: '. . . a disease, which
has hitherto hardly a place or a name in medical books.' We stress
again that Heberden's statements just reproduced were made in good
faith and in no undue exaggeration of his own achievement. We
would venture the hypothesis that the author is referring here to the
most striking clinical symptom, namely heart pain on exertion, which
he really was the first to describe as a morbid entity, and which indeed
was not explicitly brought to notice by any of his predecessors. To
make this clear we would like to quote this item in full.

> 'They who are afflicted with it, are seized while they are
> walking, (more especially if it be uphill, and soon after eating)
> with a painful and most disagreeable sensation in the breast, which
> seems as if it would extinguish life, if it were to increase or to
> continue; but the moment they stand still, all this uneasiness
> vanishes.'[26] (1802 ed., p. 364).

The last quotation depicts the so-called ambulatory angina where
walking uphill or any similar exertion is the most common provocative
factor of the attack. Some authors are even inclined to call this form the
classical Heberdenian angina. However, the further we study the text,
both in the first and the later version, the more we learn that Heberden's
concept becomes steadily more embracing. It already includes features
commonly belonging to organic lesions in the myocardium, even to a
degree of real infarction. Heberden attributed them to later stages of
angina pectoris, which is clinically sound in some cases but not in all,
since myocardial infarction may also occur without evidence of any

[25] However, on p. 62 (1772) he writes, 'I consulted an able physician of long experience, who told me that he had known several ill of it'.
[26] See, however, Morgagni's report quoted above (p. 78). in Epistle 26.31.

previous history of precordial pain. In fact Heberden speaks of 'the most usual appearance of this disease', admitting that 'some varieties may be met with.' He noted 'periodical return every night', which is not brought on by motion and he referred to 'one or two persons in whom the pain has lasted some hours or even days', a form later called *état angineux* by Huchard. In his exposition he also included cardiac insufficiency which is now known as a possible sequel of long-standing coronary disease. On p. 366 of the 1802 edition he referred to a man who,

> 'in the sixtieth year of his life began to feel, while he was walking, an uneasy sensation in his left arm. . . . After it had continued ten years it would come upon him two or three times a week, at night, while he was in bed, and then he was obliged to sit up for an hour or two before it would abate [orthopnoea]. . . . He died suddenly without a groan at the age of seventy-five.'

This report goes much beyond a so-called Heberdenian angina.

The fatal outcome, which Heberden calls in a mild and gentle way 'the termination of the angina pectoris', betrays the grave prognosis of the disease. 'For if no accident intervene, but the disease go on to its height, the patients all suddenly fall down and perish almost immediately.' This reminds us of the ancient description of cardiac syncope. The clinical picture becomes even more embracing with the statement that 'its attacks are often after the first sleep,' which would probably indicate cardiac asthma.[27]

Heberden was probably aware of additional symptoms in this 'distemper', as is implied by his words: 'it is not to be denied.' We quote fully:

> 'Yet it is not to be denied that I have met with one or two patients, who have told me they now and then spit up matter and blood, and that it seemed to them to come from the seat of the disease.'

The signs given here belong rather to a thrombo-embolic process or at least pulmonary oedema. Even cases of sudden death without any clinical history were known to our author, a fact proved by his reference to a patient 'who fell down dead, without any notice.' Later, especially in the German medical literature, they were sometimes called angina pectoris without angina, meaning without anginal pain, and were included in the picture of the so-called 'Sekundentod.'

---

[27] Cf, Paul Wood (1968), *Diseases of the Heart and Circulation*, 3rd ed., p. 304.

As to the clinical symptomatology of the classical form, Heberden noted variants in which the pain was located only in the left arm and not in the breast, or in which the seat of the pain was the right arm. He knew that 'males are more liable to this disease.' He chose the name 'angina pectoris' for 'the seat of it, and the sense of strangling and anxiety, with which it is attended.'

We have had the opportunity of discussing the question of 'pain versus dyspnoea' several times in this study. It seems that in long-standing cases accompanied by what we would now call cardiac insufficiency, Heberden would not have hesitated to include shortness of breath in the symptomatology of his 'distemper'. In fact he mentions on p. 366 of the *Commentaries*, quoted above, a patient who 'was obliged to sit up for an hour or two', which denotes respiratory distress. However, Heberden stresses that 'the patients are, at the beginning of the disorder, perfectly well, and in particular have no shortness of breath; from which it is totally different.'

This is an important point, which led Heberden to single out the disease from other heart conditions. Historically this has had a great influence on the medical profession, which became aware of the anginal pain as a clinical entity. Subsequent observers perceived the peculiarities and variants of the disorder, including shortness of breath, especially in the later stages, but sometimes also as an equivalent of anginal pain (see below p. 101). In all other respects, later observers were unable to add much to the clinical features which Heberden established.

One observation (p. 368) can be explained only conjecturally. Heberden had some ideas about coagulability and fluidity of the blood, when he described 'opening the body of one who died suddenly of this disease', his only reference to a post-mortem. The patient was 'Dr. Anonymous', and according to the clinical data death was due presumably to acute coronary thombosis. The quotation from the Commentaries runs as follows:

> 'In this person, as it has happened to others who have died by the same disease, the blood continued fluid[28] two or three days after death, not dividing itself into crassamentum and serum, but thick, like cream. Hence when a vein has been opened a little before death, or perhaps soon after, the blood has continued to ooze out as long as the body remained unburied.'

The peculiar condition of the blood noted here has not, as far as we

[28] Already in 1586 Petrus Salius Diversus called attention to this phenomenon! (see page 60).

know, been hitherto discussed in the historical appraisal of Heberden's work, and will be commented upon later.

Heberden's first printed account of 1772 lacked any anatomical investigations of the deceased persons. Indeed he remarks on p. 65: '... but I have never had in my power to see any one opened, who had died from it; the sudden death of the patients adding so much to the common difficulties of making such an enquiry, that most of those with whose cases I had been acquainted were buried before I had heard that they were dead.'[29] However, in the posthumously-published *Commentaries*, one post-mortem, namely that of the last-quoted case with blood thick as cream, has been reported. The result of the autopsy was quite negative, as Heberden puts it in the following words: 'a very skilled anatomist could discover no fault in the heart, in the valves, in the arteries, or neighbouring veins, excepting some small rudiments of ossification in the aorta'. The case is remarkable enough on account of the human qualities of the patient, himself a physician, and the excellent self-description of his disease contained in his letter to Heberden. We quote the title: 'A letter to Dr. Heberden, concerning the Angina Pectoris; and Dr. Heberden's Account of the Dissection of One,[30] who had been troubled with this Disorder. Read at the College, Nov. 17, 1772.' (*Medical Transactions, College of Physicians*, (1785), Vol. III, pp. 1–11.)

The letter describes this doctor's suffering and contains a proposal for the examination of his body after death. The patient was fifty-two years old and inclined to fatness. He had experienced the first symptoms five years before, when he had felt pain in the left arm and in the breast, and had been obliged to stop walking. 'I attributed it to an obstruction in the circulation ... sensations which to me seemed to indicate a sudden death.' While the symptoms described in the letter are in accordance with Heberden's lecture of 1768, the patient brings in certain particulars not referred to in Heberden's famous lecture. In this connection a passage about his sensations during rest is noteworthy.

> 'I have often felt, when sitting, standing, and at times in my bed, what I can best express by calling it an universal pause within me of the operations of nature, for perhaps three or four seconds.'

[29] The quotation shows that Heberden was not unaware of the importance of pathology in elucidating his cases.

[30] A recent publication by K. D. Keele (1966) first brought to light the identity of 'Dr. Anonymous'. Studying John Hunter's unpublished 'Dissection of Morbid Bodies', in the transcript of William Clift, Hunter's assistant, K. D. Keele was able to identify the person we discussed at length, and who is referred to in the historical literature as 'Dr Anonymous'. It was Dr. Haygarth of Chester.

Earlier he mentions the sensations as 'not being concomitant with the above-mentioned disorder.'

> 'I suspect they [patients who died suddenly] were subject to what I delineated, as I think that much more likely to occasion a sudden death, than either of the causes to which you attributed.'

The anonymous letter, written on 16th April, 1772, was, as previously mentioned, published in full by Heberden in 1785. Heberden adds a short comment which includes a reference to the fatal outcome of his correspondent's disease, death occurring during an attack three weeks after he had sent the letter. The attack came on suddenly during a walk, and death intervened in less than half-an-hour. The dissection was performed by John Hunter within forty-eight hours after decease. The report of the post-mortem mentioned no findings in the heart vessels and valves, 'except some few specks of a beginning ossification upon the aorta. . . . The left ventricle of the heart was remarkably strong and thick.' Nothing extraordinary could be perceived in the brain. It is to be noted that according to Jenner (see below p. 95) the coronary arteries were not examined. Keele (1966), in his paper on 'John Hunter's contribution to cardiovascular pathology', hints that Hunter showed more interest in the coronary vessels after his own first attack of angina pectoris, about 1773. He certainly dissected the coronary vessels in a case of Fothergill's in 1775 (see below p. 92).

The remark quoted above regarding the fluidity or coagulability of the blood had originally a slightly different form in the publication of 1785. Since it precedes the *Commentaries*, it is interesting to quote this first version.

> 'The blood . . . did not coagulate even after being more than two hours exposed to the air; but at the same time could not be called perfectly fluid, being of the consistency of thin cream; but there was no separation of any of its component parts.'

Heberden goes on to say: 'The sensation, described in the letter, of an apparent suspension of life for a few seconds, is what I do not remember to have ever heard mentioned by any patient besides this.' Since death intervened suddenly while the patient was walking and not during rest, Heberden felt it less probable that he lost his life through circumstances connected with this particular sensation, cautiously adding: 'but this must be decided by future experience.'

Having quoted both versions of the text on the state of the blood after dissection, we shall try to give a plausible interpretation of this phenomenon. The very introduction of this problem seems to have originated rather through John Hunter's curiosity than that of Heberden himself. Haematological investigations were close to Hunter's mind, as evidenced by his *Treatise on the Blood, Inflammation, etc.*, which was published posthumously in 1794. We put forward a suggestion which was kindly given by a consultant in pathology.[31] Blood remaining fluid is not uncommon in sudden deaths occasioned by shock, or by brain disorder. In these conditions blood is rich in fibrinolysin. The expression 'thick like cream', or in the second version, 'being of the consistency of thin cream', may be readily explained by hyperlipaemia, where the plasma may look creamy.

An expert in haematology[32] has given us the following opinion. In the light of present knowledge it is conceivable that the incoagulability of the blood, forty-eight hours post mortem, was the result of fibrinogenolysis and fibrinolysis activated possibly by cardiogenic shock. This condition is known to be associated with the activation of the fibrinolytic system. It is also possible that the patient examined was severely polycythaemic with a particular increase in red cell mass.

The third opinion we asked for, was that of a specialist[33] in forensic medicine. Without rejecting the former views, he felt that a possibility might be admitted that the blood had been coagulated, but became later liquefied: a subsequent post-mortem change due to putrefaction.

The comments proposed above would fit in quite well with our diagnosis: fatal infarction leading to sudden death by shock; arteriosclerosis with concomitant rise of lipids in the blood. The tentative interpretation shows once more the wealth of medical information given by Heberden when focused in the light of more modern concepts.

As to the sensations described by 'Dr. Anonymous', Dr. H. N. Segall,[34] a cardiologist much interested in historical medicine, has suggested that the patient 'may have died of paroxysmal ventricular tachycardia which ended in ventricular fibrillation' (p. 106). This interesting interpretation opens an entirely new outlook for the appraisal of the case. It also gives full credit to Dr. Anonymous' acuity of self-observation and to his conceiving the 'sensations' as possibly threatening life. His idea preceded its clinical and experimental confirmation which came more than one hundred years later.

[31] Personal communication by Professor H. Ungar, Head of Pathology, Hebrew University, Jerusalem, Israel, 4th September, 1967.

[32] Professor G. Izak, Head of Haematology, ibidem, 14th December, 1967.

[33] Professor H. Karplus, Head of the Institute of Forensic Medicine, Hebrew University, Jerusalem, Israel, 10th June, 1968.

[34] Harold N. Segall (1945), cf. Bibliography; the letter by Dr. Anonymous is reproduced on pages 103–4 of this paper.

Disturbances in the heart rhythm could not have been diagnosed during the eighteenth century, as they were then beyond existing medical knowledge of cardiac diseases. Sclerotic changes, however, in the coronaries and even in the myocardium, were nearer to the concept of several investigators at that time and even earlier, as we have already pointed out.

To return to purely clinical material, Heberden is very precise in underlining the higher rate of occurrence of angina pectoris in males compared with females. In fact, by the close of his life he was able to observe one hundred cases, with only three females among them. The greater incidence in the male population is now a well-established fact. However, the rate indicated here by Heberden is extremely high. To explain this statistical disproportion (97:3), we must take into account the average life span, which was quite low in the eighteenth-century, though Heberden himself was blessed by a long life of ninety-one years. Current statistics show that in younger and middle-aged people coronary disease is more frequent in males, whereas in older people there is little difference in the morbidity rate from this disease.

To conclude the evaluation of Heberden's work a few considerations as to the way he chose to communicate his findings might be added. His reluctance to quote previous authors, or to refer (with one exception) to anatomical findings, and his rather casual mentioning of disturbed physiology of the myocardium, appear incompatible with a work of such magnitude. The explanation, which we have alluded to already in the introduction, is that Heberden concentrated on giving an unsurpassed description of a purely clinical nature. His full awareness that there is a great deal more behind the disease which he simply calls 'pectoris dolor', has been exemplified by our analysis of the phenomena implicitly contained in his papers, but which became firmly established only in the subsequent evolution of medical knowledge. To quote Heberden again (1772, p. 67), when he speaks about the short-comings of the therapy then available he opens his statement with the words, 'time and attention will undoubtedly discover more helps against this teazing ailment'. Thus he knew that time would be needed to elucidate the mysteries of this disease, and he called upon future generations to devote much more attention to it. He limited his own aim to the description of those manifestations which he could unequivocally delineate.[35]

[35] After completion of this chapter we have been privileged to read the paper 'William Heberden's contribution to cardiology' (1968) by D. Evan Bedford. We draw special attention to this contribution by a writer who (together with Parkinson) was the first to describe in detail coronary thrombosis in England (*Lancet*, 1928).

Stimulated by Heberden's original paper, the medical profession, in Britain especially, continued intensive research into coronary artery disease, but paying more attention than hitherto to anatomical findings. This activity was already under way in the later part of Heberden's life, though he himself did not participate in this new trend. He may, however, have been alluding to it in the final phrase of the preface to his *Commentaries*, which we quoted earlier. This active group of investigators tried to find an anatomical localization, stressing especially the sclerotic changes in the coronary arteries. Until the name arteriosclerosis was coined, authors had used such descriptive expressions as ossified, calcified, ligamentous, tendinous and bony, for the changes in the vessels.

Perhaps the first to mark this trend was the Quaker physician John Fothergill (1712–80). His observations were read in 1774 and 1775 and published in two papers during the year 1776.[36] Being quite early reports, they may be referred to rather more fully. The first was entitled 'Case of an *Angina Pectoris*, with Remarks'.[37] The patient was a man of fifty-eight, disposed to corpulency. In July 1773 he suffered from spasms in the breast, chiefly when he walked uphill. He was first visited by Fothergill in the autumn of 1773:

> 'I soon suspected angina pectoris, a disease which I had too often met with. I saw the patient in the evening; he described a stricture surrounding his chest, sharp pain (breast, elbow left), difficulty in breathing. Death very suddenly in the morning. Postmortem: mediastinum loaded with fat, under the lungs a quart of water in each side. Heart; near the apex, a small white spot, as big as a sixpence, resembling a cicatrix.'

The next report with a dissection is contained in the paper 'Farther Account of the *Angina Pectoris*' (pp. 252–58) in the same volume. Here the patient was a man of sixty-three, whose complaints began three to four years before his death. 'In a sudden and violent transport of anger he fell down and expired immediately.' The salient features of the report on the post-mortem performed by John Hunter in March 1775 are: Cartilages of ribs ossified; in the cavity of the chest a full quart of bloody serum. Heart: substance paler, of a ligamentous consistence, in many parts of the left ventricle almost white and hard, the two coronary arteries from their origin to many of their ramifications upon the heart, were become one piece of bone. A few small

[36] See C. C. Booth (1957).
[37] *Medical Observations and Inquiries*, By a Society of Physicians in London, Vol. V, pp. 233–51.

stones in the gall-bladder (as in John Hunter's own case!). The blood had not in the least coagulated in any part of the body, nor did it coagulate upon being exposed.

This case requires a few comments: the stressing of anger and emotion as factors directly provoking the attack, a view already expressed by Harvey in 1649, the finding of ossified cartilages of ribs, not belonging to the coronary artery disease proper, but significant as a historical parallel to Rougnon's view, which we shall discuss later; the mentioning of pleural effusion as part of concomitant cardiac insufficiency; the attention given to the state of the myocardium, picturing its lack of adequate blood supply resulting in the pale colour of its substance; some parts of it, especially in the left ventricle, being white, hard and ossified, which suggests previous infarctions; and the large amount of calcification in the coronary arteries, parts of them being 'transformed into one piece of bone'. Our last comment concerns the fact that 'the blood had not in the least coagulated'. We discussed this particular point in the case of Dr. Anonymous' dissection, also performed by Hunter. Its re-appearance in Fothergill's post-mortem report clearly shows that it was a favourite subject with John Hunter.

A remark at the end of Fothergill's paper (p. 258) reveals views on the etiology and prevention of the disease which were later to become generally accepted. He advises on the first appearance of the disease a plan of restricted food, which 'might greatly retard the progress of the disorder, and to restrain excesses of passion and anxiety, which perhaps contribute more to the increase of this disease than a combination of all other causes'. This foretells the more recent ideas and measures in the etiology and prevention of coronary artery disease.

Among the authors who furthered the coronary theory of angina pectoris, Edward Jenner (1749–1832) has quite a prominent place. Jenner's fame is of course based on his immortal *Inquiry into the Causes and Effects of the Variolae Vaccinae*, but he must also be remembered for his contributions to a better understanding of our subject. Jenner was instrumental in provoking an active interest in coronary disease by his many contacts and letters.[38] As was usual in his time, most of the dissections were performed by surgeons, and Jenner was sometimes invited to help them in the examination of the bodies. In his letter to Heberden of 1778 [39] he referred to such a case in the following words:

[38] In the popular book, *Public Characters of 1802–3* (p. 21), we read: 'We may also refer our readers to a late publication by the ingenious Dr. Parry, of Bath, wherein it appears that the discovery of the cause of that dreadful malady, the anginy (*sic*) pectoris, originated with Dr. Jenner'.

[39] See John Baron, *The Life of Edward Jenner*, vol. I (1838), 39, 47; H. B. Jacobs (1919), 742–43.

'Mr. Paytherus, a surgeon at Ross, in Herefordshire, desired me to examine with him the heart of a person who had died of the Angina Pectoris a few days before. . . . But what I had taken to be an ossification of the vessel itself, Mr. Paytherus discovered to be a kind of firm fleshy tube, formed within the vessel, with a considerable quantity of ossific matter dispersed irregularly through it. This tube did not appear to have any vascular connection with the coats of the artery, but seemed to lie merely in simple contact with it. As the heart, I believe, in every subject that has died from Angina Pectoris, has been found extremely loaded with fat, and as these vessels lie quite concealed in that substance, is it possible this appearance may have been overlooked? The importance of the coronary arteries, and how much the heart must suffer from their not being able duly to perform their functions (we cannot be surprised at the painful spasms) is a subject I need not enlarge upon, therefore shall only just remark that it is possible that all symptoms may arise from this one circumstance.'

It is remarkable that in this letter Jenner not only refers to calcifications, which others had noted before him, but goes so far as to mention a structure formed in the vessel which today would probably be recognized as a recanalized thrombus[40] leading to death from occlusion. He stresses the importance of this anatomical finding and it is tempting to consider it as one of the earliest descriptions of coronary thrombosis.[41] A further comment concerns Jenner's correct diagnosis of John Hunter's disease made not by medical examination proper, but merely through impressions gathered from a chance meeting with Hunter at a spa: 'When I had the pleasure of seeing him [John Hunter] at Bath last Autumn I thought he was affected with many symptoms of the Angina Pectoris'. Jenner paid close attention to the disease and all the 'famous cases', among them that of 'Dr. Anonymous'. In his letter reproduced on pp. 3–5 of Parry's book, which we will discuss later, he referred to the autopsy of the above physician performed by Hunter. He notes that the condition of the coronary vessels is often overlooked on post-

[40] See O. F. Hedley (1938). The date of Jenner's letter may have been 1786 (Le Fanu, 1951). According to Sir Thomas Lewis (1941) this letter remained unsent. It seems to us that Jenner may have held back the letter in order not to hurt Heberden, who was himself dissatisfied with the fact that he was not able to provide anatomical evidence of the 'distemper' of which he gave his unsurpassed description. See our quotation (p. 85) from Heberden's Commentaries. This is a sign of Jenner's thoughtfulness towards others, (see also p. 95).
[41] For Crell's case (1740) see p. 76–77.

mortem examination and, with reference to the above case, he states bluntly: 'The coronary arteries were not examined'.

At that time John Hunter's disease became a concern of his doctor friends. To quote Parry again (1799, p. 109): 'Dr. Jenner conversed with myself, and many of his friends, on the symptoms of Mr. Hunter, and foretold diseased coronaries.' Referring to Hunter's symptoms, Jenner, in his letter to Parry (p. 4), remarks: 'and this circumstance prevented any publication of my ideas on the subject'; or in his letter to Heberden (1788), '. . . and I am fearful (if Mr. H. should admit this to be the cause of the disease) that it may deprive him of the hopes of a recovery'. This humane trait of Jenner is really touching and has often been commented upon by historians of this subject.

The knowledge of angina pectoris became more widespread in the last quarter of the eighteenth century. Since medical periodicals, especially in England, became more numerous, there was more opportunity of publishing observations. Among these, many lesser-known physicians contributed remarkable descriptions of cases and post-mortem findings. In 1786 one of these authors, James Johnstone, read his paper entitled 'Case of Angina pectoris, from an unexpected Disease in the Heart'.[42] The paper is interesting for its clinical and pathological details and even for its title. The author is right in finding it 'unexpected', since myocardial infarction, the condition which he probably encountered, was a morbid entity unknown in his time. The formulation in the title is therefore quite understandable. This early example shows that even at the end of the eighteenth century the name and concept of 'angina pectoris' did not cover the whole range of the disease. Incidentally, even Osler in 1897 and 1910 included well-described and anatomically-proven infarcts under the general title 'Angina pectoris', conceding, however, that they represented grave forms of the disease.

To return to Johnstone's case, the details are reported as follows: A man of seventy began in June 1785 to suffer from

> 'shortness in breathing, pain in his chest, and across to his arms, on ascent; symptoms returned till the fatal attack. On 2nd August 1785, after being some time in bed, he complained he was ill; early in the morning of 3rd August his wife was roused by the noise of his expiring groan; dead in an instant.'

The body was opened on the 4th August by Mr. Gunter, Surgeon: 'The heart very putrid, admitting my fingers passing through it with very little pressure'. Johnstone commented that,

[42] *Mem. med. Soc. Lond.*, 1792, **i**, 376–88.

8

> 'The symptoms arose from defect of power in the heart.
> Inteneration [from the Latin *tener*, meaning tender, softening]
> of the heart from putridity has been the occasioning cause of
> sudden death, by rendering the ventricles liable to rupture, as in
> the case of King George II, and it was described by Morand in
> 1732.'

Both references have already been discussed.

Another lesser-known author is Samuel Black of Ireland, who
continued the studies in coronary disease both clinically and anatomically. The patient discussed in his first report[43] was a man of fifty-five.

> 'In March 1794, while walking, sudden pain below the left
> mamma, anxiety and oppression in the chest. About five months
> the disease was manifested in walking. . . . Then attacks in the
> night with excruciating pain; the paroxysms came usually
> about two o'clock in the morning, during sleep, and lasted
> about one hour. On the 22nd March the patient was attacked
> by a most dreadful paroxysm: constant pain, dry cough,
> agony, death in two and a half days'.

The post-mortem was made forty hours after death: 'Cartilages of the
ribs became quite osseous [cf. Rougnon], heart large, and on being
handled unusually tender and lacerable. Both coronary arteries showed
complete ossification'. In the evaluation of this case Black seems to
single out 'mechanical pressure', apparently meaning heart failure
with congestion, as against angina pectoris proper. It seems that Black
paid due attention to the later stages of the disease which became complicated by heart insufficiency ('The effusion of fluid is an effect of a long-
standing disease'). This point was to be clarified by Leyden in 1884.

Black reported another rather typical case, also accompanied by a
dissection, in a paper read in 1796[44]; the case is noteworthy in that the
patient first showed symptoms of the disease at the early age of thirty-
two. In the last twelve years of his life the symptoms increased in
intensity and the patient experienced more prolonged attacks, which
anticipate the so-called 'status anginosus' described by later authors.
Two months later, 'while sitting in the evening drinking some chocolate, he fell suddenly off his chair and instantly expired'. At the post-
mortem an extensive ossification of the coronary arteries was found,
and 'even the small ramifications were indurated and inflexible. There
was also a pericardial effusion'. Black's attempt at a physiological
explanation of sudden pain through muscular exertion must be noted,

[43] 'Case of angina pectoris, with remarks', *Mem. med. Soc. Lond.*, 1795, **4**, 261–79.
[44] Ibid., 1805, **6**, 41.

though the mechanism as he conceived it is not valid in the light of modern knowledge. Incidentally, Black's work has been thoroughly discussed and evaluated in a recent paper by R. E. Siegel.[45] However, the title naming him as responsible for the 'Discovery of coronary sclerosis as a cause of angina pectoris' is questionable, if due regard is paid to Fothergill's and Jenner's contributions to the same subject.

At the very close of the eighteenth century there was published in Bath a slim volume with the title *An Inquiry into the Symptoms and Causes of the Syncope Anginosa, commonly called Angina pectoris; illustrated by dissections* (1799). Its author, Caleb Hillier Parry, is known for his sagacity and observational acuity, which among other things led him to produce the first observation on exophthalmic goitre. His is the first volume exclusively devoted to our subject which also deals with the anatomy and pathophysiology of the myocardium.[46] Much influenced by Jenner, whose letter he quotes in the introduction, Parry is also a strong adherent of the coronary hypothesis. In a 'dissertation' which he read in 1788, he states, 'Angina Pectoris is a disease of the heart, connected with mal-organization of the coronary arteries' (p. 5).

Chapter 2 is entitled 'Cases and Dissections'. Three cases were described in greater detail, all of them showing a more protracted type of disease, though death, when it occurred eventually, was sudden. The post-mortem findings refer to ossification and partial obstruction of the coronaries, and to gross pathology of the aorta. No morbid changes of the myocardium are reported. However, the description of the clinical features is extraordinarily well presented.

Chapter 3 begins with a historical survey. Seneca's case[47] is mentioned first, but the author regards it rather as a disorder of respiration—a view shared by modern historians. As to Morgagni, Parry found the case discussed in his Epistle 26 (13) the only one bearing a relation to any example of the disease before Heberden's time. He doubts whether Morgagni's cases 16 (43) and 17 (17) belong to the angina pectoris group, since they are complicated by other diseases of the pericardium, aorta, and so on. He quotes further authors, such as Wall, Fothergill, Percival and Black, and discusses all their reports of the symptoms belonging to our subject.

[45] R. E. Siegel (1963); cf. Bibliography.
[46] It was preceded by William Butter's *Treatise* (1791), but he attributed angina pectoris to 'the diaphragmatic gout'. See, however, J. E. Seegmiller (1966) on possible correlation between the presence of hyperuricaemia and the development of myocardial infarction.
[47] His observations on himself are found in Epistle 54. A monograph on Seneca's illness is now in course of preparation by Professor Roselaar of Jerusalem.

Unlike Heberden, Parry, together with Black, Wall and others, found a diminution in the strength of the pulse. In an effort to enlarge the range of the morbid manifestations implied, Parry proposed a new name: 'syncope anginosa', thus reviving the notion of the ancients,[48] and at the same time preparing the grounds for the new understanding of myocardial infarction.

> 'All the circumstances in the Angina Pectoris preceding the actual syncope are approaches towards it: and in every uncombined and recent case, like those I have described, the patient probably dies with no other symptoms than those which show an irrecoverable diminution of the motion of the heart' (p. 60).

It seems that Parry truly grasped the importance of myocardial damage as contrasted with angina pectoris proper.

To quote him again,

> 'the Angina Pectoris is a mere case of Syncope or Fainting, differing from the Common Syncope only in being preceded by an unusual degree of anxiety or pain in the region of the heart, and in being readily excited, during a state of apparent health, by any general exertion of the muscles, more especially that of walking' (p. 67).

As already stated, Parry was not able to report anatomical lesions in the myocardium, but he brought the disturbed physiology in the heart muscle to the very centre of his deliberations when he spoke of the causes of the so-called syncope. He used his literary sources of information discriminately. Referring to Hoffmann's work (discussed earlier, p. 82), Parry quotes him to the effect 'that one of the causes of Syncope is the want of a proper influx of good blood through those vessels [the coronaries] into the muscular substances of the heart, though Hoffmann was totally unacquainted with the phenomena of ossified coronaries'.

In order to explain the onset of attacks Parry says, 'and though a quantity of blood may circulate through these arteries, sufficient to nourish the heart . . . yet there may be probably less than what is requisite for ready and vigorous action' (p. 113). A few years later Alan Burns took up this track with greater emphasis on facts and experiments.

The etiology of the disease which is now regarded as due to arteriosclerosis was unknown to Parry, but he did speculate upon it when he said 'It would be an object, valuable in a more important view than

---

[48] See our note explaining the term 'syncope' (p. 31).

that of mere philosophical curiosity, could we discover the cause of that ossification . . .' (p. 132).

What we now call myocardial damage in coronary artery disease did not escape Parry's attention. He devotes the whole of chapter VI to defining the processes which he calls 'Accidental Symptoms attending the Syncope Anginosa'. He writes, 'As induration of the coronary arteries probably depends on causes which may alike operate on every other part of the heart and large vessels, there is no reason why it may not be accompanied with any of those organic injuries which have been described before'. He supposes that the coronaries may be 'so obstructed as to intercept the blood, which should be the proper support of the muscular fibres of the heart, that the organ becomes unequal to the task of circulation'. Parry lists many signs and symptoms due to muscular insufficiency of the heart. Again he comes quite close to the more current estimation of myocardial damage in the disease he describes.

To conclude the discussion of Parry, attention may be drawn to a short and informative essay on him by Sir Thomas Lewis, an authority on coronary artery disease, and himself a victim of myocardial infarction. An appreciation by a man like Lewis is no small tribute to Parry's historical position.

A study of the eighteenth-century contribution to our subject would not be complete without mention of the French physician, N. F. Rougnon (1727–99), whose importance has been minimized by certain historians while over-rated by others. If we consider only the chronological data, we find that Rougnon's famous letter on his patient, sent to Monsieur Lorry,[49] was dated 23rd February, 1768, thus preceding Heberden's paper read on 21st July of the same year. The above date is that given by William Osler in 1897. Rolleston (1937), however, quotes the date as 18th March, and mentions that the letter was abstracted in July 1768 in the *Journal de Sçavans*; he reproduced the title page of the printed pamphlet of 55 pages on page 210 of his paper. We are not interested in the chronological dispute but in the interpretation of the letter. While wider opinion does not identify Rougnon's description with angina pectoris at all, regarding the disease as related to a respiratory and not an anginal disorder, some authors are strongly inclined to consider it as related to coronary artery disease. The controversy has lasted until very recently.

In view of the difficulty in laying hands on Rougnon's letter, we shall refer to a French historical paper by Cariage in 1960, where the letter

---

[49] A.-Ch. Lorry (1726–83) a well-known Paris physician and dermatologist.

is partially reproduced. According to this writer it was published on 26th February, 1768. The patient, M. Charles, a retired Captain in the Dauphin's regiment and son of the Professor of Medicine in Besançon, was fifty years old when he fell victim to an attack. His past history over a few years showed difficulty in breathing on slight physical exertion. He was rather obese. Several members of his family had died from apoplexy. As his disease progressed, M. Charles could not walk more than a hundred steps rather more quickly than normal without feeling a kind of suffocation, especially when trying to speak. However, the attack subsided when he stopped walking for a few moments. He was rarely affected when he walked slowly. 'Six weeks before his death he complained of a strange discomfort over the whole anterior part of his breast, as if by a breast-plate'. During silence and rest he hardly experienced this disorder. One evening, after a meal with his friends, he was in a hurry to be at a party in another house; in his haste he climbed quickly up two flights of stairs. Reaching his place at the table he sat down, but died immediately.

The post-mortem reported by Rougnon is not very clear or convincing. He noted only: heart large, coronary veins enlarged prodigiously [?!] and excessive ossification of the cartilages of the ribs. In the evaluation of the case we wish to quote Osler's comment (1897) in full:

> 'I cannot agree with Professor Gairdner, "there was no trace of anything like a clinical description of angina pectoris in M. Rougnon's letter (*Lancet*, 1891, **i**, 604)". The suddenness of the attacks, the pain in the region of the heart, the abrupt termination, and the mode of death—during exertion after a full meal—favour the view that the case was one of true angina'.

In his biography of Rougnon, Cariage (1956) is not too explicit in the interpretation of the letter. He considers the fatal outcome to have been possibly caused by acute pulmonary oedema, rejects his own supposition on the grounds that the autopsy of the lungs did not show any pathological changes, but does not exclude the probability that sudden death could have been occasioned by 'une crise d'angine de poitrine'.[50] The opposite view, that there is nothing like angina pectoris in the clinical description by Rougnon, was elaborated by H. Kohn in 1927. However, we are inclined to favour Osler's interpreta-

[50] Allbutt II, 216, note i: 'it is fair to say that although Heberden named the disease and gave by far the better description of it, yet the first precise discernment and description of it was in a letter by Rougnon to Lorry, published at Besançon by J. F. Charmet in 1768'.

tion of 'true angina', more specifically of myocardial infarction or coronary thrombosis. Unlike Heberden's paper, Rougnon's pamphlet of 55 pages, partly reprinted in a journal, had no influence on the development of investigations into angina pectoris. On consulting Rougnon's two-volume work, *Considerationes pathologico-semeioticae* (1786–88) we were unable to find any reference to angina pectoris or ischaemic heart disease, and it seems that the author himself did not realize the possible impact of his letter of 1768. Otherwise the work is quite interesting, especially in the chapter, 'De arteriis sanguiniferis' (I, 147 ff.), where Rougnon refers to aneurysms, rupture, and ossification, adding that they give occasion to palpitations, difficulty in breathing and sometimes lead to a lethal orthopnoea. Speaking of vascular obstruction, he allots it to an inflammatory process. In the chapter 'de vasibus' (I, 138), a vague statement as to 'a cardiac polyp pushing the precordial vessels' can be found; the expression is not clear, nor does Rougnon give any clinical data.

It was the opinion of the cardiologist L. Gallavardin, expressed in a personal communication to Cariage in 1956, that the description resembles the phenomenon named by Gallavardin 'blockpnée d'effort', where the respiratory distress during walking is similar to that experienced by an anginal patient but in which the cardiovascular examination is essentially negative. He found that drugs such as nitroglycerine which alleviate anginal pain are likewise effective in this kind of respiratory distress, and went so far as to call the entity a painless equivalent to typical angina pectoris.[51]

To summarize the eighteenth century, which has been termed in a rather derogatory fashion as one of 'theorizing systematizers' (Garrison), it is evident that it advanced the knowledge of our subject in many ways. The clinical picture became more firmly established and included part of later more clearly formulated notions of myocardial damage. This does not deny that the foundations were laid before that time, as the former chapters show. Apart from the great names familiar to all those interested in medical history, we have been able to mention valuable contributions to our subject by otherwise not well-known authors. Again, we would emphasize the spread of medical periodicals in propagating the knowledge accumulated in this century. Special monographs devoted exclusively to heart diseases also contributed to increase interest in this field. In the light of more modern knowledge some of the observations, as well as notions arrived at by eighteenth-century authors through pure reasoning, acquire new meaning in

[51] This interesting conception was recently discussed in an Editorial of the *American Heart Journal*, 1967, **73**, 579–81.

historical perspective; these were almost overlooked by readers of that period for lack of the concepts established much later in the history of medicine. Heberden took the lead in establishing the diagnosis of angina pectoris, while our analysis has shown his scope to include almost all later developments. Knowledge of the anatomy of the disease made great strides, though the coronary hypothesis did not give an adequate answer to all the problems which arose. However, firm steps towards recognition of myocardial changes were already being taken. The disturbed physiology had been included in many observations, but was incomplete until more accomplished methods of investigation were introduced into this field. There was even some speculation about the last cause of the disease, namely arteriosclerosis, before a clear outline of those changes evolved (see p. 98).

Psychological factors moreover—the influence of stress and emotions in coronary artery disease—were noted in some of the case reports and comments of the period. As early as 1649 Harvey was very explicit in this respect when he referred to two clinical cases in his famous letter to Riolan. Fothergill, commenting on the dissection of his patient H. R. Esq. in his paper of 1776, which we have already quoted, considered not only the factor of disturbed physiology, but also the possible effect of the emotions. He gave his opinion in the following words:

> '. . . under such circumstances it is impossible to bear with impunity the effects of sudden and violent agitations, whether they arise from gusts of passion, or suddenly accelerated muscular motion' (l.c. p. 257).

John Hunter, whom we have mentioned repeatedly in connection with our subject, himself suffered in the last twenty years of his life from severe attacks of angina pectoris. His biographers reported that these were usually provoked by anger; so that he would remark that his life was in the hands of any rascal who chose to annoy or tease him. His death occurred in 1793, at a meeting of the Board of St. George's Hospital, when, during a violent dispute, Hunter suddenly stopped speaking; struggling to control his temper, he hurried into an adjoining room and died in a matter of minutes. The biographical notes, which include an account of his death, were brought to notice by his brother-in-law, Sir Everard Home, along with the post-mortem showing degenerative changes in the coronary vessels and scars in the myocardium. In considering the circumstances of Hunter's disease and death, his contemporaries and biographers had a tendency to stress the emotional factors precipitating the attacks.

In his *Life of John Hunter* Everard Home (1794) adds:

> 'It is a curious circumstance that the first attack of these com-
> plaints was produced by an affection of the mind [read emotion],
> and every future return of any consequence arose from the same
> cause'.

The more severe attacks were brought on by emotion much more than
by bodily exercise.

As to the autopsy, Home repeats Hunter's own observations that
'the blood has not been completely coagulated.'

A few years before his death Hunter experienced an attack of two
hours' duration and of unusual severity. Similar attacks would explain
the post-mortem finding of myocardial scars: 'Two spaces nearly an
inch and a half square which were of a white colour, entirely distinct
from the general surface of heart'.

In the very informative paper (1966) by K. D. Keele, the manuscripts (in the transcript of William Clift) kept at the Royal College
of Surgeons of England are examined. Likewise many pathological
specimens of John Hunter's collection are evaluated, and some reproduced, among the latter (Fig. 4b) a cardiac aneurysm. The legend
points to 'the changes of anterior cardiac infarction, the typical apical
aneurysm, inside which is ante-mortem thrombus'. The patient
was General Herbert who died in April 1757. Hunter's description of
the autopsy is most illuminating, 'the apex forming itself into a kind of
aneurism; becoming very thin. That part was lined with thrombus
just the shape of the pouch in which it lay' (Hunter, Ms. e).[52]

Post-mortem reports were often influenced by predilections and
changing fashions of the dissectors. This was the case with the bony
cartilages of the ribs (Rougnon, Hunter's report of Fothergill's patient
(H. R. Esq.), and Home's of John Hunter).

It seems that the fluidity of the blood due to cardiogenic shock,
or to delay of autopsy, was more emphasized by John Hunter and his
pupils than by later pathologists when they performed autopsies on
patients with coronary artery disease.

Home's remark: 'the internal membrane of the aorta lost entirely
its natural polish' corresponds to the identical description by Scarpa in
1804.

---

[52] For a historical review of cardiac aneurysm see: John Thurnam, *Med.-chir. Trans.*
1838, **21**, 187. This has 74 references from the literature, beginning with the mid-
seventeenth century (Appendix, p. 262). Eleven cases of his own are the main topic of
Thurnam's paper (pp. 187–262), preceding his list of references in the appendix. Incidentally, the case of General Herbert is described in detail (pp. 210–13) compiled from
the Hunterian MS, *Account of Dissections of Morbid Bodies*, vol. III, No. 32, p. 20.

CHAPTER V

The Nineteenth Century

1. During this period progress in the knowledge of coronary artery disease does not appear to be continuous. Accordingly, some historians have questioned whether it was not halted and even neglected in favour of other interests in which investigators were more actively engaged. Indeed, pathological anatomy, refined methods of physiology, surgery, anaesthetics and the rise of bacteriology in the last quarter of the century absorbed much of the creative genius of the epoch. On the other hand, the development of research and methods in the above fields were instrumental in creating the type of research which, in our own subject too, subsequently led to really spectacular progress. However, this stage was arrived at comparatively late. As mentioned in the introduction, the nineteenth-century efforts were marked even in the earlier and middle years of the period by the introduction of the notion of arteriosclerosis and its anatomical verification and, secondly, by the emergence of the important concept of thombosis. These two attainments, along with an ever-increasing amount of clinical work, paved the way to a better understanding of coronary disease and myocardial infarction.

Proceeding chronologically, we continue with the work of Allan Burns (1781–1813). His book, *Observations on some of the most frequent and important Diseases of the Heart*, was published in 1809, and contains a special chapter 'Observations on Disease of the Coronary Arteries and on Syncope Anginosa' (pp. 136–162). From the title of the volume it is evident that angina pectoris and 'syncope anginosa' were already considered 'frequent diseases'. Apparently the medical profession became more conscious of them during the short period which had elapsed since the publications by Heberden and the other authors of the late eighteenth century. Owing to the brevity of Burns' life, and his engagement in too numerous tasks and appointments, such as directing a new hospital 'on English lines' in St. Petersburg and lecturing on anatomy and surgery, he was not able to conclude his studies in our subject. James B. Herrick, the grand old man of American cardiology, was so attracted by Burns that he devoted to him a detailed paper entitled, 'Allan Burns, anatomist, surgeon and cardiologist'.

Though Burns was also an adherent of the coronary hypothesis, he enlarged it by emphasizing the disturbed physiology and proceeding to the myocardial ischaemic theory of angina pectoris. He tentatively explained anginal pain as being due to the inadequacy of the blood supply through a partial occlusion of the vessels. When he applied a tourniquet around the arm, he partially shut off the circulation in the limb. The result was weakness and fatigue by voluntary motion of the hand. By this experiment Burns meant to imitate the mechanism of angina pectoris in those cases where no complaints are manifest during rest, and he continues,

> 'If, however, we call into vigorous action a limb, round which we have with moderate degree of tightness, applied a ligature, we find that then the member can only support its action for a very short time; for now its supply of energy and its expenditure, do not balance. A heart, the coronary vessels of which are cartilaginous or ossified, is in nearly a similar condition. . . .'

Burns leaned heavily on Parry's theory and he successfully reinforced it by effective experiments of his own. Though an anatomist himself, Burns was not completely satisfied with the accepted interpretation of calcified coronaries as the immediate causative factor and tried to explain the pathophysiological processes involved. This was also the case with the pathologist Julius Cohnheim in 1877, who, after performing extensive dissections, was disappointed by his failure to find purely anatomical evidence and explanation in many cases of death from this disease.

A similar critical approach to the problem, which contrasts with the firm conviction and assured statements characteristic of many previous authors, is found in a paper by the Bostonian surgeon, John Warren (1753–1815), the earliest American we have been able to quote in connection with our subject. He was fully acquainted with the English authors from Heberden onwards and quotes Fothergill, Percival, Johnstone, Black, Parry and Charles Bell, most of whom we have already discussed. His paper, 'Remarks on Angina Pectoris' was published in 1812 and reprinted on the occasion of the 150th anniversary of the *New England Journal of Medicine* in 1962. Warren says, 'That all cases which Heberden had noticed were instances of angina pectoris, is by no means probable'. He was already fully aware that the condition which Heberden described as angina pectoris had a wider scope and meaning. Probably he had in mind the pattern later conceived as myocardial infarction. As regards Parry, he felt that he had brought 'under the same description cases essentially different from the true angina pectoris.' He continues, 'If it should be proved that ossification is the cause, it will probably be difficult to explain why it should produce its effects in this particular form, rather than that of a continued disease.'

Warren refers to four cases under his own observation and on which he performed dissections. Though he was able to find ossification in some of the autopsies, and declared that he had 'no intention of controverting the principal doctrines of Dr. Parry,' he concludes that the ossification theory is 'apt to simplify too much'. We have referred in some detail to Warren's paper because it displays his critical attitude and common sense. His son, John Collins Warren, and his successor in the professorship of anatomy and surgery at the Harvard College, was also interested in angina pectoris. He published quite early, in 1809, a small volume entitled *Cases of Organic Diseases of the Heart, with Dissections*. He shows the same critical approach as his father in remarking that in some of his own dissections a number of people who had not suffered from angina pectoris showed ossification of the coronaries.[1]

Incidentally, John Warren's interest in our subject may be partly explained by the fact that from the age of thirty he was occasionally affected with an uneasiness in the breast, as his biographers report. Many later investigators into the anginal syndrome also suffered themselves from this disease.

Our mention of Warren is indicative of the problem which arose in presenting a satisfactory theory of what was then known as angina pectoris. In fact, from that time on, many authors pondered on a possible theory, and when in 1899 the French cardiologist Huchard summarized the different opinions, he was able to list eighty mechanisms in eight groups.

It is evident that the weak point in understanding the anginal syndrome lay in the insufficient knowledge of its pathogenesis, which eventually found an answer by a deeper insight into the degenerative processes in arteries. We were fortunate to find an early investigator of arteriosclerosis, the Italian surgeon and anatomist Antonio Scarpa (1752–1832), whose name is not sufficiently stressed in his connection. The relevant material is to be found in his book *Sull' Aneurisma, Riflessioni ed Osservazioni Anatomico-chirurgiche* (Pavia, 1804).[2] We feel that it is the first anatomo-pathological description of arterial

---

[1] See also F. L. Kreysig's work (1814–17), expecially vol. II, p. 534, 'cases of angina pectoris without ossification and those of ossification without angina pectoris'.

[2] We have used the Italian original, and also taken advantage of the English translation by J. H. Wishart, 2nd ed., Edinburgh, 1819.

wall degeneration presented in full detail and well-illustrated. However, it was not Scarpa who coined the word arteriosclerosis but Lobstein, in 1833, whom we shall discuss later.

While making extensive use of the older literature, and quoting Bonet, Lieutaud, Morgagni, Haller, Lancisi and Crell, Scarpa is the first to foretell the later development of the research into the pathology of arteriosclerosis.

Scarpa's book is basically a surgical treatise and deals with ligature of the principal arteries of the extremities. Only one chapter is relevant to the theory of arteriosclerosis: chapter V, 'On Aneurism in General' (Engl. ed. pp. 54–127); and especially the paragraphs 20–22.

Scarpa opposes the view that dilatation of the aorta is the intrinsic cause of the pathology, ultimately leading to rupture; rather the 'slow morbid ulcerated, steatomatous, fungous, squamous degeneration of the internal coat of the artery' (V, par. 20, p. 84 Engl. ed.), is responsible for it.

One paragraph (p. 88) refers to similar processes in the heart, concluding, 'These diseases, which sometimes soften the substance of the heart and dispose it to ulceration and rupture, are likewise common in the arteries.' Scarpa is very precise in his exposition of the various anatomical changes. He stressed their chronicity and gradual development, proceeding from 'a slow internal cause'. These last words show his anticipation of the essential source of these changes, a subject later explored and found to involve endless factors and possibilities. In his historical remarks he quotes (p. 22 of his original edition) Crell's dissertation (see pp. 76–77) to the effect that the artery did not show any changes externally, but seemed hardened in the interior to a 'corpus durum'. Scarpa adds:

'... and especially the internal coat is subject from a slow internal cause, to an ulcerated and steatomatous disorganization, as well as to a squamous and earthy rigidity and brittleness. We have cases ... of ulcerated corrosions of the heart, from internal unknown causes' (English trans., p. 85).

Thus we infer that 'disorganization' of the internal coats as a factor responsible for arteriosclerosis had been formulated at the very beginning of the nineteenth century.

In publishing his research Scarpa gives credit to his predecessors. The case of conversion of the coats of the aorta into a steatomatous tumour had been illustrated by figures in C. G. Stenzel's *Dissertatio de Steatomatibus Aortae* (1723). According to Scarpa, ulceration of the heart was mentioned by Bonet, Johnstone, and Morand, authors whom we have already had occasion to discuss. Of course 'steatomatous disorganization' was to lead to a more modern identification of lipids and other factors in the etiology of atheroma.

Scarpa's contribution, which we have here brought again to notice, was not overlooked by those almost contemporary with him. D. Craigie, in his *Elements of General and Pathological Anatomy*, Edinburgh, 1828, gives credit to him, although with some reservations; cf. p. 90: 'Earthy degeneration of Scarpa'; p. 97: 'Steatomatous degeneration of Scarpa'; on p. 98 he quotes his words: 'The inner coat of the artery loses its fine polish.'[3]

Scarpa's emphasis on the 'steatomatous [fatty] disorganization' proved fruitful. It has been revived in the modern word atherosclerosis, in which 'athero' depicts the fatty nature of the degeneration. As regards the cardiac findings, the term 'ulcerated corrosions' replaced the older designation 'abscess of the heart'. Actual abscesses of the heart substance occur occasionally in pyogenic myocarditis, but are extremely uncommon. Scarpa radically changed the older theory of an inflammatory process, replacing it by a more pronounced metabolic meaning. He conceived this as a 'slow' structural change, which takes years to become apparent and clinically significant. The peculiarity of the arteriosclerotic process was also acknowledged when Scarpa denoted it as arising from 'an inner unknown cause.' In fact the etiology, according to more recent investigations, is a rather complicated one: nutritional, hereditary and metabolic.

It might be well to include some etymological notes on the terms mentioned. The word 'atheroma' is of course a very old one, derived from Greek and meaning 'groats' or 'porridge'. In medical usage it encompasses a great variety of morbid appearances, from the harmless tumours in the skin, especially on the head, to the destructive and life-threatening processes in the inner coats of the arteries. The Leipzig pathologist Marchand, in 1904, appears to be the first to use the term atherosclerosis instead of arteriosclerosis to designate the degenerative process in the intimal coat of the arteries. As to the term 'steatomatous', this has also a respectable pedigree. The Greek word steatoma, a kind of fatty tumour, is mentioned in Pliny (26, 87, par. 144). Celsus (7.6) writes the word in Greek, since in his time it was not yet widely used in medical Latin. In the same chapter he likewise mentions the atheroma, meaning a swelling on the head or a tumour filled with matter. As in other branches of medical terminology, these words frequently underwent changes of meaning.

---

[3] Craigie is helpful also in giving the precise location of Stenzel's dissertation in Haller, *Disputationes ad Morborum Historiam*, Tom. II, p. 527, Art. 65.

We have given attention to Scarpa's work mainly for its detailed and almost modern approach to the problem of arteriosclerosis, though Scarpa did not term it as such. We would like, however, to recall the numerous descriptions in older literature which do not have this quality. As mentioned before, from Leonardo da Vinci onwards there was often reference to tortuous and calcified vessels. To supplement the information already given, we would like to cite Malpighi's report on his post-mortem examination of Cardinal Bonaccorsi (aortic sclerosis), and Wepfer's (1620–95) work, *Observationes Medicopracticae de Affectibus Capitis internis et externis*, published posthumously in 1727. However, all the older authors refer to the artery as a whole, while Scarpa is precise in considering tissue pathology, which had just been introduced by Bichat, in his *Anatomie Générale* in 1801.

The term abscess does not need explanation, but its frequent use in older literature concerning heart pathology is noteworthy and has been repeatedly referred to in earlier chapters (Sénac and others). The term occurred already in the sixteenth century. To quote only a few of the authors, we recall Benivieni's case 89, 'Abscess in the left part of the heart ventricle, redundant with pus'; Nicholas Massa in his *Anatomiae liber introductorius* (1536), ch. 28, 'De anatomia cordis'; and Jean Fernel, *Pathologia*, Book I, ch. 12, 'De Corde',[4] where he described three ulcers in the heart. A number of these cases can be interpreted as softening processes due to myocardial infarction.

The next developments in defining the nature of arteriosclerosis may be attributed to the Strasbourg pathologist J. F. Lobstein (1777–1835). His book, *Traité d'Anatomie Pathologique*, appeared in two volumes, the first in 1829 and the second in 1833. Arteriosclerosis[5] is referred to only in the second volume, while the first bears on general pathology but not on vessels.[6] In his description of the diseased arteries Lobstein refers to their thickening as well as to their hardening. Giving precise figures in the old French measure 'ligne', which corresponds to approximately 2.25 mm, he found the coats of the diseased arteries, apart from ossification, to be $1\frac{1}{2}$ 'lignes' as against the normal measurement of $\frac{1}{2}$ 'ligne'. The inner surface appeared uneven, warty, and the colour was yellowish or brownish-red. Lobstein conceived arteriosclerosis as a non-inflammatory process, due to unnatural nutrition of the vessels and their morbid 'plasticity'. He noticed that often the lumen is not narrowed, but is usually wider than normal.

---

[4] I am indebted to Dr. W. Pagel for drawing my attention to some of the sources in this context.

[5] French original, pp. 550–53, 'De l'épaississement des artères, ou l'artériosclérose'.

[6] We have used the German translation, 1834–35.

In the chapter on obstruction of the arteries he opposes the view of the English authors that ossification may be regarded as a cause of angina pectoris. We did not, incidentally, find in his writings special references to arteriosclerosis in the coronary vessels. In the chapter on 'Diseases of the heart substance', Lobstein used the term cardiosclerosis and also, significantly, the term cardiomalacy, the latter anticipating the more accurate use by Ziegler towards the end of the nineteenth century. He also mentioned partial aneurysms of the heart, especially at the apex, and found them more often in men than in women. However, no coronary findings appeared in this description. The word 'cardio-malacy' is derived from *malacus*, meaning soft. The chief merit of Lobstein's book is that it describes arteriosclerosis in general and coins the name.

Clinical and anatomical contributions to coronary artery disease continued to make their appearance during the nineteenth century. Robert Adams (1791–1875) wrote in 1827 a remarkable article, 'Cases of diseases of the heart accompanied with pathological observations'.[7] This author, famous for one of the first descriptions of heart block, now called 'Stokes-Adams syndrome', came quite close to the idea of acute coronary obstruction as a cause of myo-cardial softening (p. 401) when he described rupture of the heart muscle. His patient suffered from severe anginal pain and from a peculiar pulse anomaly named after Adams. The post-mortem revealed that 'muscular fibre was remarkably soft in its structure, so as to admit of being broken down between the finger and thumb; death had been due to haemopericardium.' In another case, of a man of sixty-eight with severe pain in the chest, he found at the autopsy aortic stenosis of a senescent degenerative type, and the heart 'large, flabby, and of a yellow colour from fatty deposition; coronary arteries completely ossified.' In another context Adams proposes the following speculation:

> 'When we reflect that the heart can derive no supply from any other source than its coronary vessels, it will not appear then so extraordinary that partial paralysis [8] should be the immediate consequence of the complete obstruction of these channels.'

This is a fine specimen of clinico-pathological investigation with a balanced judgement. However, Adams did not proceed to a definitive conclusion that it is softening that is the consequence of coronary

---

[7] *Dubl. Hosp. Rep.* **4**, 353–454.

[8] The word paralysis, as applied to the heart, was already used by Caelius (see p. 38).

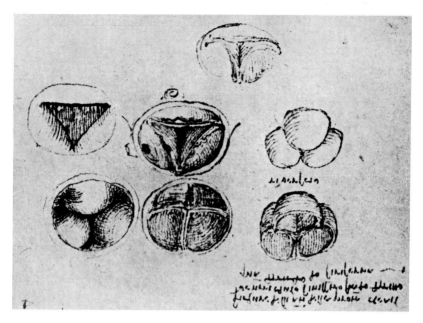

Plate II First depiction of the origin of the coronary vessels from the coronary sinus.
Leonardo da Vinci (1452–1519), *Quaderni d'anatomia*, 1911–18, vol. II, folio 9 verso,
figures 4–9.

34 *Exercitatio Anatomica* I.

Poterat hic addere doctissimus
vir, tertiam circulationem brevis-
simam, è siniftro nempe ventricu-
lo cordis, ad dextrum, circuma-
gentem portionem sanguinis per
arterias & venas coronales, suis ra-
mulis per cordis corpus, parietes,
& septum distributas.

*Qui admittit, inquit, unam circu-
lationem non potest alteram repudiare.*
Ità addere potuisset, non potest
tertiam denegare. Quorsum enim
pulsarent arteriæ coronales in corde, si non sanguinem eo impul-
su impellerent? & quorsum venæ
(quarum officium & finis est sanguinem ab arteriis ingestum reci-
pere) nisi ut sanguinem è corde
tranarent? Adde insuper, in venæ
coronalis orificio valvulam (ut ipse
vir doctus fatetur lib. 3. cap. 9.)
sæpissi-

de Circulatione Sanguinis. 35

sæpissimè reperiri ingressum pro-
hibentem, egressui reclinantem:
ergo tertiam certè non potest non
admittere circulationem, qui alteram universalem & per pulmones
quoque & cerebrum (lib. 4. c. 2.)
sanguinem transire admittit. Neque enim, in singulis partibus cu-
juscunque regionis, fieri similiter
à pulsu ingressum sanguinis & per
venas regressum, omnesque pro-
inde particulas circulationem re-
cipere, haud potest denegare.

Ex his verbis ipsissimis itaque
viri doctissimi clarè patet, qualis
ipsius est sententia, tum de circui-
tu sanguinis per universum corpus, tum per pulmones cæteras-
que omnes partes; nam ipse, qui
primam circulationem admittit,
apertè patet reliquas non repudiare.

Plate III William Harvey, *Exercitationes duae anatomicae de circulatione sanguinis. Ad
Johannem Riolanum filium* (etc.), Rotterdam: A. Leers, 1649; pp. 34–35.

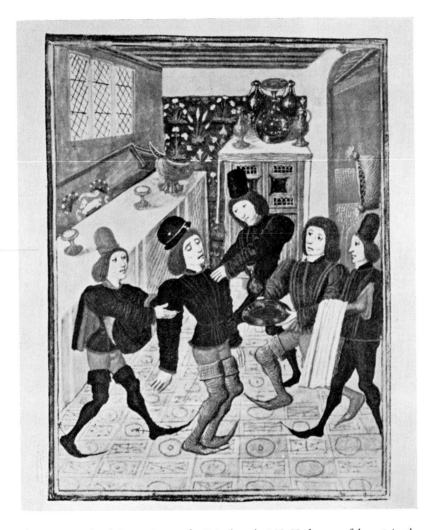

Plate IV   Death of Count Gaston de Foix (1391). MS Harl. 4379 fol. 126 in the British Museum.

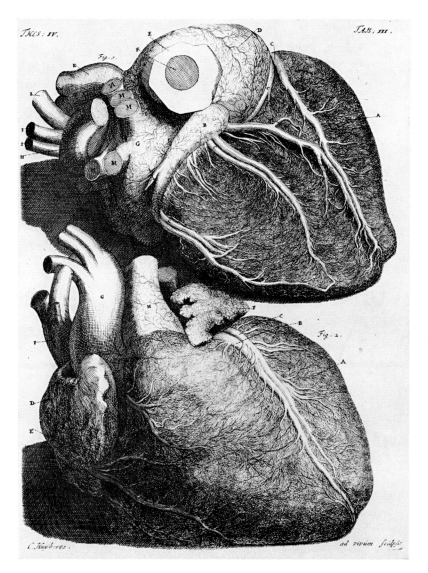

Plate V   Heart injected with red wax showing the finest ramifications of the coronary
vessels. Frederik Ruysch (1638–1731), *Thesaurus anatomicus quartus*, Amsterdam, 1704
(Tab. III).

On page 45 Ruysch remarks: 'English magnates preserve the embalmed hearts of
deceased members of their families in golden or silver boxes, and thus my art flourishes
(et sic ars mea vigeret).'

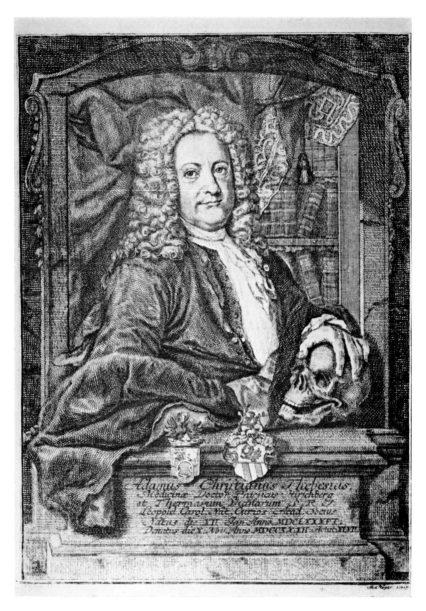

Plate VI   Portrait of Adam Christian Thebesius (1686–1732). Engraved by A. Hoger after M. Tyrnoff. From a copy in the Royal College of Physicians of London.

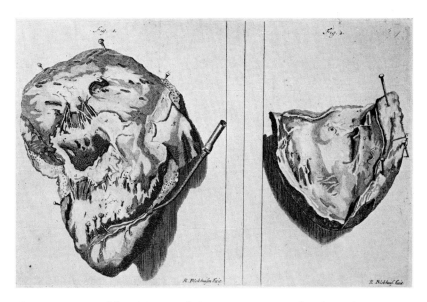

Plate VII   Dissected heart. A. C. Thebesius, *Dissertatio medica de circulo sanguinis in corde*, Leyden, 1716 (1st edition 1708).

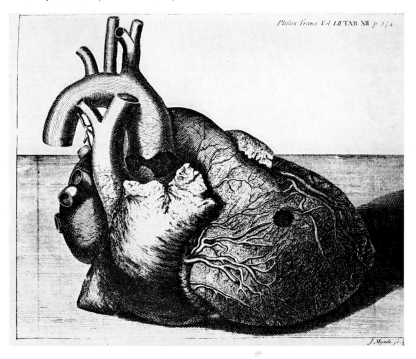

Plate VIII   Ruptured heart of King George II 'having the orifice in the right ventricle, and the extravasation covering the fissure in the aorta'. Frank Nicholls, 'Observations concerning the Body of his late Majesty, October 26, 1760.' *Phil. Trans. R. Soc. Lond.*, vol. 52, pt. I, 1761, pp. 265–275.

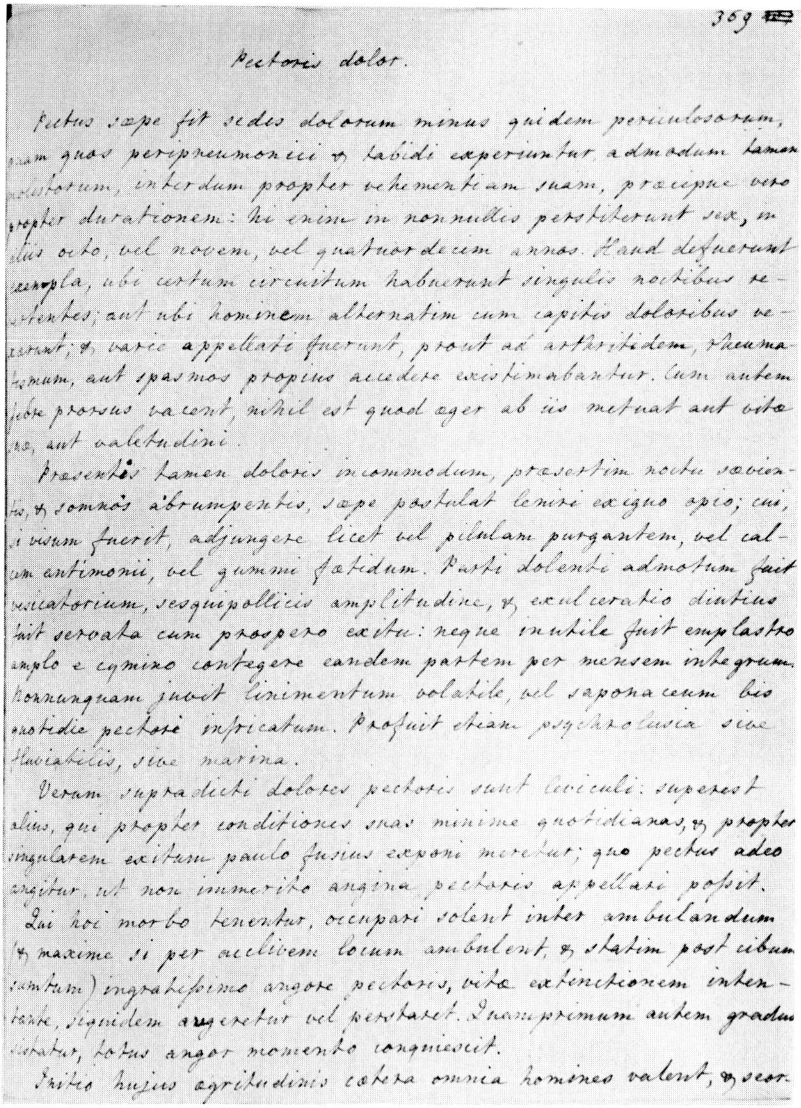

369

Pectoris dolor.

Pectus sæpe fit sedes dolorum minus quidem periculosorum, quam quos peripneumonici & tabidi experiuntur, admodum tamen molestorum, interdum propter vehementiam suam, præcipue vero propter durationem: hi enim in nonnullis perstiterunt sex, in aliis octo, vel novem, vel quatuordecim annos. Haud defuerunt exempla, ubi certum circuitum habuerunt singulis noctibus redeuntes; aut ubi hominem alternatim cum capitis doloribus vexarunt; & varie appellati fuerunt, prout ad arthritidem, rheumatismum, aut spasmos propius accedere existimabantur. Cum autem febre prorsus vacent, nihil est quod æger ab iis metuat aut vitæ, aut valetudini.

Præsentis tamen doloris incommodum, præsertim noctu sævientis, & somnos abrumpentis, sæpe postulat leniri exiguo opio; cui, si visum fuerit, adjungere licet vel pilulam purgantem, vel calcem antimonii, vel gummi fœtidum. Parti dolenti admotum fuit vesicatorium, sesquipollicis amplitudine, & exulceratio diutius fuit servata cum prospero exitu: neque inutile fuit emplastro amplo e cymino contegere eandem partem per mensem integrum. Nonnunquam juvit linimentum volatile, vel saponaceum bis quotidie pectori infricatum. Profuit etiam psychrolusia sive fluviatilis, sive marina.

Verum supradicti dolores pectoris sunt leviculi: superest alius, qui propter conditiones suas minime quotidianas, & propter singularem exitum paulo fusius exponi meretur; quo pectus adeo angitur, ut non immerito angina pectoris appellari possit.

Qui hoc morbo tenentur, occupari solent inter ambulandum (& maxime si per acclivem locum ambulent, & statim post cibum sumtum) ingratissimo angore pectoris, vitæ extinctionem intentante, siquidem augeretur vel perstaret. Quamprimum autem gradus sistatur, totus angor momento conquiescit.

Initio hujus ægritudinis cætera omnia homines valent, & scor-

Plate IX First page of William Heberden's autograph manuscript *Pectoris dolor*, in the Royal College of Physicians of London, conforming to his paper published in English in 1772.

SULL'

ANEURISMA

RIFLESSIONI ED OSSERVAZIONI ANATOMICO-CHIRURGICHE

DI

ANTONIO SCARPA

P. Professore di Notomia, e Chirurgia pratica nell' Università di Pavia, Membro dell' Istituto Nazionale della Rep. Ital., Socio della R. Acad. di Berlino, della R. di Londra, della Cesar - Leopold. natur. curios., della Imp. medic. chir. di Vienna, della Società med. di Parigi, di Edimburgo, di Mompelieri ec. ec.

PAVIA. ANNO 1804.

NELLA TIPOGRAFIA BOLZANI.

Plate X   Antonio Scarpa (1747–1832), *Sull' aneurisma. Riflessioni ed osservazioni anatomico-chirurgiche*, atlas folio, Pavia, 1804. Title-page.

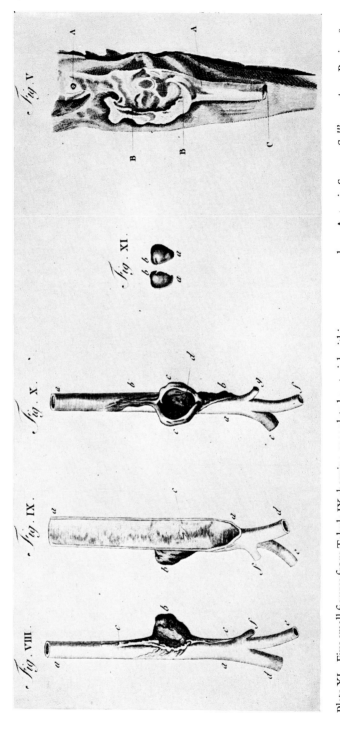

Plate XI   Five small figures from Tabula IX showing coagulated material within an aneurysmal sac. Antonio Scarpa, *Sull' aneurisma*, Pavia, 1804.

DISPUTATIONES
AD MORBORUM
HISTORIAM ET CURATIONEM
FACIENTES.

QUAS COLLEGIT, EDIDIT ET RECENSUIT

ALBERTUS HALLERUS.

TOMUS SECUNDUS.

AD MORBOS PECTORIS.

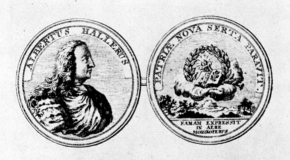

Joubert Sc.

LAUSANNÆ,

'Sumptibus MARCI·MICHAEL. BOUSQUET & Socior.

MDCCLVII.

Plate XII   Albrecht v. Haller (1708–1777), *Disputationes ad morborum historiam et curationem facientes. Tomus secundus: Ad morbos pectoris*, Lausanne, 1757. Title-page. The volume consists of a collection of tracts and medical theses on diseases of the chest from the earlier 18th century.

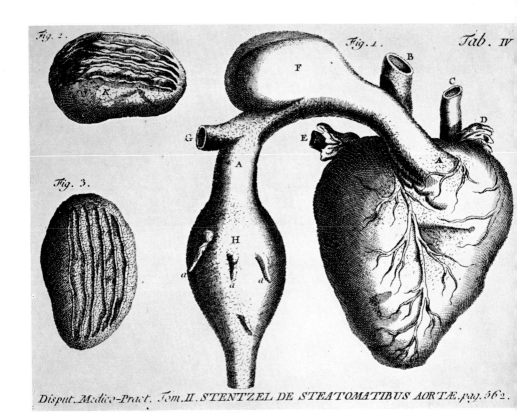

Plate XIII   Heart and vessels showing multiple aortic aneurysms and thrombi removed from the aneurysmal sacs. Christian Gottfried Stenzel (1698–1748), *Dissertatio de steatomatibus aortae*, 1723. In: Albrecht v. Haller, *Disputationes ad morborum historiam et curationem facientes. Tomus secundus; Ad morbos pectoris*, Lausanne, 1757, facing page 562.

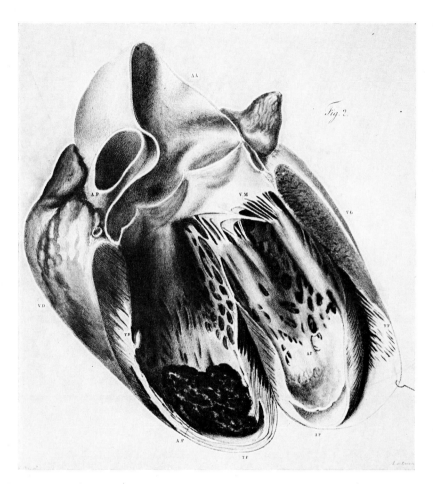

Plate XIV Partial aneurysm of the heart occupying the apex of the left ventricle.
Jean Cruveilhier (1791–1874), *Anatomie pathologique du corps humain*, Paris 1829–42,
t. II, 22° livraison, planche 3, figure 2.

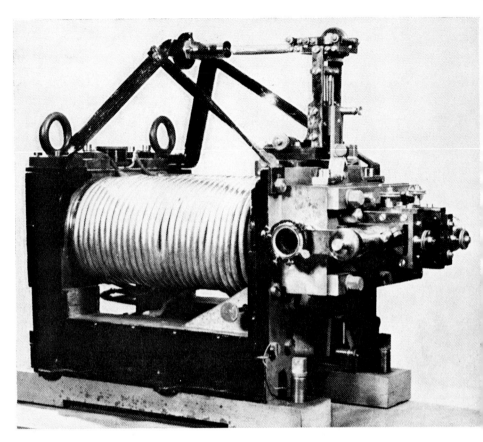

Plate XV   String galvanometer, 1903, of William Einthoven (1860–1927). From: *Some Dutch contributions to the development of physiology.* (Souvenir of the 22nd International Congress of Physiological Sciences.) 1962, p. 35.

obstruction, and speaks only of 'partial paralysis', obviously because of absence, as yet, of a generally-accepted pathological concept.

Prior to the establishment of the doctrine of thrombosis, Jean Cruveilhier (1791–1874), founder of modern pathology in France, was able to produce important contributions to our subject. In his *Anatomie Pathologique du Corps Humain*, (1829–42) he included a fine reproduction in colour of a myocardial infarct (1835). Cruveilhier did not relate his finding to coronary artery disease, though many details in the chapter on heart diseases (6 pages) also point to sequelae of this disease, for instance to partial aneurysm at the apex of the heart. The illustration we are referring to is perhaps the most beautiful one in the history of the medical illustration of our subject. It pictures an infarcted area of the left ventricular wall and is outstanding in colour, besides being precise anatomically. It is reproduced in the 22nd fascicle ('livraison') on plate 3, being the upper figure on the sheet, and is entitled 'Apopléxie du coeur'. The figure beneath it is that of a partial aneurysm with a thrombus at the apex, faithfully depicted, but not named as such. Commenting on the first figure, Cruveilhier found it remarkable that this heart contained 'extravasations of blood' in the depth of its wall not leading to rupture of the organ. He noted also the yellowish discoloration and the fragility of the corresponding part of the myocardium, but did not ascribe the pathology to coronary artery disease. The infarct is represented in two different planes: longitudinal section on the right, and transverse on the left side, a fine didactical contrivance. The red colour marks haemorrhage, while the yellow indicates necrosis. It is of historical relevance that a faithful observation and visual representation could be given without relation to the underlying ultimate cause of the process. In one biographical sketch,[9] Cruveilhier is reported to have said: 'Les systèmes passent, les faits restent.'

When R. T. H. Laënnec (1781–1826) published his classic book *Traité de l'Auscultation Médiate* in 1819, he did not mention there angina pectoris or myocardial pathology of coronary origin. In fact these items did not provide much material for his study of auscultatory phenomena. Since, however, his work proved to be much more inclusive than the title implies, he included in the second edition a full description of angina (vol. II, 1826, pp. 745–52). Laënnec found

---

[9] In *Les Biographies Médicales*, Paris, 1927–36, vol. III, p. 293. Edited by P. Bisquet; biography written by M. Genty; the writer antedates Cruveilhier's work to 1828, but this refers probably only to the first fascicle (cf. Callisen, IV, 429).

the disease to be rather common and mentions its milder manifestations as well as a specimen of a grave attack. On page 746 he gives a graphic and unusual description of the latter, comparing it to that of 'iron nails or the claw of an animal tearing asunder the front of the chest'.[10] The author rejects the coronary hypothesis and explains the disease as 'neuralgia of the heart'; he conceived it to be 'a spasmodic affection'. He thinks the disease may originate in the sympathetic nerves of the heart (II, 749). It may be added that he was interested in the coagulation process in the heart and the vessels (II, 615–16) and summarized his deliberations in four conclusions in which some ideas have been implied about phenomena which later led to the concept of thrombosis.

The continuous flow of reports and descriptions in our subject in the first half of the nineteenth century contributed greatly to a deeper knowledge of coronary artery disease. In some respects these publications followed the trend of the eighteenth-century investigators. However, the findings regarding the diseased myocardium leading to necrosis of its substance, as well as its relationship to coronary disease, came more into focus. Myocardial infarction as an entity was still not yet delineated, but the reports gave clearer indications towards this diagnosis. The authors were more consistent in their autopsy records, not only marking calcified coronaries but also describing morbid changes in the heart muscle. This correlation is quite typical of the earlier nineteenth-century descriptions. A few examples will follow.

Joseph Hodgson (1788–1869) described in his *Treatise on the Diseases of Arteries and Veins* (1815) a typical case of angina pectoris followed by sudden death. Though primarily written from the standpoint of a surgeon, this comprehensive volume also contains some data on the coronary arteries of the heart (e.g. p. 36). Hodgson makes the critical remark that 'deposition of calcareous matter does not, however, exist in every case of angina pectoris and syncope anginosa.' Case 6 describes coronary sclerosis combined with changes of the heart muscle; 'the parietes of either ventricle soft and tender.' Case 8 gives the clinical history with excruciating pain in the region of the heart,

---

[10] We have used Rolleston's translation of the above quotation (1937, p. 211). The French original reads: 'Quelquefois, et surtout lorsque l'attaque est courte et vive, il semble au malade que des ongles de fer ou la griffe d'un animal lui déchirent la partie antérieure de la poitrine.' We should like to correct a small misprint in the bibliographical reference in Rolleston's very informative paper: instead of '1819, II, 706' it must be: 1826, II, 746. His assertion that 'Laennec had had two attacks' is questionable. We found only at the very end of the second volume, pp. 768–69, a self-observation by the author of his feeling 'the contractions of his heart', which is difficult to interpret as attacks of angina pectoris. This passage has a strong human touch, when the dying author is writing down his own medical symptoms with full self-command and seeming unconcern.

and the post-mortem finding of a rent in the apex of the left ventricle, while the coronaries were found 'incrusted'. Here the author goes into a historical digression about obstruction of the arteries, which 'was noticed many years ago by Cowper.' He has also much to say about collateral circulation. In one case the necropsy report was: marked calcification of a main coronary artery leading to a partial aneurysm of the heart with an intraventricular thrombus (p. 84).

Even more specific is the report by Charles J. B. Williams (1805–89). In his book *The Pathology and Diagnosis of Diseases of the Chest*,[11] he gave a description of what would now be termed myocardial infarct, clearly relating it to coronary disease. Describing the heart muscle, he came very close to a modern concept when he noted that:

> 'A pallid yellowish appearance of the substance of the heart is not at all an uncommon accompaniment of other lesions of the organ, especially adhesions of the pericardium and accummulation of fat; but I should be inclined to refer this to an altered state of the nutrition of the organ, owing perhaps to partial obstructions in the coronary vessels, rather than to the immediate influence of inflammation.'

At the same time the designation of softening, hitherto unspecified, was replaced by attempts at a more substantial definition. Some authors began to stress the finding of fatty degeneration in the myocardium, which recalls the steatomatous changes mentioned by Scarpa and other investigators. Richard Quain (1816–98) wrote 'On fatty diseases of the heart' in 1850.[12] He was also able to show that the myocardial changes corresponded to the region supplied by a coronary artery which was extensively ossified. This comprehensive article must be regarded as a classic, providing much information on the subject. Quain cited eighty-three cases and provided illustrations of macroscopic and microscopic specimens. While regarding fatty degeneration at times as due to general or constitutional causes, he singled out another group, where it was due to a 'local modification of nutrition'. He stressed that ossified coronary arteries interfered with the nutritive function of the artery and thus produced the softening which was attended by pain on exertion. We would not speak nowadays of fatty degeneration, but of anaemic infarcts or necrosis and of thrombi inside the vessel,[13] and of

---

[11] We have been able to consult only the fourth edition, 1840.

[12] Cf. A. D. Morgan, 'Some forms of undiagnosed coronary disease in nineteenth-century England', *Med. Hist.*, 1968, **12**, 344–58.

[13] In a later paper, however, in 1871, a thrombus in the coronary artery was clearly mentioned in a post-mortem report of a case of 'angina pectoris'. (See Bibliography.)

later effects represented by scars in the myocardium. Quain's paper had a favourable response and stimulated subsequent investigators. Generally, the nutritional changes in the myocardium occurring in coronary artery disease became better known and investigated during the first half of the nineteenth century.[14]

Along with the clinical pathological endeavour, some steps were made towards the revival of experimental studies. This was mainly achieved by experimental ligation of the coronary arteries to study the results of tying-off the blood supply in dogs. As discussed previously, some crude experiments were made by P. Chirac towards the end of the seventeenth century. Incidentally, Galen had already performed experimental ligation of heart vessels, which he reported in his *De Anatomicis Administrationibus* (in Singer's translation, pp. 194–95). To quote Galen: '. . . put the ligature round the vessels springing from the heart . . . It can be done round the base of the heart, but the animal dies at once.' As evidenced by the Galenic text, the case was a ligature of a pulmonary vein.

We refer next to the surgeon John Erichsen, 1818–1896, teacher of Lord Lister. In his paper, 'On the influence of the coronary circulation on the action of the heart'[15] he reported well-planned experiments on two dogs and seven rabbits, applying artificial respiration after the heart had been removed. He gives exact figures as to the ensuing gradual decrease in the heart rate. After twenty-one minutes the action of the ventricles had ceased, while the auricles continued to act for some time longer. He concluded:

> 'First, that arrest of the coronary circulation produces a speedy cessation of the heart's action. Secondly, that an increase in the quantity of blood sent into, or retained in the muscular fibre of the heart, produces a corresponding increase in the activity of that organ.' In his comment he explained the clinical implications: 'either directly as in ossification of the coats of the coronary vessels, or indirectly, in cases of extreme obstruction or regurgitant disease of the aortal or mitral valves.'

Erichsen's contribution[16] preceded the more detailed and complicated investigations performed in the second half of the century by Panum, Bezold and Cohnheim, who are to be discussed later.

[14] An early author to describe myocardial necrosis from a clot ('coagulum') in a coronary artery was William Baly (1814–61), who microscopically demonstrated 'fatty degeneration' in the affected part of the ventricle. (*Trans. path. Soc. Lond.*, 1850–52, **3**, 264.)

[15] *Lond. Med. Gaz.*, 1842, n.s. **2**, 561–64.

[16] See Dahl-Iverson (1961).

To return to the clinico-pathological reports, it becomes clear that not every worthy contributor to our subject can be referred to. One must deliberately avoid over-coverage of the topic. It would seem valuable, however, to name and describe contributions presenting a peculiar feature or an interpretation which furthered the recognition of what is now called coronary thrombosis and myocardial infarction.

Thomas B. Peacock (1812–82) gave a concise description of partial aneurysm of the left ventricle.[17] The clinical data are complicated by chronic bronchitis, but the sudden death after pain in the precordium one day before is peculiar to a coronary event. The post-mortem describes

> 'a protuberance about the size of a pigeon's egg, at the outer part of the base of the left ventricle, which was found to be formed by an aneurysmal dilatation of the left coronary artery. The sac contained laminated coagula. A portion of the coronary artery was converted into a complete cylinder of bone. The walls of the left ventricle were unusually thin [heart aneurysm?], cavity dilated, more especially towards the apex, where a clot was adherent'.

Peacock remarked that the specimen was quite unique. He could find only three previous references to similar observations, however, with rupture of the heart. While partial aneurysms of the heart have been described more often, that of the left coronary artery is a rare finding.[18]

One of the most remarkable cases, coming very close to modern descriptions of myocardial infarction, was reported by H. P. Malmsten and Düben, of Sweden, and published in the Swedish periodical *Hygiea* (**21**, 629–30) in 1859. The date has been sometimes quoted by later writers as 1861.[19] The concise case-report has been reproduced and translated into German by E. J. Warburg in his exhaustive paper of 1930. Warburg justly stressed the share of the pathologist G. W. J. Düben in this joint publication, which is much more important than Malmsten's clinical report. A man of sixty-six became deeply depressed for three months following his wife's death. An attack came on at night, and next morning precordial pain and restlessness were noted. On the seventh day of the illness the patient was in a state of prostration, with small pulse, very strong pain, fear of impending death, weak heart sounds; death one hour after Malmsten's visit.

---

[17] *Trans. path. Soc. Lond.*, 1846–48, **1**, 227–30.

[18] See also the paper by Ian H. Porter (1962) and the list of Peacock's writings which follows.

[19] I am greatly indebted to Dr. W. Kock of Stockholm, who indicated the correct date (letter of 18th September, 1961).

The information revealed in the post-mortem examination by Düben goes far beyond a ruptured wall, long familiar through Harvey's case of Sir Robert Darcy's post-mortem finding in 1649. Düben describes the clot in some detail. He applies the word necrosis, which conforms to modern usage, and then proceeds to the microscopic appearance of the muscle fibres. It is appropriate to quote the main points of his report: Two 'librae' of blood in the pericardial space; rupture of the left ventricle, near the apex and the septum. At the ruptured wall was a clot, partly firm, partly purulent. The adjacent wall of the heart was softened into a pulpous mass measuring one and a half 'zoll' (approximately an inch); here the muscle fibres were destroyed. Their microscopic appearance showed derangement of structure, and replacement of the fibres by detritus, by granulated, slightly fatty tissue and, in some spots only, by connective tissue. The necrotic changes were more pronounced at the seat of the rupture. As regards the left coronary artery, the anterior branch contained an old canalized clot beginning near the area of softening. Düben's concluding comment is:

> 'The canalized clot must have been formed a long time ago, and is the cause of the softening, slowly progressing and without symptoms. The period of Mr. Malmsten's observations was restricted to the last stage of the illness when the rupture appeared.'

Microscopy, Düben's outstanding contribution to this case, was used comparatively late in the research into coronary artery disease. This technique is much older than its application to our subject. The emergence of cell-studies had been marked by Robert Hooke's *Micrographia* (1665); Malpighi was able to discover the capillary arterio-venous anastomoses and excelled more than any previous medical authority in discovering the finer structure of the viscera, for instance the glomeruli in the kidneys, already in the second half of the seventeenth-century. In 1674 Leeuwenhoek[20] had observed red blood cells through his one-lens microscope. These highlights had, however, no influence on the growth of knowledge in our subject, and only the second half of the nineteenth century saw its advance by means of microscopy. Düben's microscopical findings in 1859 seem to be the beginning of this kind of research, later to be followed by Vulpian (1866), and brought to perfection by Weigert in 1880. Thus the concept of ischaemic necrosis awaited the development of microscopy as an adjunct to pathological studies.

[20] See *Collected Letters*, Part I (1939), p. 85; and also A. Schierbeck (1959), pp. 109 ff.

We thought it useful to reproduce almost in full Düben's findings and deliberations, since they reveal much more than is implied in the title of the joint publication by Malmsten-Düben, 'Fall af ruptura cordis' (A Case of Heart Rupture). Since this title was too common to arouse curiosity, the brief paper had been overlooked until much later (E. Warburg, 1930), although it merits an outstanding place in the history of our subject. We found in a recent and very informative article[21] on the history of spontaneous rupture of the heart a remark to the effect that Malmsten-Düben's paper has been translated and printed in the *Dublin Medical Press*, but we have been unable to locate this publication. As to Malmsten, whose share in the paper is not of great moment, he maintained a persistent interest in the subject, and in 1861 remarked, in discussing a case of sudden death, that one must think about thrombosis of a coronary artery. In 1876 he diagnosed *in vivo* heart rupture, though the post-mortem revealed only myomalacia and embolism of the right coronary artery.

While Malmsten-Düben's case arouses the vivid interest of the historian in view of the unusual pathological content, another case has the appeal of its most revealing presentation of the clinical course. We must not forget that many of the clinical descriptions to which we have frequently referred were sometimes marred by stereotyped phraseology and, with the particular exception of Heberden's classic, did not always contribute to a broader knowledge of the symptoms.

In quite a different category is the case in which the patient was the famous educationalist Thomas Arnold and the author, P. M. Latham (1789–1875), a clinician much interested in cardiology and especially in angina pectoris.[22] For a contemporary reader it is a classic description of a coronary thombosis, though the author did not use this term. However, he felt rightly that he had met with a special nosological entity, and stressed 'the short period that intervened between the first paroxysm and the last of which the patient died.' Moreover, Latham included in this same chapter thirty-seven other similar cases in which the disease proved fatal after an interval of fourteen days, ten days, and three hours respectively.

While paying due attention to his comments on this and similar cases, we may conclude that Latham indeed felt he had found something new and which had not been clearly described before in the literature

---

[21] A. Levene, 1962.
[22] The report appears in Latham's *Lectures on Subjects connected with Clinical Medicine, comprising Disease of the Heart* (1846, Vol. 2, pp. 373–79.)

on angina pectoris.[23] We are aware of the 'doctor's dilemma' in his rhetorical question on p. 380:

> 'Is there any form of organic disease which can be regarded as the efficient cause of angina pectoris absolutely and at all times?'

However, Latham, as a busy practitioner much concerned with making his reports pleasantly readable, did not enter into greater depth to elucidate this problem. What is most attractive in his deliberations is his particular care to give a more precise classification when he came across an unusual and unfamiliar course of this disease. This can be seen from his remark on p. 382:

> 'These cases, so new and interesting in their details . . . taught us much, very much, . . . if we regard them as constituting *the* disease.'

These short quotations and a statement (p. 373) that the case 'had one extraordinary circumstance belonging to it' show Latham's conviction that the disease which he specifically described stood out from the motley conditions included at his time under the name of angina pectoris. Latham could not expound his case fully since the concept of thrombosis had yet to come.

Latham's case was noted by the medical profession only later, when it was realized that the term 'angina' was too limited to cover all the manifestations. This was already the case before myocardial infarction and coronary thrombosis had become generally-accepted and easily-diagnosed entities.[24] Latham's report was cited, apparently for the first time, by Sir William Osler in his *Lectures on Angina Pectoris and Allied States* (1897), pp. 34–36 (from a later edition, 1876), in the chapter on 'Death in the first well-marked paroxysm.' Here again it appears that Osler was not completely satisfied by the old term, angina pectoris, which did not cover all the manifestations of ischaemic heart disease. He hesitated, however, to adopt the nomenclature of myocardial infarction or coronary thombosis even at a time when the notion of thrombosis was in current use and many excellent papers on the subject (e.g. by Weigert, 1880) were already published. More recently, the case of Thomas Arnold has again been reprinted by T. East[25] and by P. F. M. Wrigley in a survey on ischaemic heart disease in the nineteenth century.[26]

[23] Latham brings his case into a chapter (II, 359 ff.) entitled 'Affections of the heart, consisting in a certain assemblage of symptoms, not in express forms of disease', a heading which gives the historical setting for the concepts of his day.
[24] Cf. Warren's criticism as early as 1812 (see above, pp. 105–6).
[25] *The Story of Heart Disease* (1957), pp. 109–11.
[26] *Oxford Med. Sch. Gaz.*, 1962, **14**, 159–73; pp. 163–64.

Nevertheless, this report is not available in the current source-books (such as R. H. Major's *Classic Descriptions of Disease*, and *Cardiac Classics* by Willius and Keys), and therefore we shall include it in its unabridged form. Incidentally, the patient was not seen by Latham himself, but the report, signed by J. Hodgson of Birmingham, was communicated to him in a letter by the attending physician Dr. Bucknill. This must have been the renowned Joseph Hodgson to whose contributions we have referred earlier (see p. 112). He was presumably responsible for the post-mortem, since at that time he worked as surgeon at the General Hospital and Eye Infirmary in Birmingham. This fact, not noticed elsewhere, may give a special flavour to the report and is a further reason for its inclusion, despite the vagueness of its pathological description.

'T. A. was within a day of completing his 47th year. Up to a very few hours before his death, both body and mind seemed equally to give proof and promise of health. He still took his accustomed pleasure and refreshment in strenuous exercise. His thoughts were still busily employed upon the highest subjects, conceiving and composing with wonderful ease, rapidity and power. He retired to rest at midnight on the 11th of June 1842, feeling and believing himself to be in perfect health. At a quarter before seven the next morning his medical attendant was called. What had previously occurred and what followed I will give in the words of Dr. Bucknill who was with him during the short remaining period of his existence.

'On my entering his room he said that he was sorry to disturb me so soon; and that he had not sent for me before, thinking that it would go off. He added "I have had very severe pain in the chest since five o'clock at intervals, and it gets worse I think." This pain was seated at the upper part of the chest towards the left side and extended down the left arm. He had been rather sick. He then asked me what the pain was. "What is it?" He was now almost free from pain. His pulse I could scarcely feel. The tongue was clean. There was cold perspiration over his face. The feet and legs were cool. The breathing at this time not troubled. I gave him immediately some hot brandy and water, and having ordered a mustard plaster for his chest, till this was ready I applied hot flannels and had his legs and arms rubbed, and the feet wrapped up in flannels wrung out of hot water and mustard. The pulse became natural, the extremities more warm and he was free from pain. The mustard plaster was brought and put on. It was not large enough and I ordered another. The pain then returning I gave him more brandy and water, and it soon left him. And now he asked me again what the pain was. I told him I believed it was spasm of the heart. He exclaimed, "Ah." I asked him whether he had ever fainted in his life? "No, never." I then asked him, if any of his family had ever had any disease of the chest? "Yes, my father had; he died of it." He inquired if disease of the heart was suddenly fatal? I answered that it was. "Was it a common disease?" I said not very common. "Where do you find it most?" "In large towns I think." "Why?" "Perhaps from anxiety and eager competition among the higher, and intemperance among the lower classes." He was then quiet and free from pain and I proposed to leave him for a minute or two. He had no pain whatever in my absence. On my return the perspiration was still in drops upon his forehead. The pulse was again feeble and I gave him more brandy and water and had the flannels with mustard renewed. An attack of pain was coming on. He said, "I must stretch myself." I took one of his hands and held it until the pain was gone off. It was of short duration. I said, is it gone? He answered, "Yes entirely," adding that he "could scarcely bear it if it were as severe as it had been." He then asked me "what was the general cause of this kind of disease."—He then said, "is this likely to return?" I answered that I was afraid it was, but that, as the attacks had been less severe and less frequent, I hoped they would pass off. He next asked me if the disease was generally suddenly fatal. I said generally (for those who knew him were aware that it was impossible not to tell him the exact truth). I then asked him if he had any pain. He said, "none but from the blister; one can bear outward pain, but it is not so easy to bear inward pain." I was now dropping some laudanum into a wineglass, when he inquired what I was going to give him. I told him laudanum, Hoffman's anodyne and camphor. And, while I was preparing the mixture and before I had finished, I heard a rattling in the throat and a convulsive struggle. I called out, and turning to him I supported his head, which was thrown back, on my shoulder. His eyes were fixed and his teeth set, and he was insensible. His breathing was very laborious, his chest heaved and there was a severe struggle over the upper part of the body. His pulse was imperceptible, and after deep breathings at a few prolonged intervals all was over. He died in little more than half an hour after I first saw him.

'The examination of the body was made forty-eight hours after death, the weather being very hot. Its external appearance evinced rapid decomposition. It was discoloured and very livid in many parts. The skin was tightly distended with air, which was found in the cellular tissue throughout every part.

'When the right cavity of the chest was punctured a great quantity of air rushed out. The lungs on this side were healthy but their posterior part was gorged with blood and serum, and about eight ounces of bloody serum were found in the cavity of the pleura. On the left side were some old but not extensive adhesions of the pleura and about the same quantity of bloody serum was in this cavity as in the right. The lungs on the left side were healthy but more extensively gorged with blood and serum than on the right. Posteriorly they resembled soft spleen.

'The pericardium was healthy. It contained about an ounce of serum of a straw-colour. The heart was rather large. The external surface was healthy. It was very flaccid and flat in its appearance. It contained but little blood, and that was fluid. There were no coagula of any kind in it. All the valves were quite healthy, and so was the lining membrane throughout. The orifices of all the great vessels were quite natural. The muscular structure of the heart in every part was remarkably thin, soft and loose in its texture. The walls of the right ventricle were especially thin, in some parts not much thicker than the aorta, and very loose and flabby in their texture. Its cavity was large. The walls of the left ventricle too were much thinner and softer than natural. All the muscular fibres of the heart generally were pale and brown. The aorta was of a brown-red colour throughout its internal surface, probably from putrefaction. A few slight atheromatous deposits were observed in the descending thoracic aorta. The pulmonary artery was of the same brown-red colour with the aorta. There was but one coronary artery, and, considering the size of the heart, it appeared to be of small dimensions. It with some difficulty admitted a small director. It was slit open to the extent of nearly three inches. Its internal surface was red but healthy with the exception of a slight atheromatous deposit situated about an inch from the orifice of the artery. This however did not appear to diminish its cavity.

'The liver was pale and rather small; the gall bladder was distended with yellow bile; the spleen was very soft and bloody.

'The stomach and intestines were distended with air. The kidneys were soft and rather bloody, and their surface presented in some degree the mottled appearance known by the term "Bright's kidney."

'The head was not examined. From the absence of all symptoms of disease in the brain to the last moment of existence there was no reason to believe that any thing unhealthy existed in the head.

(Signed)   'S. BUCKNILL
          'S. B. BUCKNILL, M.D. } Rugby
          'J. HODGSON, Birmingham.'

From this case-history we learn first that an acute attack of ischaemic heart disease was observed in 1842, and then recorded in 1846, without clear acknowledgement of the diagnosis which appears to us obvious when seen in retrospect. Latham was fully aware that the case had 'extraordinary circumstances belonging to it,' but was reluctant to acknowledge 'an express form of disease'. In his perplexity as to the true interpretation he concludes with the following supposition: 'Probable cause was spasm of the heart, or a first attack of angina pectoris.' Secondly, the description is unusually lively. The many details and the clever conversation between patient and physician—whenever there was a short respite from the attacks—are attractive features and give the appearance of leisurely talks even in such gloomy circumstances. The minute account is unusual in comparison with similar reports and the reason thereof seems to be the attending physician's high esteem for his respected patient. The conversation throws light even on etiological factors of heredity, as when the patient reported that his father had suffered from 'disease of the chest.' The last item was emphasized by Osler (1897), who referred to three generations of the Arnold family who died from coronary occlusion. Thirdly, Latham in commenting on this case and two others finds them to be 'uncomplicated'. In fact many complicating circumstances do appear in Thomas Arnold's case—such as earlier changes in the heart, pulmonary oedema, Cheyne-Stokes respiration, etc. Fourthly, the short duration of the final illness and the frequent recurrence of attacks are to be noted, while the phrase 'could scarcely bear it if it were as severe as it had been' recalls Heberden's wording. Fifthly, the relatively young age of the patient, in his forty-seventh year, may explain the lesser degree of arteriosclerosis in the post-mortem, since it is stated that only a few slight atheromatous deposits were found. In contrast to many other reports the emphasis is laid not on the ossified coronaries, but on the softening of the heart and its dilatation. The remarkable anomaly that 'there was but one coronary artery' points to the impossibility of collateral compensation, which explains the fatal outcome even more clearly. The artery was rather narrow, and when it was slit open a deposit was found situated one inch from the orifice, but this, however, did not 'appear to diminish its cavity' nor did it cause a complete occlusion. Our consultant pathologist felt the atheromatous deposit in the lumen of the coronary artery a significant feature; while post-mortem fibrinolysis may have dissolved a possibly established thrombus. Sixthly, the importance attached to the necropsy report can be assessed by the signatures of the three gentlemen involved in the case and present at the examination of the body.

It seems that Latham's case report, unnoticed by the profession for more than half a century until Osler brought it to light again in 1897, continues to arouse the interest of scholars for its manifold features.[27]

2. It might be permissible to deviate from the sequence of chronological presentation by adding briefly the conclusions drawn by Pickering. He estimated that calcification is not necessarily connected with clinical symptoms and signs, as indeed Thomas Arnold's case clearly demonstrates. This statement had already been pronounced much earlier, e.g. by John Warren in 1812, as mentioned before. The nomenclature of the degenerative process in the arteries underwent some changes and variations: from the name atheroma by Haller, 1755, through Lobstein's arteriosclerosis in 1833, to the 'Endarteritis deformans sive nodosa' of Virchow in 1856, to be discussed later, followed by the term 'Nodular arteriosclerosis', coined by Councilman in 1891 and adopted by Osler. Finally, Marchand's 'atherosclerosis' in 1904, found widest acceptance, but failed to be adopted by all modern authors.

Before passing on to the broader conception of thrombosis by Virchow, attention may be drawn to F. Tiedemann, a physiologist in Heidelberg (1791–1861), whose name is mentioned only casually in surveys on our subject. Of his many works on anatomy and physiology of the arteries, one is of special interest to us, since it contains chapters exclusively devoted to coronary arteries. Besides, it includes very extensive information and a bibliography of historical references.

[27] E.g. Sir George Pickering in his lecture on thrombosis, 13th March 1963 in Jerusalem; Saul Jarcho (1965) discusses Latham's views on angina pectoris but does not mention the case of Arnold.

This work, *Von der Verengung und Schliessung der Pulsadern in Krank-heiten* (On narrowing and occlusion of arteries in diseases) was published in 1843.[28] While the most important historical data are concentrated in a chapter beginning on p. 33, Chapter 17 (pp. 293–309) deals with the 'Effects of narrowing or partial occlusion of the coronary arteries of the heart, and the ensuing symptoms.' Later developments, especially thrombus formation, have not been defined, but deposits of fibrin, plaque formations, and concretions in the coats were adequately described. The most valuable aspect of Tiedemann's publication is its usefulness as a guide to this history and bibliography of our subject up to the year 1843.

One of the most important methods in the study of disease is the correlation of clinical and pathological findings. Historically, coronary artery disease was treated in much the same way, and the earlier authors were very eager in their attempts to explain the clinical phenomena by assiduous anatomical investigations. In former times physicians themselves performed the opening of the bodies, and were often helped by surgeons or anatomists. The second half of the nineteenth century saw the emergence of pathology as an independent academic discipline. During this period pathologists took over the lead, and consequently the investigations became more detailed and scientifically based, though the clinical features were more casually presented. We referred to this fact earlier while discussing the great works preceding this period, such as those by Bonet and Morgagni. There were assiduous efforts to find close correlation between clinical and post-mortem findings, but full correspondence between bedside observations and the results derived from the post-mortems could not be achieved in many cases.

Still the deeper knowledge of our subject gained new ground with the development of pathological anatomy. Not only was this progress furthered by special publications regarding the coronary vessels and their diseases; even greater importance is to be attributed to new concepts and to the fuller study of vascular pathology, which subsequently shed further light on the coronary pathology.

Rokitansky (1804–78) and Virchow (1821–1902) were considered as the leading authorities of their day in pathology. Neither of them paid much attention to coronary disease, especially when we take into account the enormous bulk of their literary output and the great number of autopsies they performed. Indeed, when in 1901 a bibliography of Virchow was published it listed about 1,000 of his publications,

---

[28] Incidentally, this historically-important work has not been listed in the detailed entry on Tiedemann in Hirsch's *Biographisches Lexikon*, (2nd ed., vol. 5, pp. 586–87, 1934).

while Rokitansky's signature appeared against 30,000 autopsies. With this great amount of work done in pathology it is astonishing that we cannot point to any specially illuminative case-report on our subject. However, the work done by Virchow, especially on occlusion of arteries, thrombosis and infarcts in general, is really overwhelming. It led to a changed attitude and to a more precise definition of processes which under the somewhat diffuse denomination of 'obstruction' had already figured in Egyptian and Greek antiquity. Morphology and general biological ideas were intimately connected in the works of these masters of pathology, when Rokitansky, the morphologist, tried unsuccessfully to revive the ancient idea of dyscrasia. Rokitansky's share is much smaller than that of his Berlin colleague and critic who comes closer to our theme by introducing the concepts of thrombosis, infarct and embolism in general.

With regard to arteriosclerosis, Rokitansky, in his *Manual of Pathological Anatomy* (1841–46), is quite definite in dismissing inflammation as an etiological factor, a theory which Virchow tended to accept. Rokitansky says that 'the deposit is an endogenous product derived from the blood, and for the most part from fibrin.' He knew of the vascularization of the plaque from the lumen and described the system of fine canals in aortic plaques, resulting from partial resorption in the deposit, which he regarded as fibrinous in origin. He considered the degeneration of the connective tissue cells below the lining endothelium as unknown in origin, much as did Scarpa in 1804.

The dramatic events of a coronary occlusion did not seem to attract Rokitansky's interest, though he remarked that fatty degeneration of the heart is very frequently associated with ossification of the coronary arteries.[29] As late as the date of Rokitansky's death (1878) the diagnosis of coronary heart disease was not appreciated either by him or by his medical advisers, as is tragically evident from his own Autobiography, in which he refers to his last illness, an obvious case of this disease, explaining it as 'neuralgia'.[30] His attending physicians diagnosed the case as bronchiectasis with cardiac enlargement or aortic aneurysm with neuralgic manifestations (*Allg. Wien. med. Ztg.*, 1878, **23**, 306); no post-mortem was made.[31]

Virchow's extensive studies on thrombosis began early in his career,

[29] See English translation by George Day (1852), pp. 173–206.

[30] This stands in striking contrast to the clear perception and presentation of his own illness by 'Dr. Anonymous', quoted previously in the section on Heberden.

[31] See E. Lesky's scholarly edition of the Autobiography (1960), especially pp. 71–72, and note 97. We are indebted to Professor Lesky for a photocopy from the above journal (1878) and for the comment in her letter of 8th January 1969 on the diagnosis of Rokitansky's attending physicians.

with a paper on 'Occlusion of the pulmonary artery' in the year 1846. Some of his publications contain interesting historical references to his predecessors. At all times he had a tendency to modify his theories. In this connection we may bring to mind his most famous work, *Die Cellularpathologie* (1858) which was eventually formulated after many faulty attempts—after expressing, for example, the erroneous idea of cell generation from the 'blastema', the very reverse of his famous dictum 'omnis cellula e cellula'. He devised an appropriate nomenclature, mostly derived from Greek and Latin sources, making use of the terms 'thrombosis' and 'embolism'.

The Greek word 'thrombos' occurs in Galen (e.g. Kühn VII, 726); the old Latin translation of thrombos was 'grumus' (a little heap, hillock of earth). Galen uses the word mostly for a concretion of blood under the skin, in the sense of a subcutaneous haematoma. The latter usage is to be found already in Hippocrates (Littré VI, 127, par. 4).

A few introductory remarks on the historical material which preceded Virchow's definitive concept of the thrombotic process, place this advance in its proper setting. Galen was the first to mention 'a disease which is called thrombosis', referring to it as follows (Kühn XVIII B, 446):

> 'The tunic of the vessels is crushed or bruised, for bodies that are crushed lose the physical unity, being torn in many small places. The places which surround the vein take up this blood which has poured out, but in receiving it they do not leave it as they received it, for it becomes black in course of time. ... and the disease originates, which is called thrombosis. Therefore when the disease has originated in the blood, the blood is called a thrombus and is a thrombus.'

In another work, *De locis affectis* (IV, 11) Galen clearly mentions a vascular obstruction, though here he does not use the word 'thrombosis'. The case in question does not belong to coronary pathology, as the disease is concerned with the pulmonary arteries, and is generally interpreted as mitral stenosis.[32] What is of interest in our context is that Galen explained the disease by supposing 'an obstruction caused by viscous and dense humours, or by formation of a crude tubercle.' So a thrombo-embolic phenomenon, such as Virchow was able to demonstrate, is already alluded to in a Galenic text.

---

[32] This is one of Galen's rare case-histories and concerns his patient Antipater, himself a physician. We have found some twenty references to this case, starting with Maimonides, through Diversus (sixteenth century), and particularly in the seventeenth and eighteenth centuries.

The root 'thrombus' in the classical literature does not always mean an intravascular structure, but sometimes simply clotted blood. This can be seen in Caelius Aurelianus (Drabkin's edition, p. 573), when the urine discharge from the bladder is suppressed by particles of clotted blood.

We have already had occasion to refer to obstruction in the blood vessels, as described by earlier authors. Attention may now be drawn to the historical shift in nomenclature and the ultimate clarification through Virchow's work. Thanks to his contributions the term 'thrombus' describes a stoppage or clot in a vessel, while 'infarct' refers to the resulting change in the heart muscle. As to the Latin verb *infarcire* (to stuff into), authors of the seventeenth century used this to signify a structure which blocked up an artery or filled the heart chamber; this word was used, for instance, by Bonet (I, 845), in the title which he gave to the report of Vesalius' case, mentioned earlier.

That authors previous to the establishment of the thrombo-embolic doctrine had been conscious of thrombotic phenomena in the vessels is shown by two additional references. J. W. Wedel (1645–1721) brought cardiac arrhythmia into causal connection with a blood clot found in the lumen of a vessel (*intra vasa e coagulo sanguinis*), which is analogous to Diversus' (1586) speculations, as well as to Dr. Anonymous' (1772) forebodings,[33] and also to the more modern pathological demonstration by J. F. Payne (1870, to be discussed later) of a 'dark-red clot completely blocking the coronary artery'. Wedel's patient had suffered from 'fluttering action of the heart'. Again Wedel refers to Galen's account of the physician Antipater.

Another author to be referred to is P. A. Michelotti (1673–1740) who devoted a treatise exclusively to diseases of blood vessels, *Tractatus Universalis Morborum Sanguinis Ductuum* (1731).[34] This author spoke of solidification, densities, lesions of the inner surface of the vessels, and cruor (p. 418). He also refers (p. 424) to an earlier observation by the French physician Alexis Littré in 1703, where mention is made of a mass in the heart which entered a pulmonary artery. Littré's observation as quoted by Michelotti aroused our curiosity, since it could have been regarded as an anatomically-proven early description of pulmonary embolism. From a study of the original text (*Mémoires de l'Académie Royale des Sciences*, 1703, pp. 90–94) it appears that the observation by Littré referred to an abdominal malignancy with cardiac metastasis. The post-mortem showed a 'polyp' in the heart, more precisely in the right heart, whence it extended to the lungs

---

[33] 'I attributed it to an obstruction in the circulation' (Heberden, 1785).
[34] We have used the second edition of 1748.

10

through the pulmonary artery, following its ramifications. Thus the description shows the spread as common in pulmonary embolism from the right heart. Indeed such cases, though of different etiology, are listed in modern text-books of cardiology, as, for instance, in Paul Wood's *Diseases of the Heart and Circulation* (3rd edition, 1968, p. 943) in chapter 17 on pulmonary embolism, where one of the causes is: 'Infiltrative—as in cancer'. So we have been able to explain Michelotti's inclusion of Littré's observation in his comprehensive volume on the diseases of the blood-vessels; an unexpected but not inappropriate prelude to Virchow's important studies on embolism.

The other term which Virchow used and skilfully adapted to modern pathology is 'embolus', of Greek origin and with the same meaning in Latin. The Latin version was used in mechanics for the piston of a pump, while 'embolium' meant 'something thrown in'. This is equivalent to the pathological meaning of sudden obstruction of a vessel through an abnormal particle circulating in the blood.

With these two words coined from classical languages, Virchow embarked on extensive pathological research, beginning, as mentioned previously, in 1846. Part of this research has been conveniently arranged and republished in two small volumes in 'Sudhoff's Klassiker der Medizin' under the title, *On Thrombosis and Embolism*. More about this subject is found in Virchow's *Gesammelte Abhandlungen zur wissenschaftlichen Medizin* (1856), a substantial part of this volume (pp. 219–732) consisting of papers grouped under the heading 'Thrombosis and embolism'. Thrombosis, according to Virchow, is based on three requirements: increased coagulability of the blood, sluggishness in the blood circulation, and a lesion in the coats of the vessels. This conception of thrombosis is closely related to Virchow's views on the arteriosclerotic processes. He considered atheroma as a chronic inflammatory disease of the intima, while in his opinion the cholesterol formation was a late manifestation of atheroma. In 1856 he observed a gelatinous swelling of the intima, preceding atherosclerosis. On the basis of his theoretical conceptions Virchow was able to describe thrombosis and embolism in the lungs, liver and spleen, but no particular or more detailed investigations bearing on our subject are to be found. At one stage in his long career Virchow was interested in thrombosis of pyaemic origin, especially when it inclined towards embolization.[35] However, he was not very interested in coronary thrombosis, which hardly occupies any place in his numerous writings. His great importance to our theme is based on his elaboration of the general concept of

[35] As for instance in his *Cellularpathologie* (1858), pp. 176 ff.

thrombosis. From here his pupils were able to continue their special studies on coronary pathology, which ultimately led to the establishment of a clear-cut diagnosis. This is also the reason for having given him a prominent place in our text, which aims to trace the development of thought on our subject rather than to provide an encyclopaedic presentation. We have therefore considered the work of Virchow and his predecessors more fully than is usual in surveys of this topic.

The most significant contribution by a pathologist to our subject must be credited to Carl Weigert (1845–1904), a pupil of Cohnheim until the latter's death, and from 1885 onwards director of pathology at the Senckenberg Foundation in Frankfurt-on-Main. Apart from his famous work on staining microscopical preparations, he wrote a paper 'On pathological processes of coagulation' (Über die pathologischen Gerinnungs-Vorgänge) in 1880, in which the following statement appears:

> 'With atheromatous changes of the coronary arteries thrombotic or embolic occlusions of their branches not infrequently occur. If the closures occur slowly, or more important still, in such a way that the collateral channels, even though insufficient for nourishment, exist, there follows a slower atrophy with disappearance of the muscle fibres, but without injury to the connective tissue. These destroyed muscle fibres are then replaced by fibrous tissue and the so-called chronic myocarditis is nothing else but such a process.
>
> 'If, however, a very sudden complete cutting off of the blood occurs in certain parts of the heart, yellow dry masses entirely similar to coagulated fibrin result. Here also, however, microscopic examination reveals almost no fibrous exudate . . . but all muscle fibres and all connective tissue are devoid of nuclei.'

This quotation not only provides a general description of myocardial changes following a coronary thrombosis, but also includes a very important detail, namely that of the destruction of cell nuclei. Likewise it stresses also the clinical history, since pathological findings largely depend upon the time-factor: sudden closure produces a very different effect from that following a slower process. These ideas were used four years later by the clinician E. Leyden in his most informative paper on coronary thrombosis, which will be discussed later. The introduction of the time-factor into the picture would moreover explain those cases not mentioned by Weigert, in which pathological findings are absent, death having intervened almost instantaneously.

We should like to recall here the contribution by Cruveilhier, and his excellent illustration of an haemorrhagic infarct, at a period when it was not regarded as a sequence of coronary occlusion.

Weigert's remark that the patchy degenerations in the heart muscle are 'nothing else but such a process', namely a result of coronary disease, is a criticism of the clinical diagnosis of the so-called chronic myocarditis. This faulty diagnosis persisted until the early twentieth century. Incidentally, Weigert himself fell victim to coronary disease at the age of fifty-nine.

The attention of the profession to the possibility of a coronary death was often aroused by its occurrence in famous patients during the nineteenth century. This was the case, for instance, with the noted Danish sculptor B. Thorvaldsen (1770–1844) and may be regarded as a relatively early example. The sudden death took place in the theatre. The post-mortem, performed by the doctors Dahlerup and Fenger, runs:

> 'Myocardium slightly brittle, coronaries calcified, the interior showing several atheromatous plaques, one of them ulcerated and pouring the atheromatous mass into the lumen of the artery and occluding it.'

This case has been referred to by Osler in his *Lectures on Angina Pectoris* (p. 33). The often-quoted case of F. J. Talma, the French tragedian, in 1826, is less clear. The post-mortem revealed an aneurysm of the heart apex, but it seems more likely that he actually died from an intestinal obstruction, probably due to malignancy.[36]

We have already remarked that the opening of bodies for the purpose of explaining a coronary death did not in all cases unequivocally demonstrate the ultimate cause, though, on the whole, pathological anatomy did much to clarify the understanding of the underlying process. When death occurred very suddenly there was no time for the formation of visible morbid changes. Deaths resulting from an acute cardiogenic shock or from a fatal arrhythmia escaped the searching eye of the pathologist.

Experimental Approach

Some investigators turned to the experimental approach, as mentioned previously with regard to Chirac and Erichsen. In 1862 the Danish physiologist P. L. Panum (1820–85) continued this trend; however, instead of ligating a coronary artery he tried to produce an experi-

---

[36] A. Cabanès, 1920; *Chronique Médicale*, 1904, **II**, 665; H. Vierordt, 3rd ed., 1910.

mental embolism by injecting a mixture of fat, wax, oil, and soot into the coronary arteries or into the aorta of dogs. The conventional ligature of the coronaries was resumed in 1867 by the German physiologist A. v. Bezold (1826–68). He also found that the slowing-down of contractions occurred first in the left ventricle, later in the right and lastly in the auricles. He analysed too the irregularities noted during the experiment. When the ligature was loosened the heart action could be restored to normal in certain cases.

In 1881 J. Cohnheim, together with Schulthess-Rechberg, published their well-known paper on the results of an experimental coronary artery occlusion on the heart. The ligature of one of the branches of a coronary artery resulted in a progressive arrhythmia. After one hundred and five seconds the blood pressure fell suddenly, while the auricles continued to function, though at a slower rate.[37] Incidentally, similar phenomena under different experimental conditions had already been reported by Harvey at the beginning of Chapter 4 of his *De Motu Cordis*, entitled 'The Motion of the Heart and its Auricles as noted in Animal Experimentation':

> 'As indeed Galen noted, when all the rest is quiet and dead, the right auricle still pulsates'; or 'at length nearly dead, it [the heart] fails to respond to the motion, and it stirs so obscurely that the only signs of motion are pulsations of the auricle, as if just slightly nodding the head'.

Harvey's perspicacity led him to ponder on the problem of the origin and conduction of the heart beat:

> 'While the heart gradually dies, it sometimes responds with a weak and feeble beat to two or three pulsations of the auricles.'

Chauncey D. Leake was even inclined to the view that heart block is being considered here. This interesting opinion refers to an experimental procedure rather than to a clinical description of heart-block.[38]

We have already referred to Cohnheim's experiments of 1881 leading to his theory that the coronary is an 'end-artery'. In this paper the author does not adhere to the view that the heart stops through inhibition by the vagus nerve or by lack of oxygenated blood.

[37] Since the classical experiments of Cohnheim, the question of the experimental reproduction of coronary artery narrowing has not ceased to arouse the interest of researchers. In a recent paper by T. I. Malinin *et al* (1968) experimental gradual narrowing was produced in swine to simulate the slowly progressing narrowing of human disease. The authors, feeling that the pathogenesis of myocardial infarction is still ill-defined, tried to overcome the difficulties by using histochemical techniques.

[38] See Leake's translation (1928) of the *De Motu Cordis* and his note on page 40.

He is inclined to think that interruption of the blood flow causes an accumulation of toxic matters in the heart, thus impeding its action. It may be recalled that as late as 1878 Cohnheim supposed that metabolites are the ultimate cause of interruption of the heart action.[39]

In spite of the fact that Cohnheim's concept of the coronaries as 'end-arteries' did not carry weight, the paper discussed above was of great import. It established more firmly the decisive role of these vessels in supplying blood to the heart, a notion rooted deeply in the whole history of cardiology. The theory of 'end-arteries' was overthrown in face of deeper knowledge of the collateral circulation.[40] It remained, however, valid under the name of 'functional end-arteries'. Indeed, when the disease was of very short duration there was no time for collateral channels to develop and consequently, occlusion of the coronary artery immediately proved fatal.

Another item of historical value was touched upon in Cohnheim's experiments, namely the changes in rhythm, with or without bradycardia. Many of the previously-quoted records of coronary events and later those of experimental procedures, among them that by Harvey mentioned above, point to rhythm anomalies. We may recall in this connection our previous references[41] to Vesalius (*Fabrica*, 1555), and to Saxonia (*De pulsibus*, 1604), both of whom described heart block. Changes in the heart rhythm are not necessarily connected with coronary artery disease, but their occurrence is quite frequent.

To return to clinical descriptions, which in the second part of the nineteenth century were mostly accompanied by pathological findings, there is a marked shift towards the use of the terms thrombosis and infarction to denote the underlying pathological condition. First to be mentioned is A. E. F. Vulpian (1826–87) of Paris who in 1866 published a case report of rupture of the heart. As a pathological finding this subject had already been known for more than two hundred years. However, the title contains already a clear diagnosis of myocardial infarction and the sequence of events leading up to it:

> 'Infarct of the wall of the left ventricle of the heart coinciding with an old blood clot in one of the coronary arteries. Rupture of this infarct into the cavities of the ventricle and of the pericardium.'

[39] Cohnheim's independence from the conventional approach in his speciality led him to assume failure of function in those cases in which no anatomical anomaly could be found. This is exemplified by the following unorthodox remark, '. . . anatomical examination of arteries *post mortem* is so far from being a fair criterion of the extent to which they were *intra vitam* permeable' (*Lectures on General Pathology*, 2nd ed., 1882; English translation (1889) p. 38.)

[40] See our more detailed discussion of anastomoses below (p. 152).

[41] For Vesalius, p. 52; Saxonia, p. 61;

Vulpian[42] was physician to the Salpêtrière, where many arteriosclerotic patients of the capital were concentrated and from which much research into brain and cardiovascular pathology was to emerge. Vulpian's report of the cardiovascular changes can be summarized as follows. The tear in the ventricular wall is described as

> '. . . a flattened cavity hollowed out in the wall of the heart. In this area the tissue was softened and was brownish-red in colour [haemorrhagic infarct]. In the left coronary artery a decolorised and evidently older blood clot of granular appearance, and very pronounced atheroma were found while the artery was completely occluded for the length of half a centimetre only.'

Thus a blood clot in the coronary artery as well as an infarct of the heart wall have been described. The chief characteristic of the new approach is the author's free evaluation of this case with the aid of the terms thrombosis, embolism and infarction, instead of the time-honoured nomenclature of softening and bony channels.

Another feature which indicates a more comprehensive type of report is Vulpian's addition of the microscopic examination after death. Taken from the necrotic part of the myocardium, the tissue showed broken muscular fibres, fatty granulation and some granular bodies. The histology is certainly much less detailed than the gross anatomy, which Vulpian discusses at some length. However, the establishment of microscopy as a prerequisite in a pathological report heralds the new phase in the development and investigation of the knowledge of coronary artery disease. The microscopic findings do not surpass those of Düben in 1859, since they ignore the destruction of cell nuclei, as demonstrated later by Weigert in 1880. Vulpian's report did not take the form of a well rounded-off paper provided with general discussion and conclusions; it had been intended as a case-demonstration for a meeting of the Anatomical Society of Paris. Otherwise Vulpian would quite possibly have contributed more to the understanding of coronary artery disease; but the above observations and deliberations alone grant him a prominent place in the time prior to the final confirmation of this diagnosis.

C. B. Radcliffe (1822–89), in the same year as Vulpian, described an unusual form of softening. His report, 'A case of acute uncomplicated myocarditis, in which the disease was diagnosed during life', appeared in 1866.[43]

[42] For biographical data see A. Ebner (1967).
[43] *Lancet*, 1866, **I**, 124.

A middle-aged man suffered for six weeks from occasional attacks of sharp pain at the pit of the stomach and left arm, 'evidently angina pectoris'. His illness was acute for two days; the first day, the pulse was extremely feeble, and the patient was cold; on the second, sitting awkwardly on the edge of a chair, he declared: 'I must keep as I am—I dare not stir.' For twelve hours his face was pale, large beads of sweat stood out on the forehead, the extremities were clammy and cold, and his pulse at the wrist failed altogether. His mind was clear, and he knew that he was dying. While up to pass urine in the middle of the night, after several hours' quiet sleep, the pain at the pit of the stomach returned in an unusually severe form, with cold perspiration and a feeling of deadly faintness. The pain continued for four hours until death intervened. Post-mortem: muscular structure of both ventricles soft and friable, the colour of mulberry-juice, and broke down readily under the finger; when the heart was lifted by a portion of the right auricle, the muscular substance broke down, and tore like wet paper under the weight of the heart itself. Radcliffe's conclusion is: sudden failure in the action of the heart.

This case offers a vivid description of the clinical features and displays an uncommon degree of softening in the post-mortem examination. Our pathological consultant, however, questioned the validity of the anatomical report, and found the softening of 'both ventricles' a decomposition which took place after death. The word 'uncomplicated' may be explained by the absence of coronary pathology. Infarction is not an acceptable anatomical diagnosis since no circumscribed lesion was found, both ventricles being soft and friable. Cases of softening reported in historical literature may sometimes be interpreted as infarctions, and were often incorrectly termed myocarditis, especially towards the end of the nineteenth century. In Radcliffe's case the true nature cannot be explained by the post-mortem report since no microscopic examination was performed, but the clinical picture is that of an acute coronary event.

Here we may appropriately refer to another small contribution to our subject. Although the learned author did not use the term coronary thrombosis, the report gives undoubted evidence of it. J. F. Payne (1840–1910), physician, pathologist and medical historian, published a brief paper[44] concerning the sudden death of a man of sixty-seven after

'. . . occasional attacks of dyspnoea and fluttering action of the heart, [post-mortem:] . . . coronary arteries thickened, calci-

---

[44] *Brit. med. J.*, 1870, **i**, 130.

fied and narrowed, especially the left main branch hardly to admit a fine probe; the right contained a dark-red clot, and was completely blocked.'

Payne concludes that nutrition of the heart had stopped immediately, and fatal syncope was the result. The case is quite an early specimen of acute coronary thrombosis, together with probable acute arrhythmia, described at a time when auricular fibrillation, flutter, and other arrhythmias had hardly been investigated, and well before the advent of electrocardiographic studies.

On the whole the diagnosis of thrombosis and occlusion remained a matter of pathology, since physicians were still not able to diagnose it in a living patient. Probably the first author to make such a diagnosis was Adam Hammer (1818–78), a German physician who left his country in 1848 after participating in the revolution, and settled in the United States, in St. Louis. His report of 1878 on 'A case of thrombotic occlusion of one of the coronary arteries of the heart'[45] was published in English translation in the same year in the *Canadian Journal of Medical Sciences* in Toronto[46]—an indication of its importance— and later included by R. H. Major in his *Classic Descriptions of Disease*, omitting the prefatory passages and beginning with the case-report itself.

Hammer attributed considerable importance to the fact that the diagnosis was made during the patient's life, and added in brackets after the title the words 'Am Krankenbett konstatiert' (established at the bedside). In the prefatory passages the author lists a large number of arterial diseases 'already known in pathology and often enough proved, including thrombosis and infarctions.' Feeling uncertain about the diagnosis, he investigated the whole literature in order to be sure that no such diagnosis had ever been made during a patient's life. Passing through New York in the spring of 1877 he interviewed several physicians, but 'even Dr. Jacobi, who was held to be a kind of living medical dictionary, was not able to give me any information'. When Hammer arrived on the Continent he discussed the matter with eminent physicians, among them Kussmaul in Strasbourg, and Bamberger in Vienna. All of them declared that they had met no such case, nor read about it. 'This being so, and the gentlemen urging me not to withdraw the case from the public, I was led to make the following report'.[47]

[45] 'Ein Fall von thrombotischem Verschlusse einer der Kranzarterien des Herzens', *Wiener med. Wschr.*, 1878, **28**, 97–102.

[46] 1878, **3**, 353–7; here the words 'diagnosed during life' are added to the title.

[47] The report is condensed, but Hammer's terminology is retained.

On 4th May, 1876, at 9 a.m. Hammer was taken by a young colleague to see a patient whose case he could not understand. The patient was thirty-four years old and had suffered for a year from frequent attacks of articular rheumatism. Improvement set in gradually, and he had recently completed a convalescence. His pulse-rate was 80 to the minute. The morning before, he had insisted on getting out of bed. At 1 o'clock the patient suddenly collapsed in his chair. The attending physician came and found the pulse weak, only 40 beats to the minute, slight dyspnoea but absolutely no pain. At 6 p.m. the pulse was slower, only 23 beats to the minute; at 10 p.m. the pulse was 16. By the time Hammer arrived the pulse was 8 beats to the minute; face and skin of the entire body pale, cool and covered with sticky sweat. 'The patient had no idea of the seriousness of his malady.' No murmur could be heard, on examining the heart, but after each beat 'a clonic spasm of the heart' was noticed, 'which lasted exactly five seconds, and then ceased as if cut off.'

In view of the sudden appearance and the steadily progressive course, Hammer thought 'that the supply of blood to the heart muscle had been cut off. Such an obstruction could be produced only by a thrombotic occlusion of a coronary artery.' The patient lived 19 hours longer and died early on 5th May. Permission was given by the relatives to remove only the heart but not to disturb any other organ. The post-mortem was carried out 29 hours after death. It stated

> 'that the right auricle and ventricle were filled with thick coagulated black blood, containing massive clots of fibrin and globular vegetations. The right aortic valve was stretched by a mass which not only filled the right sinus of Valsalva but also bulged out like a half-sphere. On removing this mass it was found that the upper layers from above, down to the origin of the coronary arteries inside the sinus were composed of fresh, coagulated, jelly-like, whitish-yellow material mixed with blood. On the right and left valves there were fresh, white, soft, endocarditic excrescences.'

Hammer gives the following comment:

> 'So long as the thrombus did not reach the level of the exit of the coronary artery, the patient felt relatively well, but with the beginning occlusion of the lumen of the artery collapse appeared. The constant diminution of the pulse-rate was directly caused by the constant growth of the thrombus until complete closure appeared.'

The author concludes with the remark:

> 'This case will interest particularly the clear-sighted and clever
> Cohnheim, as he wrote in his *Lectures on General Pathology*,
> which appeared in print at the end of the year 1877 on p. 24:
> "In fact Bezold, by closing the coronary arteries with a clamp,
> and Panum, by producing an embolus in the same with a thin
> wax emulsion, were able to stop the heart; but whether a similar
> event in human pathology will ever be observed, is to me
> improbable enough." He did not know, and indeed also
> could not know, that this occurrence had indeed been observed
> 18 months before.'

This report seems to be the first diagnosis of a coronary occlusion
made during the life of the patient, and has been constantly referred to
in subsequent historical writings and in surveys of cardiological history.
However, the type of occlusion it represents is quite different from the
usual picture of an arteriosclerotic coronary thrombosis. In his survey
of 1962 on the history of myocardial infarction William Dock remarks: 'This report should be perhaps in the section on infections,
endocarditis, or on complete heart block.' Certain features indeed do
not belong to our subject, such as a recent history of rheumatic fever,
the pathological finding of vegetations on two cusps of the aortic
valve, and the unusual complete absence of pain in the clinical
history. Despite the peculiarities of this case, Hammer's contribution
takes its place in the history of thrombotic occlusion of the coronary
vessels.[48]

One of the most instructive papers ever written by a clinician deeply
versed in pathology, was that of E. von Leyden (1832–1910), a pupil of
Traube and Frerichs in Berlin. His comprehensive paper, 'On the
sclerosis of the coronary arteries, and the morbid states arising from
them', was published in 1884. With it appeared two pathological
tables depicting on one the degenerated heart wall, a spherical bulging
of the apex and aneurysm of the heart; and on the other an almost
complete occlusion of a coronary artery. The paper reveals meti-
culous attention to clinical detail, and a deep insight into the different

[48] 'Coronary arteries may rarely be blocked by emboli or by aortic valve vegetations
in bacterial endocarditis' (Paul D. White, *Heart Disease* (4th ed., 1951) p. 526). The third
edition of P. Wood's textbook (1968) mentions that 'the clinical features of coronary
embolism are indistinguishable from those of coronary thrombosis' (p. 22). In the light
of this information, attention is drawn to a letter to the Editor (*J. Amer. med. Ass.*, 1954)
by S. Bober: According to the writer, the first case of coronary embolism in which the
diagnosis was made before death and confirmed by autopsy was described by Korczinski, professor in the University of Cracow, in 1867.

types that a coronary artery disease may include. It also presents a historical view of the problem, while the clinical and pathological features are well balanced. In his critical review of the literature, Leyden regrets that authors were neglecting the evaluation of physiological disturbances and paying too much attention instead to the physical signs and symptoms, much to the detriment of the knowledge of coronary artery disease. He recalls that Stokes warned the profession not to overrate the physical signs, which do not always reveal the underlying pathological conditions. As to the phenomenon of coronary occlusion, Leyden found Tiedemann's book[49] of 1843, 'exhaustive, critical and clear, so much so that the standpoint of the textbooks of today would appear backward by comparison.' On p. 293 of Tiedemann's work the sequelae of occlusion had already been mentioned: thinness of the heart wall and atrophy, while the muscle fibres become brittle and soft and show fatty degeneration. Leyden recalls that gangrene of the heart was mentioned by Potain, as quoted by his pupil Pelvet in a Paris thesis of 1867. As a corroboration of his views, Leyden presents a case of his own in which a 'necrotic infarct had led to softening and rupture.' Leyden considered the first microscopic examination to be that made in 1850 and 1851 by Quain, who had also proved that the necrotic foci corresponded to the area supplied by the diseased artery. However, Leyden found that the term 'fatty heart' was not explicit or accurate. He gave credit to Ziegler, who compared the foci with brain softening, and named them 'myomalacia cordis'.[50] We may recall our earlier statement that a similar term had been used by previous authors, for instance by Lobstein.

Leyden divided coronary sclerosis into four groups according to the pathological anatomical findings:

1. Sclerosis or ossification without concomitant changes in the heart muscle, in which the coronaries are already diseased but the sclerosis is regarded as an accessory finding.

He explains that in a case of sudden death an occlusion can take place without degeneration of the heart muscle.

2. Acute thrombotic softening or haemorrhagic infarct of the myocardium, following a sclerotic thrombosis of a coronary artery, usually the left one. This corresponds to Ziegler's myo-

---

[49] See above, p. 124.
[50] See *Virchow's Archiv*, 1882, **90**, 211; and the many editions of his textbook, English translation by D. Macalister, 1885–97 (several editions). For data on Ernst Ziegler's life and work see C. Hodel and H. Buess (1966).

malacia cordis as well as to Cruveilhier's heart apoplexy. Micro-scopy reveals the breakdown of the muscle fibres and fatty de-generation with softening or rupture.

3. The chronic variety, in which fibrous degeneration of the heart muscle represents the sequel of an acute event. The later develop-ment often leads to dilatation and hypertrophy, or to the so-called disseminated myocarditis, or aneurysm, the decisive feature being loss of muscle substance. Acute cases can be compared with encephalomalacy, and chronic ones with arteriosclerotic con-tracted kidney.

4. The combined type: fibrous degeneration, plus a recent and acute softening leading to death within days or weeks. Here the sclerotic changes are characterized by their recurring appearance.

In the clinical analysis of his own cases, which included post-mortem evidence, Leyden distinguished three groups:

(a) *Acute cases with sudden death*: as described already by Forbes, Tiedemann and others. The most serious cases do not always feature angina pectoris, but are often marked by collapse, heart insufficiency or acute pulmonary oedema.

(b) *Subacute cases*: including various transitional stages from an acute to a protracted course of disease. As an example Leyden de-scribed a case of angina pectoris which was, however, accompanied by moderate oedema and dyspnoea. The post-mortem revealed an atheromatous ulcer in the descending branch of the left coronary artery, leading to a complete thrombotic occlusion. The anterior part of the left ventricle resembled an infarct, i.e. softening with fatty degeneration of the muscle, but not a complete necrosis, from which fact he deduced that collateral vessels had already been supplied. Recurrent thrombosis therefore belongs to this second category. The cases are quite numerous but difficult to ascertain during life.

(c) *Chronic cases*: this group had not previously been conceived as coronary artery disease, but had been described as chronic fibrous myocarditis, dilatation of the heart, or aneurysm. From his own ex-perience Leyden brought the example of a patient suffering from cardiac asthma and dropsy, in which the clinical diagnosis was dissemi-nated fibrous myocarditis and heart insufficiency, but the anatomical finding was coronary sclerosis, with patchy foci in the heart muscle. The disease was of ten years' duration, and accompanied by faintings attacks.

Another case with a twelve-year history showed the rare manifestation of a very slow pulse of 30. The last example to be extracted
from Leyden's paper is concerned with cardiac asthma, dropsy and
nephritis, with a dilated left ventricle. In this case the anatomical
findings were heart aneurysm, excessive fibrous degeneration, and left
coronary arteries totally occluded.

The author draws attention moreover to the different stages that
may be displayed in the course of the disease. In the first stages, attacks of
angina pectoris may last for a longer period of time, the heart circulation
remaining unimpaired, while later on heart insufficiency becomes the
most prominent feature. It may be recalled that this conception of
subsequent stages in the medical history of the patient had already been
outlined in the last years of the eighteenth century, by Black and
by Parry.[51]

Leyden's comprehensive paper of seventy pages is an example of the
great progress in the knowledge of coronary sclerosis which had been
attained by the leading clinicians. Thus, by 1884 almost all the pertinent
clinical and anatomical material had been assembled, but the ultimate
diagnosis of ischaemic heart disease had yet to await the beginning of the
twentieth century, and at least a further twenty years to become an
established, easily-diagnosed clinical entity.

In the last decades of the nineteenth century a few more important
clinical contributions were made to our subject. Among them we
would like to stress secondary pericarditis, which sometimes accom-
panies a coronary event. The earlier authors, however, did not appreciate sufficiently the connection between pericarditis and coronary
occlusion, but their observations are valid and interesting.[52] Thus
Christian Bäumler gave in 1872 the following account:

> 'Pericarditis may occur in a very restricted area of the peri-
> cardial surface; such a partial pericarditis usually clears up in a
> few days. The main symptoms in such cases are: precordial
> pain, difficulty in breathing and pains radiating to the throat,
> the back and the left arm. The heart action is accelerated and is
> influenced by muscular activity much more than in a healthy
> person. The body temperature is increased only slightly, and a
> pericardial friction can be distinctly heard; but no signs of an
> exudate are manifest.'

Thus an association of pericarditis with anginal symptoms due to
coronary thrombosis had been described as early as this. In this con-

[51] For Black (1786) see above, p. 96; and for Parry (1799) see p. 99.
[52] See also G. Blumer (1936).

nection we wish to mention two other observations of the same kind made by Bramwell (1884, p. 310) and Pavinsky (1897).

We turn to the paper by Vladimir Kernig (1840–1917), generally known for "Kernig's sign" in meningitis. The paper was entitled: 'Treatment of angina pectoris', and published in German in the *St. Petersburg Medical Weekly* in 1892, and then abstracted in the *Lancet* (1892, **2**, 438–39). It is remarkable not only for a fine description of the pericardial friction, but also for its additional explicit clinical and anatomical observations:

> 'The severe and prolonged paroxysms of angina pectoris may be explained by the presence of a thrombus or embolus in the coronary arteries. Two cases conformed to this etiology in the post-mortem examination. Sudden death had followed a severe paroxysm, and well-defined softening of the cardiac muscle with incipient demarcation of the focus of disease was present. In some cases, within a few days after the paroxysm, pericarditic symptoms were observed, from which might be understood that the centre of softening had reached the pericardium.'

Incidentally, the case was quoted by Osler in his volume of 1897 (p. 55). An earlier but less explicit observation was published by Donald Hood, in the *Lancet* (1884, **I**, p. 205).

Several historians of cardiology have been astonished at the slow acceptance of the diagnosis of coronary heart disease, even after the concept of thrombosis had been established and many clinical contributions were pouring forth from different centres, often taking the form of medical theses. The latter attracted, however, very few readers. The electrocardiograph was introduced only in 1903, but this is not the only reason for the belated emergence of a clear-cut diagnosis. This method of examination was not even applied in the classic papers of Obrastzow-Strachesko (1910) and Herrick (1912). There are indeed a considerable number of medical theses which came very close to an ultimate diagnosis. Those published in France were listed in an extensive bibliography appended to the comprehensive textbook on cardiology by Huchard (1899). Medical research at the end of the nineteenth century was absorbed by the great discoveries in other spheres such as surgery, bacteriology and roentgenology, while the medical profession was yet reluctant to accept a diagnosis known chiefly through dissections. As mentioned before, the belated appearance has puzzled most historians, including J. B. Herrick in his *Short History of Cardiology* (1942).

However, a description published almost at the close of the nineteenth century deserves special mention. This was by George Dock of the University of Michigan (1860–1951), and appeared under the modest title: 'Notes on the coronary arteries', in 1896. It is prefaced by a historical introduction[53] which, incidentally, also attempts to explain the neglect of our subject by the medical profession. After enumerating some reasons, Dock concludes that 'it is not surprising that later writers allowed the subject to escape them.' Most illuminating is Case 4 of this paper, in which the diagnosis was made during the patient's lifetime, when Dock was called in as consultant by the attending physician. To quote Dock himself:

> 'The diagnosis was myomalacia following coronary sclerosis, with secondary pericarditis. This was based on the history of increasing dyspnoea and heart pain, without evidence of disease in lungs or kidneys, or other (valvular) disease of the heart, the history of the acute attack indicating infarction, and the acute onset of pericarditis without other cause.'

This concise diagnosis, logically derived, formulated in scientific terms, and made at the bedside, is one of the first clear-cut and definitive modern contributions to our subject.

The case concerned a man of sixty-four, who had never been sick until about three months before death. The first symptoms consisted of shortness of breath, and only a week before death he experienced severe pain in the heart region. Soon after this, on rising suddenly, the patient fainted, and became pulseless and very dyspnoeic. Dock saw him a week later. During the first examination he noticed a loud friction rub over the apex. (This was of course pericarditis, which accompanied the coronary event, an occurrence not always associated with, but often forming an important part of the syndrome. It was to be described at greater length by Kernig in 1905, and even more elaborately by Sternberg in 1910, who coined the term 'Pericarditis epistenocardica'[54]). Signs of cardiac insufficiency were present and

[53] Very much later, in 1939, Dock's paper, 'Historical notes on coronary occlusion from Heberden to Osler', offered a balanced survey with many references. Dock was a keen book collector and presented 1500 volumes to the library of the Los Angeles County Medical Association.

[54] Reference has been made to earlier descriptions of pericarditis accompanying coronary sclerosis by Sénac (see above, p. 113), Charles Williams (p. 76), and Bäumler (p. 140). As recently as 1959, William Dressler of New York was able to describe (following a preliminary report in 1955) a new kind of secondary pericarditis, occurring several weeks after the infarction rather than accompanying it. The 'post-myocardial infarction syndrome', which includes pericarditis, is probably an immuno-biological reaction to the necrosis. Accordingly, adrenal steroids act almost in a specific way in the treatment of the condition. Historically, Dressler's observation shows that still more recent knowledge can be added to our already established clinical entity. See also Paul Wood, *Diseases of the Heart and Circulation* (1968), p. 858.

dullness on percussion of the lungs (hydro-thorax) was found. After exertion on leaving bed, the patient expired suddenly.

The post-mortem revealed: fluid in each pleural cavity, congestion and oedema of the lungs. The heart was enlarged. The pericardium was adherent over the apex by a thin, greenish fibrinous exudate. Red thrombus was noted in the descending coronary branch. From the level of the thrombus, the muscle was dry, yellow and red. The wall of the left ventricle was the seat of a recent infarction. The non-infarcted parts of the heart showed brown atrophy, fibroid degeneration and fatty change.

Dock's comment stresses:

> 'the relation of the coronary sclerosis to the gradually developing dyspnoea and of the infarction to the acute attack a week before death. The case illustrates also the fact that a heart extensively necrosed may continue to act fairly well for some time if exposed to no sudden strain . . . It is also a fine example of atheroma limited almost entirely to the coronary vessels.'

The last remark is of historical value and explains cases where the coronaries showed a predisposition to sclerosis, while the other vessels remained almost intact. This fact recalls our earlier discussion of Thomas Arnold's case.

Towards the end of the nineteenth century (1894) a series of papers on angina pectoris by Sir Clifford T. Allbutt (1836–1925) began to make their appearance. He pursued this topic almost till the end of his life. On the last occasion he attended a meeting at the College of Physicians on May 5th, 1924, he expressed his satisfaction that his aortic hypothesis concerning angina pectoris had received that very day confirmation from K. F. Wenckebach, the guest speaker at the College. In June 1894 Allbutt brought forward for the first time his conception that anginal pain is due to disease of the first part of the aorta, and not of the coronary arteries or myocardium.

The numerous papers on angina pectoris have been collected and republished, after revision, as Section II in Allbutt's book *Diseases of the Arteries including Angina Pectoris*, London, 1915 (Vol. II, pp. 211–540). They are a mine of information and would require a special study. The Wellcome Library possesses a copy which belonged to Sir James MacKenzie, who added very many pencil notes to this section, the volumes being inscribed: 'Sir James MacKenzie, 5.12.19.' Allbutt's thesis that anginal pain originates from a disease at the root of the aorta, just above the semilunar cusps, topographically recalls Morgagni's case, Epistle 26, paragraph 31: '. . . from the very origin behind the semilunar valves' (Alexander's translation, p. 820, line 2).

In view of his aortic hypothesis, Allbutt speaks in a somewhat depre-
catory fashion of the 'orthodox coronarians' (II, 263).

Not intending to deal with the history of angina (II, 216, note 1),
Allbutt remarks (ibid., last paragraph): 'more than once the disease
had been incidentally adumbrated before [Heberden]'; the few authors
mentioned being Morgagni, E. A. Müller and F. Hoffmann. There is
truth in his introductory phrase to Section II:

> 'In this secret and fell disease there is a fascination to which no
> physician is a stranger, a fascination in its dramatic events and
> in the riddle to be read.'

The comprehensive books on cardiology at the end of the nineteenth century played their part in propagating knowledge of coronary artery disease. However, as we mentioned earlier, illuminating
discoveries in our subject were brought about by papers rather than
by books. We have referred in the Introduction to the comprehensive
work[55] by Henri Huchard (1844–1910). The confusion prevailing at
the turn of the century is characterized by the numerous theories of
angina pectoris, amounting to eighty according to Huchard's table
(pp.77–80) in which he refers to them as 'liste interminable d'opinions'.
Though unable himself to delineate the special group of coronary
thrombosis and myocardial infarction, he felt strongly that a new
approach was needed, and spoke in his preface of a 'new class of diseases', which he called 'arterial and myocardial cardiopathies.' However,
in his list of historical references (pp. 523–77) containing 185 cases,
he paid more attention to the coronaries than to the myocardium,
italicizing the former but not the latter. S. A. Levine in 1929 gives the
following comment on Huchard's three important and detailed volumes
(2168 pages):

> 'Huchard called attention to the importance of the coronary
> artery and to the frequency of coronary thrombosis, but this
> type of retrospective study did not furnish the clinician with
> the critical bedside data which might enable him to diagnose
> the condition during life.'

Huchard himself introduced the diagnosis and notion of the so-called
'status anginosus', which signified a very protracted type of attack
often leading to myocardial infarction.

---

[55] *Traité Clinique des Maladies du Coeur et de l'Aorte* (1889). We have used the last
edition (1899–1903) where the most informative part is contained in the second volume
(pp. 1–259).

The equally-important volume by Osler in 1897 has already been mentioned several times. In the same year as G. Dock's publication, a medical thesis was published in Paris by René Marie, 'L'Infarctus du Myocarde et ses Conséquences, Ruptures, Plaques, Fibreuses Anevrismes du Coeur.' It is one of the most informative treatises yet to have been presented for a degree in our subject. Marie surveyed the work done previously in this field, added his own material (which is very close to modern knowledge) and arranged it systematically. Later writers found Marie's pathological study a splendid description of the post-mortem changes of coronary thrombosis. However, this process was not clearly associated with a definite clinical symptomatology until some time later.

CHAPTER VI

The Twentieth Century

1. In approaching the twentieth century we find that much can be
learned about the existing knowledge in our subject from a book which
made its appearance just at the onset of the century. The author, L.
Krehl (1861–1935), was a leading figure in German medicine, and much
interested in heart diseases. Through long personal contact with him,
we are able to appreciate his vast knowledge of, and interest in, the
problems of internal medicine, and we may assume that even in his
earlier years he truly represented the medical knowledge of his time.
His book may therefore be regarded as featuring the knowledge then
available. The work is called, *Die Erkrankungen des Herzmuskels*
(Diseases of the Myocardium), and was published in 1901. Of the 462
pages which it comprises, only a few (pp. 367–72) are devoted to a
chapter on 'Occlusion of the coronary arteries', a fact which shows
that in those times the disease was not thought to be as significant as it
is now. Despite its brevity, this chapter contains much important information, as for instance: 'Occlusion is compatible with survival;
the patient survives, unaware of the abyss which he has crossed.'
As will be discussed later, the classical paper by Herrick also made a
point of the possibility of survival, in contrast to the old notion of
immediate death from coronary occlusion. Another pertinent remark
is that 'intact coronary arteries and intact hearts seem to be more
vulnerable'. This probably means that preceding pathological processes
give some protection to the heart by developing a collateral circulation.
In describing the cases of instant death, Krehl remarks that people die
in the same unusual posture of the body as they were during the last
moments of their life. We remember Krehl referring in his lectures to a
case where early in the morning a man was found dead on a park
bench sitting crouched over the shoe-lace which he had been tying.

This volume reveals a full knowledge of myocardial infarction but
little attention is paid to the clinical diagnosis. The index does not
include the term 'myocardial infarction'. The work ends (pp. 456 ff.)

with a short history of cardiology, containing many appropriate references. Krehl was not over-enthusiastic about the standard of historical
research in cardiology in his time, and comments:

> 'As to the major part of these historical remarks, I did not gain
> the impression that they had originated from actual knowledge
> or from accurate judgement.'

The range of Krehl's historical references is fairly wide: from Aretaeus'
saying, 'Syncope is a disease of the heart,' to a doctoral thesis from
Marburg, as late as 1887, by Sternberg, 'On diseases of the myocardium
following disturbances in the coronary circulation.'

In the course of our investigation it has become evident that observations leading to deeper insight had become increasingly over-
lapping and more difficult to separate. In fact, coronary thrombosis,
as shown already, had been repeatedly presented in the literature by
most impressive descriptions. The papers now to be discussed, however, must be singled out as classics, even if one finds that part of the
information they contain exists in earlier descriptions. As mentioned
in the Introduction, neither Obrastzow nor Herrick claimed to be
'discoverers' of coronary thrombosis, and both referred extensively
to their predecessors.

W. P. Obrastzow (1849–1920)[1] and N. D. Straschesko (1876–1952),
two Russian clinicians of Kiev, jointly published in 1910 an important
paper which they had presented at the first Russian Congress of
Internal Medicine held in Moscow in December 1909. Its subject was
the diagnosis of coronary artery thrombosis of the heart.[2] Three cases
of coronary thrombosis were described in detail, in two of which the
diagnosis was made while the patient was living, the first case having
been seen already in 1899. Two other cases were added, in which the
same diagnosis was made but no post-mortem performed. The authors
stressed that the attack was in most cases precipitated by physical
exertion or emotional upset, and classified the clinical symptoms into
three groups:

1. An almost continuous retrosternal pain, which they called
   'status anginosus', a term already used by previous authors.
2. Severe and prolonged difficult respiration, which they termed
   status dyspnoeticus, or asthmaticus. The authors felt strongly

---

[1] I am indebted to Professor B. D. Petrov, of Moscow University, for verifying the
year of birth.

[2] It appeared in Russian, in a little-known journal *Russkii Vrach*, then later in the same
year in *Ztschr. klin. Med.* ('Zur Kenntnis der Thrombose der Koronararterien des
Herzens'). The paper was republished in *Klinicheskaia Meditsina* (*Moscow*)in 1949, **27**,
p. 15, but with the omission of the bibliographical notes.

that dyspnoea can be regarded as an equivalent of anginal pain. We have frequently referred to this view in the course of our survey of the older literature (cf. Bartoletti, Rougnon).[3] The problem of pain versus dyspnoea is a major one, since in the older descriptions coronary disease is often disguised by the clinical predominance of respiratory distress.

3. Pain and pressure are sometimes localized in the upper abdomen, 'status gastralgicus', instead of the chest, a fact described previously, for example, by Huchard; in these cases an acute abdomen had been wrongly suspected, the ultimate diagnosis being coronary occlusion.

A further aid to the differential diagnosis between angina and thrombosis is, according to the authors, the appearance of cardiac insufficiency in the latter. Incidentally, cardiac insufficiency need not always accompany myocardial infarction, though it often does. In more chronic cases cardiac failure had been often described, from Parry to Leyden. With regard to coronary thrombosis, Obrastzow and Straschesko stressed the point that the heart provided an insufficient volume of blood, with the result that the pulse in the limbs is either impalpable or very weak. They called the condition 'Mejopragia cordis', a term which sounds a little awkward, and was not generally accepted in medical usage. The derivation, however, is sound: *meion*, meaning 'less', and *prasso*, 'I do', which means diminished functional activity in a part.

Measurement of blood-pressure and the low readings that are usually obtained in cases of coronary occlusion were mentioned in only one case in this paper, where the decrease was so marked that the pressure could not be determined. The rise in temperature, now regarded as due to necrosis, was also mentioned in only one case and misinterpreted as an inflammatory condition. It is worth noting that one diagnosis of coronary thrombosis, without a post-mortem being made, had been arrived at as early as May 1883, this time with the help of a consultant, F. F. Mering, of Kiev University (not to be confused with J. von Mering, the colleague of O. Minkowski in the production of experimental pancreatic diabetes). Highly impressed by his recollection of this heart case, Obrastzow carefully studied analogous patients for the next twenty-five years in order to find out the clinical features leading to the catastrophe.

When we regard this paper and Herrick's of 1912 as classics, we are referring to their endeavour to establish the diagnosis based on bedside

---

[3] For Bartoletti see above, p. 69, for Rougnon pp. 99–101.

observations, often confirmed by autopsies, but primarily aiming at clinical recognition during the patient's life.

From a historical point of view, the number of references in this article to previous research in the field is quite remarkable. It would take too long to try to reproduce the full list of references assembled by Obrastzow and Straschesko, even though all their references are limited to the last three decades before the publication. However, the coverage of the literature of this period can be regarded as almost exhaustive. Devoting the greatest part of their endeavour to a diagnosis *intra vitam*, the authors did not omit mention of Hammer's case. They remarked that it was extremely difficult at that time to arrive at a bedside diagnosis, and referred to the publications by Krehl in 1901 and Romberg in 1909, which expressed the same view.

A rare example of diagnostic acumen was given, however, as early as 1911 by H. Hochhaus of Cologne in his paper, 'Diagnosis of sudden occlusion of the coronary arteries'. Four cases are described in great detail, two of them having been diagnosed *intra vitam* and confirmed by autopsy. Hochhaus can be classed as one of the pioneers in this field. Sudden onset of pain and dyspnoea, progressive heart failure, pericardial involvement and abdominal symptoms were noted. The pathology of old and fresh thrombosis was clearly delineated, but no attention was paid to histological investigation. A case complicated by occlusion in an artery of one leg is referred to, recalling that described earlier by Vesalius, which we have discussed in a previous chapter.[4] The very informative details cannot easily be abstracted, and the reader would gain much from a perusal of this paper.

The other classic to be mentioned is that of James B. Herrick (1861–1954) of Chicago, which is generally better known than that by his Russian colleagues of 1910. The paper is entitled: 'Clinical features of sudden obstruction of the coronary arteries',[5] which differs only slightly from that of the Russian authors, as 'sudden obstruction' is used instead of 'thrombosis'. It is evident from the first two words of his title that Herrick also wanted to stress the clinical course of the disease. Again, we wish to point to the large place he gave to historical references, as did his colleagues of Kiev.

It is often the case that important insight emerges more organically once planted in the fertile soil of history. Discoveries do not make their appearance abruptly, and they stand out even more prominently when seen against the background of past endeavour. Herrick covered most

---

[4] See above, p. 53.
[5] *J. Amer. med. Ass.*, 1912, **59**, 2015–20.

of the publications of his predecessors within the limited scope afforded by an article in a journal. In his paper, not only are clinical observations and anatomical findings adequately presented, but also experimental work, the important role of collateral circulation, and the physiological basis of signs and symptoms. This is achieved in the first part of the paper, before the actual presentation of cases. It cannot be regarded as a historical introduction, but forms an integral part of the whole content, occupying slightly less than half of the paper. As mentioned in the Introduction, Herrick's paper of 1912 did not meet with any response in the medical world. Only his publication of 1919, which already included electrocardiographic tracings, was able to arouse the interest of a select group of medical readers.

In his autobiography, *Memories of Eighty Years*[6] (1949), Herrick speaks of his work on coronary thrombosis. He refers good-humouredly to the little attention shown by the medical profession to his paper of 1912:

> 'The publication aroused no interest. It fell like a dud. Recognizing the radical nature of the view I held . . . I doggedly kept at the subject, doing what I called "missionary work" . . . I hammered away at the topic. When in 1918 I showed lantern slides and electrocardiograms [of coronary obstruction], physicians in America and later Europe woke up [to the diagnosis which was] later to become a household word translated by the layman into "heart attack".'

More autobiographical material is to be found also in his 'Intimate account of my early experience with coronary thrombosis'.[7]

In contrast to the previous authors who were much impressed by the relation between coronary disease and sudden death, Herrick first tries to dispel the dogmatic adherence to this view. His thesis is that occlusion is not necessarily lethal. He tried to support it by older observations and mentioned Osler's reference to the fact that the patient may live for some time after obstruction. Likewise he quotes Krehl (1901) to the effect that in man occlusion is compatible with a continuance of life.[8]

[6] Pages 196–97 and 200.

[7] *Am. Heart J.*, 1944, **27**, 1.

[8] Paul D. White (1967) has noted the good prognosis in some of his coronary patients followed up for 50 years. A few of his optimistic sub-titles are: 'Myocardial infarction at the age 52—Death from pneumonia at age 90—with good health in between' (p. 183); 'Good health at 78 despite deeply inverted precordial T-waves for 27 years' (p. 194); 'Edema of the legs cleared by walking at age 103' (p. 309). In the last case, the autopsy revealed (inter alia) moderate coronary atherosclerosis with an old recanalized (and symptomless) occlusion of the right coronary artery.

In Herrick's view the symptoms and end-results are influenced by the blood-pressure, by the condition of those parts of the myocardium which are not immediately affected by the obstruction, and by the ability of the remaining vessels to carry on their work. Sudden overwhelming obstruction is likely to be followed by a more profound shock than gradual narrowing through sclerosis with the increased likelihood of anastomosis formation. The differences in course and outcome may be classified according to the four groups mentioned by Herrick:

1. Sudden death group, as described by Krehl, in Nothnagel's System XV, 369, seemingly instantaneous and perhaps painless.
2. A group represented by anginal attack, with severe pain and profound shock, in which death follows in some minutes.
3. Non-fatal group, with mild symptoms, but without the usual causes (such as walking) precipitating an attack. This group generally shows obstruction of small coronary twigs. Such obstruction in small vessels may produce symptoms differing chiefly in degree from those causing obstruction of larger arteries.
4. Group showing severe symptoms, usually fatal, but not immediately, and perhaps not necessarily so. To the clinical features of this last group Herrick directs attention in the following case.

A man aged fifty-five was seized with severe pain in the lower precordial region. The attending physician found him cold, nauseated, with small rapid pulse, and suffering extreme pain. The pain did not cease until three hours had passed; from this time, the patient remained free from pain, but the pulse continued rapid and small. When Herrick saw him twelve hours after the painful attack he found a feeble pulse of 140, very faint heart sounds, and temperature sub-normal, later rising to 99°F. It was remarkable that in spite of the very bad state of his circulation, the patient was able to indulge frequently in active muscular effort without evident harm. A few hours before death the patient described a slight pain in the heart region. Death followed 52 hours after the onset of the attack. The post-mortem revealed a red thrombus completely obliterating the left coronary artery, and well-marked areas of yellowish and reddish softening in the wall of the left ventricle. An acute fibrinous pericardial deposit was found over the left ventricle, which probably explains the slight pain complained of a few hours before death.

Herrick's first case is remarkable in that there were relatively long periods of painlessness, and for the abdominal features which led at first to the misinterpretation of this case as a gastric condition.

He refers to five other cases of coronary thrombosis, though no autopsy control confirms this opinion. All of them showed sudden development of a weak pulse and failure of the heart muscle, the final attack being described by the patient as the severest and most prolonged in his experience. Herrick took note of the time-interval between the obstruction and death: in one case, three days; in another, seven; in two, twelve; and in the last, twenty days. The same attention to the days of survival was shown by Latham in 1846.[9] There is, however, a difference in the motives of the two authors. Latham was striving to differentiate coronary thrombosis, as it is now termed, from the usual type of angina pectoris, and for this reason drew attention to the short interval between the onset and the fatal outcome. Herrick's motive was rather different, tending to stress the fact that the disease is not immediately fatal.

Various atypical features such as predominant gastric and abdominal symptoms, or cases with little or no pain, and the differences in pulse-rate from very slow to very frequent, were represented in this paper. Though the pulse-rate is often specified, no exact figures are given as to blood-pressure: the typical fall was not overlooked, though expressed only in a few words: 'blood-pressure is low.' Dock's case of occlusion had been mentioned very briefly at the beginning of the article and Obrastzow's towards the end. As noted, the complication by a second-ary pericarditis also came under consideration.

In 1918 and 1919 Herrick elaborated on his earlier work, including also electrocardiographical investigations. He differentiated cases due to anaemia and not to the usual coronary sclerosis. He paid more attention to the lowering of blood-pressure, which tended to become still lower in 'unfavourable' cases. He referred to the experimental work done by Fred. M. Smith on dogs: according to the branch ligated, electro-cardiographic tracings were compared with those taken from patients with symptoms of coronary thrombosis. In two or three cases with necropsy, the only significant vascular sclerosis was in the coronary arteries. The observation reveals the relative independence of the process from generalized arteriosclerosis.

The question of possible anastomoses in coronary artery occlusion has often been referred to in the course of our study and may well be summarized at this point. For this purpose Louis Gross's book, *The Blood Supply of the Heart* (1921), which includes a special chapter on this subject (pp. 77–92), is very useful for its historical references. We have discussed earlier the first experiments by Chirac in 1698 on the

9 See above, p. 117.

effects of tying off an artery in a dog. No light was then thrown on the question of anastomoses, nor was any unanimity reached subsequently in this matter. Thebesius in 1708, followed later by Haller, Morgagni and Sénac, came to the conclusion that anastomoses exist between both coronary arteries. Caldani's dissections in 1810 revived this claim, particularly as regards the root of the pulmonary artery, while Cruveilhier again described the so-called wide anastomoses. We have already referred at greater length to Erichsen's experimental ligations performed in 1842, which brought about a more modern trend of investigation.

On the other hand, Hyrtl in 1855 categorically denied the existence of wide anastomoses. This was also the view of Henle (1866) who stated, however, that capillary anastomoses do occur. On the whole Erichsen's conclusions gained recognition, especially from Panum, von Bezold and later Samuelson,[10] all of whom experimented with dogs and were able to demonstrate the intercommunication between coronary arteries. In 1880 Langer showed an even wider range of intercommunication by proving that anastomoses exist between the coronary arteries and those of the pericardium and, through these, with the arteriae mammariae internae.

The greatest obstacle to the general acceptance of anastomoses, at least in experimental animals, was Cohnheim's paper of 1881, which carried weight because of the author's high reputation. His view was invalidated by subsequent experimenters.[11] That the author was not completely apodictic is shown by his remark: '. . . If any anastomoses exist they may consist of fine capillaries.' The problem was taken up again by the Scandinavian Kölster in 1892 in a paper in which he gave an accurate description of the process of infarct formation and healing by scarring.

In his summary Gross emphasized the great diversity of results after the obliteration of coronary branches: from almost instantaneous death, to complete absence of clinical signs, the condition being recognized only incidentally through post-mortem examination after some intercurrent disease.

In order to overcome the difficulties in evaluation Jamin and Merkel introduced a method of radiographing the injected coronary arteries in anatomical specimens. This method was instrumental in establishing the fact that anastomoses do exist in the human heart, as was confirmed by Spalteholz in 1907, by Miller and Matthews in 1909 and by many

[10] See Bibliography (1881). Concerning the experiments which he began after the age of sixty, see B. Naunyn, *Erinnerungen* (1925), p. 274.

[11] However, in 1945 C. J. Wiggers found in the dog that if an extensive collateral circulation has not developed prior to the total occlusion, the muscle in the affected zone is not likely to survive (see Bibliography).

subsequent investigators. On clinical evidence Herrick, in 1912, came to the conclusion that gradual obliteration allows the heart to adapt itself to the new condition. He suggested that the vessels of Thebesius might serve as accessory nutritive channels in such cases. Gross's book is illustrated by beautiful roentgenograms of his own. We may recall Krehl's dictum that younger hearts are more vulnerable in cases of coronary occlusion. Gross reaches the similar conclusion that

> '. . . in the average young adult's heart, the intricate systems of anastomoses are not prepared to act suddenly as entirely adequate compensatory agents. When the obliteration occurs in a relatively older individual's heart, the patent and free anastomoses can often amply supply the affected area so that the myocardium can be completely spared.'

Gross' competent and well-documented volume gives the historian an opportunity to demonstrate how much valid material is already contained in the observations and deliberations of the former investigators in our field.

As Gross' book appeared, electrocardiography was only just coming into clinical use, although Einthoven had devised his instrument some eighteen years earlier. Today this is of course one of the most important diagnostic procedures used in the study of coronary artery disease, and especially of myocardial infarction. The dramatic discovery of electromotive activity in living tissue had begun long before the advances in physics and the construction of instruments. The torpedo fish has the power to 'narcotise the creatures it wants to catch, overpowering them by the strength of a shock which is resident in its body'. This quotation from Aristotle shows the interest of the ancient naturalists in the then so obscure properties of animal electricity. In a paper of 1957 we had occasion to refer to Galen's therapeutical trials in applying a 'live' torpedo fish to a patient's head, which can be regarded as an early specimen of electroshock therapy. The procedure was also mentioned by Scribonius Largus, about A.D. 48, and commented upon later by Avicenna. Plato in his Menon dialogue (80a) had remarked that the seafish 'narke' paralyses and makes one numb.

The understanding of the electromotive effect began with Galvani of Bologna, who demonstrated this phenomenon in the muscles of a frog's limb. The experiments have often been described, as were those of Volta (1745–1827) of Pavia, famous for the construction of the 'Voltaic pile'. It is not necessary to enter into the details of the controversy between these two authors. In 1842, Carlo Matteucci of Pisa proved the action potential of a skeletal muscle, and in the middle of the century E. Du Bois-Reymond of Berlin was able to measure with a galvanometer the electric potential of living tissues. He is often called the father of electrophysiology. As to the heart muscle, Kölliker and Müller of Würzburg, in animal experimentation, succeeded in demonstrating electromotive activity in this organ (1856). The first electrocardiograms, both of the frog's heart, were published by T. W. Engelmann in 1878 (Utrecht) and in the same year by Burdon-Sanderson and F. J. M. Page of London. Later, Burdon-Sanderson was able to record the potential variations from a tortoise's heart.

Meanwhile the capillary electrometer was devised by the physicist Gabriel Lippmann (Heidelberg, later Paris) in 1872. With the aid of this instrument, A. D. Waller of London produced the first record of the electrical activity associated with the human heartbeat, using the term 'cardiogram' which was later changed by Einthoven into 'electrocardiogram'. Since Waller's physiological experiments appear to be the first to be made on a human heart, it seems appropriate to include here a brief quotation from his paper, 'A demonstration on man of electromotive changes accompanying the heart's beat' (1887):

> 'If a pair of electrodes (zinc covered by chamois leather and moistened with brine) are strapped to the front and back of the chest, and connected with a Lippmann's capillary electrometer, the mercury in the latter will be seen to move slightly but sharply at each beat of the heart.'

Waller was critical of his results and tried first to ascertain that the electrical variation was physiological and not due to the mechanical alteration of contact between the electrodes and the chest wall. He performed accurate time-measurements on the supposition that physiological variation should precede the movement of the heart. Indeed the experiment showed that 'the electrical phenomenon begins a little before the cardiographic lever begins to rise.' Unfortunately the records obtained by photographing the movements of the mercury column were inaccurate, chiefly because of the inertia of the instrument. The tracings obtained were corrected a little later by physiologists following up Waller's initiative, especially by Bayliss and Starling of London in 1892.

Finally, in 1903 W. Einthoven (1860–1927), the Dutch physiologist, published his invention of the accurate and practicable string galvanometer. In 1894 he had begun his studies with the capillary electrometer then in use. He greatly improved upon this instrument, obtaining more accurate tracings and developing methods for correcting distortion in the curves, but on the whole remained dissatisfied with the capillary electrometer. Primarily interested in the physiological aspects, Einthoven strove also to attain an accuracy sufficient for application to human beings and to clinical practice. In 1900, he published his paper 'On the normal human electrocardiogram and on the capillar-electrometric examination of some heart patients.' Here he was able to demonstrate that tracings obtained from patients suffering from heart disease were different from those taken from normal patients. He finally abandoned the capillary electrometer which had required correction of the curve obtained, and was able to announce his invention of the string galvanometer. The paper, 'The galvanometric registration of the human electrocardiogram etc.' was published in German in the leading physiological journal of the time[12] and a brief quotation from it follows:

> 'I have tried to find a way to avoid as far as possible the construction of a new curve; in so doing I have at length devised an instrument which satisfies many requirements and is especially suitable to inscribe the human electrocardiogram directly in almost its exact proportions.
>
> The essential part of this instrument—the string galvanometer—is a thin silver-coated quartz fibre, which is stretched like a string in a strong magnetic field. If an electric current is led through this quartz fibre, the fibre shows a movement which can be observed and photographed by means of a considerable magnification, just as in the case with the movement of the mercury in the capillary electrometer. It is possible to regulate the sensitivity of the galvanometer very accurately within wide bounds by tightening and loosening the string' (p. 474).

Einthoven, who had a medical degree and never engaged in medical practice but was a physiologist all his life, became director of the Physiological Institute of Leyden University. However, he was eager to provide the medical profession with a workable and important tool to serve the needs of daily practice. His family background may well have increased his desire to see his discovery applied clinically, since he was the son and grandson of physicians.[13] This desire came to fruition

---

[12] *Pflüger's Arch. ges. Physiol.*, 1903, **99**, 472.

[13] His grandfather was a Jewish doctor in the Dutch West Indies. In the obituary in the *New English Journal of Medicine and Surgery* (1927) the statement was made for the first time in medical literature that Einthoven was 'born from Jewish parents'. Being interested in this item, after making enquiries as to the writer of the unsigned obituary, we were informed by Dr. Viets of Boston that it was written by the late John F. Fulton, with whom we had been privileged to maintain many most agreeable contacts. Unable to trace further the source of Dr. Fulton's information, we pursued our enquiry, and

step by step, as the instruments became adapted to clinical electrocardiography—through development of the audition-tube amplification,
later followed by the device of a heated stylus, the direct writing
electrocardiograph, and several other devices. The method was initially
applied for the purpose of studying the physiological conditions before
coming to a conclusion as to the pathological findings. As regards the
latter, tracings from patients with coronary thrombosis became available only much later, about 1918. In the period immediately following
Einthoven's first publications, anomalies not directly bearing on
coronary disease were given more attention, especially the analysis
of disorders of the heartbeat, such as arrythmias, atrial fibrillation,
flutter, heartblock, and so on. In due course important data about the
heart were learned from a study of the shape, direction, amplitude and
time relations of the individual waves and deflections.

For designating the waves Einthoven took the letters P, Q, R, S, T
from the middle of the alphabet, a system still in use today. He may
have chosen this method deliberately in order to leave margin for
future investigators. Such anticipation of future development links
Einthoven with Heberden, who also considered 'future experience'.

The further advances cannot be outlined even sketchily, owing to the
wealth of technical innovations accumulated over the next decades.
The great variation of the electrocardiographic leads, used for con-
necting any two parts of the body by electrodes and wires with the
recording galvanometer, is the first in a series of technical developments;
it is represented by bipolar limb leads, as well as unipolar and precordial,
all of them serving to increase our insight into the cardiac mechanism.

In studying the history of electrocardiography we have the benefit
of the informative book on this subject by G. E. Burch and N. P.
DePasquale, in 1964. Though in the preface the authors underline the
relative brevity (309 pp.) of the volume, it covers all facets of the subject
and has a documentary value in that it reproduces the original tracings
by the founders of this branch of medical diagnostics. Considering
the magnitude of electrocardiographic work on coronary artery disease,
it seems that the space allotted to it (pp. 179–91) is limited, half of these
pages being taken up by illustrations of electrocardiograms. It is of
historical interest to point out that the early electrocardiographers
achieved their brilliant results by using the relatively-simple registration
of only three leads instead of the usual twelve applied nowadays.
Some early investigators even used only one lead to attain practical

eventually discovered that Einthoven's grandfather and father had been married to
non-Jewish women; so that the statement 'born from Jewish parents' should be amended
accordingly.

results. This was the case when Nicolai and Simons in 1909 described the effect of digitalis on the T waves; however, this is not directly relevant to coronary artery disease.

We referred earlier to Fred. N. Smith who, following Herrick's advice, described the electrocardiographic changes after ligating the coronary arteries of dogs in 1918. The following year Herrick published tracings two days after ligation of anterior and posterior descending branches of the left circumflex artery in a dog, and compared them with those obtained from one of his patients with a classic syndrome of myocardial infarction. In England, Bousfield in 1918 was probably the first to publish an electrocardiogram obtained during and after an episode of angina pectoris in man.

Of great practical importance is the work done in 1920 by H. E. B. Pardee of the United States. He published serial electrocardiograms from the same patient at various intervals following myocardial infarction, thus demonstrating the variability and fluctuation in the pattern obtained. He was the first to illustrate the curved T wave, a special pattern which he explains in the following words: 'The T wave . . . quickly turns away from its starting point in a sharp curve, without the short straight stretch which is so evident in normal records.' In 1925 he described an upward convexity followed by a sharply-pointed downward peak, a feature seen in the T wave of lead 3.

Besides the clinical contributions published in the *Lancet* in 1928 by J. Parkinson and D. Evan Bedford, to be discussed later, some electrocardiographic observations were communicted by these authors in the British journal *Heart* in the same year. They were probably the first to recognize the reciprocal relationship between the S–T segment and T waves changes in leads 1 and 3 in acute myocardial infarction. They observed also that the T_1 type curve occurred in anterior myocardial infarction and the T_3 type in the posterior. These observations were extended by other investigators a year later.

In 1933 F. N. Wilson of the University of Michigan studied the QRS complex as well as the S–T segment and the T wave in myocardial infarction, and established the so-called 'Q_3T_3' type curve.

A number of investigators began to study the electrocardiographic changes on exercise in patients with suspected angina pectoris. The most popular method was the 'two-step test', developed by Master and Oppenheimer in 1929. As previously mentioned, the introduction of precordial leads increased the accuracy in the study of myocardial ischaemic conditions. This method was introduced and developed by F. Wood and C. Wolfert between 1931 and 1933.

Some of the leading cardiologists engaged in the development of cardiographic methods and, obtaining spectacular results, found it necessary to warn the profession not to neglect other accepted means of approach to the subject. We quote from P. D. White's *Heart Disease* (the 4th and last edition, 1951, p. 183):

> 'The electrocardiograph does not take the place of such other methods of examination as history taking, percussion, auscultation, and roentgenology . . . it must be realized that the electrocardiogram may be perfectly normal even in the presence of serious heart disease. This method of study should therefore be viewed modestly as helpful. . . .'

A fine example of integrating electrocardiographic method with clinical and other laboratory findings was given in the above-mentioned paper by Parkinson and Bedford, 'Cardiac infarction and coronary thrombosis' (1928). Among other observations they found that blood-pressure when first recorded is low, sometimes below 100 mm. systolic. After recovery from initial shock, the temperature rises to 99–102°F. Leucocytosis up to 20,000 is common. Embolic complications from intracardiac thrombosis are liable to occur. The authors quote Libman and Sacks (in 1927) to the effect that leucocytosis may develop as early as $1\frac{1}{4}$ hours after the onset of the attack. This particular paper by Parkinson and Bedford is presented in quite a modern way, and the unequivocal recognition of the diagnosis is clearly distinguishable from the more evasive attitude of Sir James Mackenzie in his book *Angina Pectoris* published only five years earlier.

Sir James Mackenzie (1853–1925), one of the leading cardiologists of his day, was still reluctant to include the clinical entity of coronary thrombosis, and to separate it from the classical angina pectoris. He advanced the understanding of cardiac irregularities by the use of the polygraph, and exerted a great influence on the early phase of modern cardiology, being also the teacher of Sir Thomas Lewis. Mackenzie himself suffered from long-standing coronary artery disease and was much interested in the study of this condition. In his above-mentioned book of 253 pages infarct is indexed only once, on p. 158. The patient, a professor of medicine, fifty-four years old, died after prolonged coronary illness, when he had had 'the best night for several nights'. The pathology showed 'thrombosis of one of the coronaries, with an infarct which had apparently become infected'. To quote S. A. Levine (1929, p. 6), 'Mackenzie never made the clinical distinction between angina pectoris and coronary thrombosis.' We may call attention to the paper, 'Sir James Mackenzie's Heart', by D. Waterston, 1939, which reports that the first infarction occurred in 1908 and the final and lethal one in January 1925. At the end of the paper is appended the opinion of Sir Thomas Lewis, together with that of Dr. Grant. The comment is quite up-to-date, with a full appreciation of myocardial infarction.

As to Sir Thomas Lewis himself (1881–1945), an acknowledged leader in modern cardiology, well known for his studies of auricular fibrillation and for the establishment of electrocardiography in England as early as 1909, the study of coronary diseases was not his main field of work. Attention is drawn to Chapter 11 on 'Anginal Pain' (pp. 118–26) of his volume *Clinical Signs illustrated by Personal Experiences* (1934). His comments do not add much to the historically well-known views of Burns, Parry and other earlier authors; for instance: 'anginal pain in the theory of muscular ischaemia; comparison between intermittent claudication and angina of effort, blood supply presumably inadequateto the needs of the working tissue'. Lewis' interest in the early workers on coronary artery disease is documented by his paper on C. H. Parry, (1940–41). What attracted him most in Parry's work was that 'he realized that functional efficiency rather than structural integrity of the arteries is of prime importance'. In his volume *Diseases of the Heart* (1933), the first specific disease described is 'Cardiac Ischaemia, Coronary Thrombosis', followed by a chapter on 'Angina Pectoris'. The arrhythmias and valvular diseases only come later.

Lewis suffered from coronary arteriosclerosis, had a coronary thrombosis in 1927 and again in 1935, and the third and fatal one in 1945 at the age of sixty-four.

2. With the advent of electrocardiography and later of laboratory aids, the medical profession acquired techniques to diagnose coronary disease with greater precision. It is known that even before these procedures became available the disease was often diagnosed at the bedside. As in other diseases, the emergence of graphic registration or quantitative factors concerning diseased states of secretion, respiration, blood flow, and so on, gave the medical profession a clearer approach to the interpretation of diseased states. It is even probable that the awareness of the condition and sureness in the diagnosis of coronary diseases increased in proportion to the availability of tools and methods. This explains why the condition became more often identifiable. Thus diagnosis was brought within the range of the average physician, and not left exclusively in the hands of a select group of specially interested investigators.

Among the aids to a proper identification of the disease, there are some simple procedures easily performed at the bedside, which gained recognition in establishing the diagnosis. They were valuable not so much in uncomplicated cases of angina pectoris, but more in detecting organic lesions connected with coronary thrombosis or infarction.

The decrease in blood-pressure is a common occurrence in some stages of acute coronary occlusion, though there are some exceptions. Even the simple procedure of sphygmomanometry became available relatively late, when in 1880 Samuel von Basch devised the first workable instrument for the estimation of blood-pressure in patients. Measurement of the blood-pressure in animals had been known since the famous experiments of Stephen Hales, published in 1733. Basch's instrument was improved upon by P. C. Potain of Paris and in particular by the Italian physician S. Riva-Rocci (1896), who did away with a great deal of the clumsiness of the original instrument and eventually produced one with a cuff, placed around the arm, and connected with a mercury manometer, still in current use. A further advance was made by the Russian N. Korotkov, in 1905, who applied the auscultation method. The decrease in blood-pressure was already implied in Aretaeus's impressive description of cardiogenic syncope. In modern times the fall in blood-pressure in a patient suffering from occlusion in a coronary artery was quantitatively ascertained as early as 1895, by Joseph Baylac. According to René Marie, discussed earlier, Baylac measured in his patient a blood-pressure of 15 units using Potain's instrument, as against 18 units in normal individuals. As previously noted, Obrastzow (1910) was able to measure the blood-pressure in one of his patients, while Hochhaus in 1911 referred to a decrease in two cases. Herrick, in 1918 and 1919, classified this phenomenon as one of the clinical signs of infarction.

The second point to which authors began to refer as a fairly constant symptom was the rise in body temperature due to myocardial necrosis. This phenomenon was noted by Kernig in 1905, as an occasional occurrence in the so-called 'status anginosus'. Emanuel Libman in 1916 mentioned in passing that the diagnosis of a recent thrombosis of a coronary artery can be often facilitated by noting slight fever, or moderate leucocytosis, and the signs of a local pericarditis, all of them following a few days after an attack of severe pain. Parkinson and Bedford (1928) found fever a more useful diagnostic sign of infarction than leucocytosis, which will be discussed in the following paragraph.

The first to call attention to the development of leucocytosis (as well as fever) as a part of the picture of coronary thombosis were

S. A. Levine and Ch. L. Tranter, in a paper published in 1918. They observed two cases early in the year 1916. The first male patient developed a temperature of 102°F., while the leucocyte count rose to 21,400. In the post-mortem, extensive myocardial infarction of the left ventricle, and coronary artery sclerosis were present. In the second male patient, the leucocytes amounted to 19,900, next morning 33,500. The post-mortem revealed a thrombus in the anterior coronary artery as well as old and fresh thrombi and necrosis of the myocardium. Both patients showed infarction of the heart, simulating acute surgical abdominal conditions. In 1927 Libman and Sacks devoted a special paper to the topic, stating that leucocytosis is not only a prime diagnostic sign, even more significant than fever, but that it is also of prognostic importance. They advanced the opinion that if the leucocytosis does not disappear after a few days, it signifies progressive necrosis of the heart muscle.

A further laboratory aid was added by determining the sedimentation rate of the red cells.[14] Acceleration in acute myocardial infarction is quite common and remains rapid for weeks until the healing process of the myocardial necrosis is completed. Since the method is very simple and easily performed at the bedside, it had probably been in use for quite some time; however, we could not find any literary evidence before the year 1933. It seems that Gerhard Scherk was the first to stress its importance. He used leucocytosis and increased sedimentation rate as criteria, and let the patients remain in bed until both tests showed a return to normal.

Sedimentation rate as a test was first introduced by the Polish physician E. Biernacki, who devoted to its description papers in 1894, 1897 and 1906. The first author in Western Europe to work on it was R. Fåhraeus, in his paper 'The suspension-stability of the blood' (1921), preceded by a shorter one in 1918. Fåhraeus has taken great interest in historical matters, including the earlier developments in this field. He quotes the four elements of the Pythagoreans, who explained the blood-changes in an amber vessel. He mentions also John Hunter (1786) as to rouleaux formation in the blood, quoting him to the effect that in inflammatory processes the blood has an increased disposition to separate. Likewise, he recalls H. Nasse, 1836, who correlated sedimentation with the intensity of rouleaux formation. In 1917 Fåhraeus used oxalated blood and left Westergren to devise the technique; hence the name 'Westergren method'.

A more recent development is connected with the introduction of the

---

[14] Cf. the paper by Paul Wood (1936).

glutaminoxaloacetic transaminase in the blood. The serum glutamic oxaloacetic transaminase (SGO-T) was studied by a group headed by J. S. La Due and F. Wroblewski after this enzyme was first observed in 1938 in the breast muscle of the pigeon. The next step was the examination of the quantity of enzyme in the serum after myocardial infarction, at the stage when the heart substance, which contains much of this enzyme, has become necrotic and the enzyme is poured into the blood-stream. In 1954 this group found an elevation of the SGO-T in the sera of patients with a recent myocardial infarction. The increase takes place up to 12 hours after the event, and returns to normal in a few days. A similar increase was found after experimental production of infarcts in dogs, where the level of the transaminase corresponded to the size of the area of necrosis in the heart. The test is used also in the diagnostic evaluation of liver disease. It is regarded as an important practical aid to the diagnosis of a recent myocardial infarction.

3. We have followed step by step the development of diagnostic procedures in the study of coronary artery disease. Simultaneously research was directed towards establishing the etiological factors. Arteriosclerosis, metabolic factors including the influence of diet, and hereditary disposition have been mentioned earlier. Many of these factors were corroborated by experimental methods aiming at the creation of a firm ground for theories and deliberations. Ethnological variations in mixed populations will be referred to in due course.

Emotional Factors

When we discuss the influence of emotions on coronary artery disease we have not the firm basis of an experimental approach. However, strain and stress of life and individual fluctuations of mood and mental disposition have always been considered important determinants of the disease. In previous chapters we have made frequent reference to authors who noted the role of emotional disorders in the production of the disease. An historical survey of this problem shows that heart diseases in ancient times were not sufficiently specified nor anatomically differentiated. We must therefore discard the interesting reference to psychogenesis in heart troubles, namely the so-called love-pulse as mentioned by Galen and other authors, and restrict ourselves to opinions concerning states suggesting coronary disease.

When Aretaeus in the second century gave his classical description of cardiac syncope he did not pay much attention to the etiological factors, with the exception of his statement that it is not due to a

febrile cause. However, from the stress he lays on emotional determinants of the disease in his discussion of therapeutical measures, it may
be inferred that these were given much consideration by the ancient
author. The Biblical poetry frequently associates pain in the heart
with a sorrowful state of mind. We referred earlier in some detail to
the controversial 'case-history'[15] of Nabal in the 25th chapter of the
first book of Samuel, where the great fear and anxiety of the patient
could well have been responsible for his cardiac death. During the
Middle Ages pain in the heart was often associated by the authors with
the feeling of fear and grief, as mentioned earlier. In Avicenna's
treatise, *De Viribus Cordis*, the medicaments recommended were
intended as a prescription for heart pain as well as for melancholy;
corals, ruby and most of the therapeutical measures were of a symbolic
and magical character, but the administration of opium is also mentioned. A passage from *De Viribus Cordis* is quoted also in Maimonides'
treatise, *De Accidentibus*. Vesalius' reference to thrombo-embolic
disease probably due to coronary lesion, describes the patient Immersel
as having a melancholic disposition.[16] This psychological factor was
also mentioned in the case of Hercules Saxonia, discussed earlier.[17]

The most pertinent example of the connection of coronary disease
and mental stress and emotions was presented by W. Harvey (1649)
in his second letter to Riolan. Together with the 'distressing pain in the
chest', Harvey refers to the 'unquiet and anxious life' of the patient
Sir Robert Darcy. The next case by Harvey, that of an anonymous
patient who 'at last fell into a strange distemper suffering from extreme
oppression and pain of the heart and breast', is even more impressive
for its detailed description of psychological stress. To quote Harvey,
the patient, having

> 'received an injury and affront from one more powerful than
> himself, and upon whom he could not have his revenge, was
> overcome with anger and indignation which he yet communi-
> cated to no-one . . .'.

This quotation has been included in our discussion of Harvey, but is
repeated for the depth and validity of its psychological implication.

After the diagnosis of angina pectoris had been advanced by Heberden, many more authors paid attention to the manifold environmental
and psychological aspects. Not only was the psychological history of
the patient taken into consideration, but also the role of social and

[15] See above, p. 39.
[16] See above, p. 53.
[17] See above, p. 61, and J. O. Leibowitz an D. T. Ullmann (1965).

cultural influences and emotions in general. J. N. Corvisart in the introduction to his book on the diseases of the heart (1806; English translation 1817), drew attention to the 'social state; all functions disordered by ever-agitating or ever-renewing causes'. The phrase 'ever-renewing causes' is significant in that Corvisart, followed by modern authors, apparently evaluated a prolonged state of tension as more pathogenic than a sudden manifestation of emotional disorder.[18] Corvisart also described the influence of passions on the heart, especially during the calamitous events of the Revolution, as did an American author D. Wooster in 1867, who wrote during the period of the Gold Rush. Osler, in his *Lectures on Angina Pectoris and Allied States* (1897), a work to which we have often referred, mentioned 'arterial degeneration in the worry and strain of modern life'. He spoke of 'pressure, working the machine to its maximum capacity'.

The role of specific emotional states, notably anger, was stressed by the late eighteenth-century investigators. John Fothergill, in his paper, 'Farther account of the Angina Pectoris' (1776, p. 258), was very explicit in the evaluation of psychogenetic factors. To quote Fothergill: '. . . the plan proposed (restricted food, avoidance of emotional stress, etc.) might greatly retard the progress of the disorder, by assisting to restrain excesses of passion and anxiety, which perhaps contribute more to the increase of this disease, than a combination of all other causes.' The famous case of John Hunter's fatal attack was commented upon by Everard Home: '. . . death came suddenly, in consequence of a fit of temper at a meeting of the governors of St. George's Hospital, October 16, 1793.' Another outspoken opinion in this connection was formulated by P. M. Latham in 1846: 'Death has followed mental excitement more frequently than bodily excitement.' It is evident from this historical literature pertaining to the influence of emotional factors, that these were not neglected by the earlier authors. The most acceptable and weighed opinions are those of Harvey and Corvisart, who attached less importance to sudden excitement or anger as provoking a coronary event, but more to a successive or 'ever-repeating' stress situation, thus coming nearer to modern psychological concepts. In fact, most of the fatalities in coronary artery disease occur without the immediate incitement of psychological upheaval. One casehistory, referred to earlier, describes sudden death of coronary origin in a patient who had been quietly sipping his cup of chocolate.[19]

The above discussion has been devoted to the psychological state as

[18] S. J. Kowal, 'Emotions and Angina Pectoris, A Historical Review', *Am. J. Cardiol.* 1960, **5**, 421–27.
[19] See above, p. 96.

a possible contributing factor to the disease. Another viewpoint is the influence of the disease on the psychological condition of the patient. This particular aspect is not directly within the scope of our historical studies. We might however mention M. Schrenk, who, in a historical paper on angina pectoris in 1967, has summarized (pp. 179–83) some older psychiatric considerations regarding the so-called 'Präkordialangst'.[20]

Concerning other etiological factors, a great deal of work has been done with regard to the influence of diet on the development of arteriosclerosis. From some of our previous historical references it becomes apparent that general arteriosclerosis does not always involve coronary sclerosis. The coronary vessels were found to have comparatively independent reactions to noxious factors. They may accompany the general arteriosclerotic process, or not participate at all, or in some cases they show a predilection for it, the other vessels remaining relatively untouched. Bearing this distinction in mind, the subsequent research in arteriosclerosis may be reviewed.

The first paper on experimental arteriosclerosis was that of A. I. Ignatovski, 'On the influence of animal food on the tissues of the rabbit', which was published in St. Petersburg in 1908. The author showed that rabbits fed on milk and egg yolk developed severe arteriosclerosis. Similar experiments were carred out by N. W. Stuckey in 1912 with the result that neither fish oil nor sunflower seed caused arterial lesions, and that egg yolk and brain were more probable causes than milk.

In 1913, N. Anichkov and S. Chalatov added pure cholesterol to rabbit food with the result that arteriosclerosis was produced in these animals. A summary of the research of Anichkov's school was published in 1958 by A. L. Myasnikov in a paper entitled 'Influence of some factors on the development of experimental cholesterol atherosclerosis'. As early as 1916 C. H. Bailey had given a confirmation of the experiments with cholesterol. T. Leary in 1935 stressed the opinion that atherosclerosis is a metabolic disease.

The changing conditions relating to food intake in immigrant populations gave rise to a further evaluation of the nutritional factor. Thus F. Dreyfuss of Jerusalem, in 1953, described the very low incidence of atherosclerosis among immigrants from Yemen to Israel, while Yemenites who had lived in Israel for two or three generations show almost the same incidence of this disease as the rest of the population. The same result is apparent in a study by J. Toor, A. Katchalsky

---

[20] This term had already been used in the German translation of J. B. von Helmont, (1683), p. 831, par. 7, 'Hertzens-Angst (Cardiogmus)'. It is also found in Cohnheim's paper already cited (*Virchow's Archiv*, 1881, **85**, 510).

and others, 'Serum-lipids and atherosclerosis among Yemenite immigrants in Israel', published in 1957.[21] Protection against arteriosclerosis by unsaturated fats was first suggested by I. Snapper in his *Chinese Lessons to Western Medicine* (1941) where he referred to the contrast between the diets in Holland and North China, which influenced the incidence of vascular lesions. This was followed up by J. Groen and his collaborators in a paper of 1952 in an experiment of nine months' duration on sixty normal human volunteers.

The spectacular results of experimental arteriosclerosis in rabbits do not, however, apply to the higher mammals. In 1946 T. W. Li and S. Freeman published a paper, 'Experimental lipemia and hypercholesterolemia produced by protein depletion and by cholesterol-feeding in dogs', which shows a striking difference in the production of sclerotic changes. In 1957 E. H. Ahrens showed that in man the bile daily provides as much cholesterol as five to ten eggs, and its absorption is increased when the diet is rich in animal fat; adding cholesterol to the diet has a minimal effect on the blood level. In the previously-mentioned paper of 1952 by Groen and his collaborators it is stated that in man hypercholesterolemia is not produced by cholesterol feeding, but by egg and brain supplements, foods rich in saturated fat as well as cholesterol.

The practical application of the experimental findings to the therapy of coronary artery disease has not been conclusively determined. This can be seen from an editorial by I. Snapper in 1963, significantly entitled 'Diet and Atherosclerosis: Truth and Fiction'. The paper includes the historical development of the clinical implications derived from geographical pathology. Snapper begins with a reference to the Dutch author C. D. De Langen of 1916, who observed the rarity of atherosclerosis, phlebothrombosis and gallstones among the Javanese, who are naturally disposed towards hypocholesterinemia. Another very informative editorial was provided by William Dock in 1958, illustrating the development of the problem since 1908.

Further information about the occurrence of the disease can be derived from reading the regular reports of the International Society of Geographical Pathology, the 9th Conference at Leyden being almost exclusively concerned with cardiovascular disease. Geographical pathology, as a special discipline, was furthered by the well-known book by August Hirsch in 1859–64.[22]

[21] See also H. Ungar, and A. Laufer, 'Necropsy studies of atherosclerosis in the Jewish population of Israel' (1961), and H. Ungar *et al.*, 'Atherosclerosis and Myocardial Infarction in various Jewish groups in Israel' (1963).

[22] 2nd ed. 1881–6; English translation 1883–6. This was preceded by L. L. Finke, *Versuch einer allgemeinen med.-prakt. Geographie, etc.*, 3 vols., 1792–95.

Sir George Pickering, who was mentioned earlier, makes further historical references to arteriosclerosis in a paper of 1964. He does not consider cholesterol and the lipid hypothesis to be pertinent to the pathogenesis of myocardial infarction. He quotes from Muir's textbook of pathology to the effect that fatty change is of secondary importance. It may be noted that Scarpa, 1804, one of the first who introduced the notion of fatty 'disorganization' and whose work has already been discussed,[23] has not yet been accorded a proper place in the different historical surveys of arteriosclerosis.

Social and occupational influences have also been made responsible for the emergence of coronary artery disease. It was advanced that the victims were usually males of the age of fifty, often from the better educated and higher social classes. Likewise, there was believed to be a greater incidence among the liberal professions. A paper by Ryle and Russell, 'The natural history of coronary disease', in the *British Heart Journal* of 1949 gives some idea of the occupational mortality, although the findings do not seem to be representative of the population as a whole: 368 physicians and surgeons, 218 clergymen, 20 workers in chemical processes, 32 agricultural labourers, and 40 coal miners. The high morbidity and mortality from coronary artery disease among physicians has often been noted, as, for example, by Osler in his Lumleian lectures published in 1910, stating that angina pectoris may be called 'morbus medicorum'.[24]

Among other causative factors regarding the incidence of coronary artery disease the problem of physical activity is of some importance. J. N. Morris and M. D. Crawford in a statistical study[25] found a higher incidence of disease in bus-drivers compared with conductors. The higher incidence was confirmed in other population groups. However, further investigations into this matter are needed to clarify the point.

As to the age at which the disease makes its appearance, we are again reminded of the concise Hippocratic aphorism, 'Frequent recurrence of cardialgia, in an elderly person, announces sudden death.' However, there are many exceptions to the rule, some of which were mentioned previously, in which younger persons suffered from the disease. The examples of the past have been supplemented by more recent experience In a paper of 1953 entitled 'Coronary disease among United States soldiers killed in action in Korea', W. F. Enos and his colleagues showed atheroma grossly visible in fifty per cent of the coronaries of

[23] See above, p. 106-7.
[24] For more recent occupational statistics see, *inter alia*, A. H. T. Robb-Smith, *The Enigma of Coronary Heart Disease*, 1967.
[25] Coronary heart disease and physical activity of work', *Brit. med. J.*, 1958, **2**, 1485.

Americans, average age twenty-two years. It was felt that this finding was due to the high intake of egg and milk. Indeed the Korean and Chinese soldiers, eating no milk products and little egg or meat fat, had no lipid in the intima of their coronary vessels. These interesting and unexpected findings which were revealed by autopsy presumably indicate anatomical rather than clinical changes, since the soldiers had obviously undergone physical examination before enlisting for active military service.

Incidentally, coronary intimal thickening may even be found in infancy and childhood. In a recent article by E. H. Oppenheimer and J. R. Esterly in 1966 the authors noted: 'Structural disorganization (expression used by Scarpa in 1804!) of the arterial wall resulting in obliterative endarteritis, calcification, severe endothelial plaques, and even a scar in the myocardium.' Another paper by a pediatrician revealed coronary thrombosis and myocardial infarction in a four-and-a-half year old boy. These findings, however, have been revealed in children with extensive congenital heart malformations.

4. In the history of coronary artery disease therapy[26] does not appear to have been a strong point of medical endeavour. The urgent need to reduce the violence of the attack must have been felt even in remote antiquity; obviously the measures were of a palliative nature, and directed more against the symptoms than the essence of the disease. Thus Aretaeus[27] was eager to abate the sweating accompanying syncope of cardiac origin, administering also wine to strengthen the heart, a procedure mentioned as late as 1772 by Heberden. For the treatment of shock due to the so-called 'morbus cardiacus', Celsus in the first century was sufficiently astute to think of the water-balance in the body and suggested the administration of liquids to combat depletion. If drink could not be retained by the patient Celsus advocated a barley-water enema as a last resource (III, 19.6). He was not very far from modern practice in his insistence that the physician keep watch even when the patient 'seems to be out of danger, since a rapid relapse into the same state of faintness is always to be borne in mind'.

In the Middle Ages many remedies against contriction in the breast were prescribed, for instance in the ninth-century manuscript on Anglo-Saxon magic published in 1952 by Grattan and Singer (p. 197). In our section on the Middle Ages we referred to several works, in the West as well as in the East, containing instances of therapy in cases suggestive

---

[26] See J. O. Leibowitz, *Intern. Congr. Hist. Med.*, 1966.
[27] See above, p. 32.

of coronary artery disease. The Renaissance authors, to whom we referred earlier, prescribed blood-letting, assuming obstruction in the blood vessels. The chemically-minded seventeenth-century physicians, for instance T. Willis, used volatile salts, ammonia, as well as 'cordials', supposed to stimulate the heart and raise the spirits.

Heberden was not very hopeful as to therapy:

> 'With respect to the treatment of this complaint, I have little or nothing to advance: nor indeed is it to be expected we should have made much progress in the cure of a disease, which has hitherto hardly had a place, or a name in medical books' (*Commentaries*, 1802, p. 368).

Nevertheless he was able to propose some remedies, saying:

> 'Wine and cordials taken at going to bed will prevent, or weaken, the night fits; but nothing does this so effectively as opiates. Ten, fifteen, or twenty drops of Tinctura Thebaica taken at lying down, etc.' (1772, p. 67).

These measures are also appropriate nowadays for acute attacks.

In 1867 T. Lauder Brunton[28] (1884–1916) published his paper 'On the use of nitrite of amyl in angina pectoris.' In his introductory paragraph he says:

> 'Few things are more distressing to a physician than to stand beside a suffering patient who is anxiously looking to him for that relief from pain which he feels himself utterly unable to afford.'

Incidentally, this author names dyspnoea as accompanying angina pectoris, which contradicts the classical view of absence of dyspnoea, as postulated by Heberden. Brunton did not speak expressly of coronary vasodilators as they are now conceived, and attributed the effect of amyl nitrite to a lowering of the blood pressure. In this connection it is interesting to note that the drug was first successfully administered by Lauder Brunton to a patient *without* coronary artery disease, but suffering from aortic incompetence and stenosis.

In 1879 William Murrell introduced nitro-glycerine, a drug which works more slowly but has a more lasting effect, as a remedy for angina pectoris. Vasodilators gained a permanent place in the therapy and were

---

[28] We wish to call attention to Arthur Hollman's very informative critical review (1963) on the current use of coronary vasodilators and its historical development, beginning with Sir Lauder Brunton.

also used prior to exertion in order to prevent attacks. Modern investigators in 1959, using coronary artery catheterization, showed that nitro-glycerine increased the coronary blood flow by 63% in healthy subjects, but in cardiac patients it remained unchanged or even fell.[29] This appears as a dramatic reversal of previously held notions about nitrites. In spite of these findings the clinical use remains valid, its value perhaps residing in its effect of decreasing the contractility of the heart. Older experiments by Fred. M. Smith after ligation of a coronary artery in dogs showed that administration of nitro-glycerine reduced the ischaemic area by improvement of the collateral circulation.

To combat or at least to reduce early mortality from acute myocardial infarction, intensive coronary care units were established in the early 1960s. It seems that the idea has been borrowed from the care units after open heart surgery, first organized at Minnesota University in 1958. It had been found earlier that sudden death is sometimes preceded by an arrhythmia. The idea was alluded to by 'Dr. Anonymous' and has been discussed in the chapter on Heberden. Thus continuous electrographic monitoring was introduced in order to apply life-saving measures such as external cardiac compression, or massage, electrical defibrillation and electrical pace-making. Automatic signals by means of visual and auditory warnings have been used. More details, bibliographical references and a report on 150 cases are to be found in the paper by A. J. Goble and his colleagues, 'Mortality Reduction in a Coronary Care Unit'.[30]

There were also attempts at surgical intervention in angina pectoris. In 1916 T. H. Jonnesco used cervical sympathectomy under the supposition that the anginal pain was due to irritation in the cardio-aortic nervous plexus. This operation was abandoned later.

Another surgical measure was introduced by Claude Beck in 1935, who initiated a collateral circulation to the heart by irritation of the pericardium. He thus produced pericardial adhesions in order to increase the blood supply to the heart muscle from the pericardial vessels. These procedures, and the grafting of a systemic vein into the coronary sinus, were described by P. D. White, 1951, as 'promising but still hazardous in man'.

Another surgical procedure is the so-called coronary thrombo-endarterectomy, developed by the Cleveland group, which involves the removal of the thrombus from the lumen of the vessel. This procedure, to be successful as well as favoured by prospects of recovery,

[29] R. Gorlin, et al, Circulation, 1959, 19, 705.
[30] Brit. med. J., 1966, i, 1005.

however, requires preliminary diagnostic steps, which were achieved by selective coronary arteriography, introduced by Sones in 1962. This provides data as to the exact location of the occlusion and the state of the artery behind the obstruction. The endarterotomy and patch-graft reconstruction seem to be a most promising if somewhat hazardous method of surgical intervention. In 1967 a number of patients underwent this operation which is reserved for a select group.[31]

A widely-accepted measure against complications of thrombosis and embolism was the introduction of anti-coagulant drugs. First came the use of heparin in experimental animals in 1938. From 1942 onwards, I. Wright used dicoumarin instead of heparin in man. By applying this drug at the earliest stage of acute coronary thrombosis with myocardial infarction, the complications of thrombosis and embolism could be greatly reduced. By 1948 Wright was able to report that the mortality was 13 per cent in the treated patients and 23 per cent in the controls. The administration of anti-coagulants is a preventive measure, as distinct from a remedy against an already-established disease. However, there is a considerable variation of opinion as to how long these drugs should be administered.[32] Some clinicians restrict the treatment to six or eight weeks after the attack while others continue it for years. During its administration a constant vigilance must be maintained to detect any bleeding which may result from the drug intake. Persons liable to bleeding in the inner organs, as from peptic ulcer, or from the cerebral vessels in certain elderly people, are generally excluded from anticoagulant medication.

5. Investigators interested in the historical aspects have not been unanimous as to how long coronary artery disease has been in existence. In our introduction we referred to the relatively belated emergence of clear-cut descriptions of the disease. The earlier observations were overlooked, since they did not easily fit into the existing systems of medicine. This further delayed the recognition and acceptance of the condition as a clinical syndrome. As Langdon-Brown (1932) has re-marked in another connection,

> 'So apt are we to set aside observations we cannot include in known categories. The history of science is full of such burials and resurrections.'

[31] In 1946 A. M. Vineberg first introduced implantation of the internal mammary artery, thus achieving myocardial revascularization.

[32] See J. McMichael and E. H. Parry (1960), and A. M. Masters (1961), where it is suggested that anticoagulant therapy might also have been overestimated as a *sine qua non* of treatment for coronary obstruction.

In view of the many signs and symptoms we have been able to find in the historical literature, its early existence cannot be denied though some writers do not accept this view. L. Michaels, in a historical appraisal published in 1966, puts forward the following opinion:

> 'The remarkable absence of systematic descriptions before 1768, therefore, raises the distinct possibility that angina pectoris first made its appearance to any appreciable extent, in the second half of the 18th century and had hardly existed previously.' (p. 259).

As to coronary thrombosis before 1912, he states that

> 'the possibility must be considered that it had been almost non-existent rather than prevalent but unrecognised.' (p. 263).

The author mitigates his negative attitude by the cautious words 'possibility' and 'hardly existed', which are in keeping with the sound and informative content of his paper devoted to a critical appreciation of the etiology of coronary artery disease. Indeed we are well aware that only through a very thorough and time-consuming study of sources can the earlier history of the disease be detected, although it was certainly not as common[33] in the past as it is nowadays. It is worth noting that J. N. Morris in a number of papers between 1951–59 has suggested that the incidence of severe coronary atheroma did not increase in the forty years up to 1949, but that thrombosis and heart disease did. The statement was based on 6000 autopsy records from the London Hospital for the periods 1907–14 and 1944–49.

Most historians of cardiology have in fact considered the long pedigree of the disease, though no detailed investigation has previously been made into the earlier stages of the development. Their acknowledgement of the long record of the disease is clearly seen from the relevant contributions of Herrick, Willius and Klemperer, to mention only a few.

In a paper by W. B. Bean, 'Clinical masquerades of acute myocardial infarction' (1962), the feeling is aphoristically expressed that 'Heart attacks must have occurred ever since there first were people to have heart attacks.' Bean shows how frequently the disease may be disguised and not readily ascertained even at the present time. Before the advent of modern concepts and diagnostic procedures this must have been a rule rather than an exception. Bean considers ten possibilities of 'masquerade', some of which recall our previously-mentioned

[33] See Paul D. White and H. Donovan, *Hearts, their Long Follow-up* (1967), pp. 176–77.

references to the historical literature: for instance, the absence of complaint from the patient, which previous authors called 'angina pectoris sine angina'; severe attacks of dyspnoea, to which we referred in the discussion on pain versus dyspnoea; shock without pain, re-calling Aretaeus' description of syncope; 'acute indigestion', referred to by authors of the early twentieth century, and so on. Bean concludes his paper with the words:

> 'Not every pain in the chest means myocardial infarction, and not every myocardial infarction makes itself known to its victims and to you.'

Transposed into historical terms, this paper reveals how many cases must have been obscured by atypical and inadequately-understood factors, which is also a reason for the rarity of historical references re-lating to our subject.

A number of papers produced recently discuss the influence of environmental factors on the changing incidence of coronary artery disease. The paper by H. B. Sprague (1966), gives ample acknowledg-ment to the presence of these influences in modern times. However, the philosophy of the article is built on the assumption of the long his-torical record of the disease.

> 'Certainly the disease did not suddenly leap into existence about 1920, fully armed for destruction like Athena from the brow of Zeus.'

Sprague is not even certain that coronary artery disease became more prevalent in recent medical history. He feels that

> 'excellent presumptive histories of these attacks, especially in fatal cases, may be found in medical and lay literature at least over the past two hundred years.'

He finds it reasonable to assume that the prevalence of coronary arteriosclerosis has remained much the same in Europe and the United States for more than several hundred years, relative to the population 'at risk', as determined by the average age and freedom from other causes of death, especially tuberculosis and other infectious diseases. He stresses the fact that certain families have genetic vulnerability or resistance to vascular degeneration. As to the influence of diet, he does not find the conclusions very consistent, considering that fatty meals have been the rule since colonial days. He finds that over-nutrition in childhood and adolescence may often be the greatest threat to longevity. He sees the reason for the increase of the disease over the last few decades as:

'... failure to die early of other diseases, and the delay in recognition by the medical profession of the clinical pattern of acute coronary occlusion and myocardial infarction prior to about 1920.'

An editorial in the *Journal of the American Medical Association* in 1966 summarizes present opinion and evaluates the two papers discussed above in the following way: Michaels regards these 'firsts' (Heberden—Weigert—Herrick) as true landmarks, denoting actual beginnings of disease occurrence, whereas Sprague does not share this view. The editorial concludes:

'The testimony of the past is no less vulnerable to subjective bias than the evidence of the present'.

Having indicated the views of an epidemiologist and a clinician in this controversy, we now proceed to the standpoint of an historian. Working according to the principles and methods of historical investigation we have tried to avoid in this study the pitfall of subjective bias in considering the testimony of the past. We have critically presented those signs and symptoms described during antiquity and the subsequent periods of history which are suggestive of coronary artery disease. Although the old classics do not provide a systematic and all-inclusive picture of the disease, the factual material and historical comments we have assembled can indeed be taken as an indication that 'the disease did not suddenly leap into existence' during the modern phase of medical history.

Throughout our study we have paid close attention to the history of ideas, finding for instance that concepts such as 'obstruction' in Egyptian and classical antiquity were subsequently verified, and of course improved, by modern methods of research. The idea of 'obstruction' in the vessels in ancient medicine was derived from speculation and reasoning, by way of analogy to other spheres of medical observation. Diagnosis was dependent moreover on the alertness of physicians in perceiving significant symptoms in daily practice. So it was that syncope or sudden death came to be described earlier than anginal pain, while in modern times the concept of angina preceded chronologically that of cardiogenic shock in coronary occlusion. Even circumstantial factors could promote diagnostic acumen, as in the case of Thomas Arnold, a patient whose high intelligence and power of expression helped the physician to establish a correct diagnosis.

13

Personal or historical circumstances sometimes resulted in promoting the diagnostic interest of physicians; diseases in kings and important persons, to which we referred earlier in the cases of King George II, Thorvaldsen, Amatus's abbot, Vesalius's Immersel and many more, also contributed to stimulating curiosity and diagnostic achievement. The occurrence of an increased rate of sudden deaths in Rome at the beginning of the eighteenth century was instrumental in drawing the attention of Lancisi to cardiovascular investigations. The Korean War occasioned the discovery of early coronary sclerosis in autopsies of many young victims, thus broadening our knowledge of the subject. Bearing in mind that such incidental historical constellations are not always available, nor sufficiently exploited, the flow of increased knowledge was not a continuous one, a circumstance partly responsible for the belated and interrupted progress in research.

When, later, the development of clinical medicine, physiology and pathology provided the physician with deeper insight into the morbid condition, progress was at last made. In the expansion of modern knowledge which followed, the old descriptions became obscured and so it seemed that a new disease had come into being.

Not only in modern times has it become necessary to rescue the imposing endeavour of our predecessors from oblivion. Paradoxically enough, the father of medicine, Hippocrates, already had the same task. In his book *On Ancient Medicine* (Chap. 2) he declares that medicine is not a new science, and concludes:

> 'An origin and way have been found out, by which many, and elegant discoveries have been made, during a length of time, and others will yet be found out' (translation by Adams).

Appendix

GALEN

WITHOUT a knowledge of the actual circulation and of the direction of the blood flow in the veins, Galen described the separate blood supply to the heart. He assumed that the coronary vein has the function of nourishing[1] or thickening the heart, while the coronary artery is necessary for 'refreshing'[2] the blood in the vein and in the whole of the heart. He considers that the pulmonary vein is insufficient for this task, so that the heart needs a special supply which is provided by the coronary artery. Galen's idea was taken up by Berengario (1522) and by Colombo (1559), as mentioned in the text, but only Harvey (1649) was able to create the firm physiological basis for his concept of a 'third circulation'.

(a) Galen on the nutritive and 'refreshing' functions of the coronary vessels (translation by M. T. May, I, 325; see also translation into French by Ch. J. Daremberg, I, 446).
$$\textit{De usu partium}, \text{ Book VI, Chapter 17}$$

'Since the substance of the heart is thick and dense and needs thicker nutriment, it is nourished by blood from the vena cava before it enters the heart; for when it arrives there the blood will have to become warm, thin, and spiritous. Now in this connection, although it has seemed unreasonable to some, it will be found to be most logical that the heart prepares nutriment for the lung, but not for itself; for the lung requires thin, spiritous blood, but the heart does not. The heart, being the source of its own movement, must have a strong, thick, dense substance, whereas it was better for the lung to be not heavy and dense, but light and loose-textured, because it is moved by the thorax. Since each viscus uses nutriment similar to itself, it is logical for the heart to require thick blood, and the lung spiritous blood. This is the reason why the heart does not nourish itself, and why before the vena cava is inserted into it, a part just large enough to nourish the heart [*sinus*

---

[1] τρύφειν: to thicken, to congeal, to make grow, to bring up.
[2] αναψυξιν: to cool, to revive by fresh air, to refresh (Liddell and Scott, *Greek–English Lexicon*).

coronarius] branches off to curve round the head [base] of it on the outside and be distributed to all its parts. It is reasonable too that an artery [aa. coronariae] should accompany the vein as it curves around and should branch along with it, and that this should be a branch of the great artery just as large as is necessary for cooling the vein I have just described and for preserving the proper temperament of the innate heat in the outer parts of the heart. The whole body of the heart, which is exceedingly thick and dense, could not be sufficiently cooled by the vessel inserted into it which comes from the lung [v. pulmonalis]. For, as I have also shown in my book On the Natural Faculties, material can penetrate a body itself to a certain small extent, but can go no farther without the help of a broad passageway, and it is for this reason that arteries and veins are all placed at moderate intervals not only in the heart [coronary supply] but also throughout the animal, an arrangement which Nature would not have made if it were possible for material to penetrate very far without a broad passageway.'

(b) On the natural faculties, Book III, Chapter 15 (translation by A. J. Brock, 1928).

On an independent and special coronary blood supply to the heart:
    [p. 321] 'For, the fact that the insertion of the vena cava into the heart is larger than the [p. 322] vein which is inserted into the lungs [pulmonary artery] suggests that not all the blood which the vena cava gives to the heart is driven away again from the heart to the lungs. Nor can it be said that any of the blood is expended in the nourishment of the actual body of the heart, since there is another vein [the coronary vein] which breaks up in it and which does not take its origin nor gets its share of blood from the heart itself.'

On the desirability of a nearby supply of blood to the heart:
    [p. 325] '. . . certain bodies exert attraction along wide channels . . . and attract even from a distance . . . while [others] can only do so from among things which are quite close to them [apparently coronary sinus and vein] . . .. Numerous conduits distributed through the various limbs bring them pure blood, much like the garden water-supply, and, further, the intervals between these conduits have been wonderfully arranged by Nature from the outset so that the intervening parts should be plentifully provided for when absorbing blood, and that they should never [p. 326–27] be deluged by a quantity of superfluous fluid running in at unsuitable times' [coronary flow and its regulation according to requirement?].

THE SUDDEN DEATH OF THE COUNT DE FOIX

(From: Sir John Froissart, *Chronicles*, translated by Thomas Johnes, London, H. G. Bohn, 1849. 2 vols. Vol. 2, pp. 498–99.)

IN this year, [1391], died likewise suddenly, the noble and gallant count de Foix. I will say how it happened. True it is, that of all the pleasures of this world he took most delight in the chase, and was always well provided with hounds of all sorts, having never less than sixteen hundred. The count de Foix was at this season hunting in the forest of Sauveterre, on the road to Pampeluna in Navarre, not far distant from Orthes in Bearn. The day he died, he had all the forenoon been hunting a bear, and it was late in the evening when he was taken and cut up. His attendants asked where he pleased to have his dinner prepared: he said, 'At the inn of Rion, where we will dine, and in the cool of the evening ride to Orthes.' His orders were obeyed. The count with his companions rode a foot's pace towards the village of Rion, and dismounted at the inn. The count went to his chamber, which he found ready strewed with rushes and green leaves; the walls were hung with boughs newly cut for perfume and coolness, as the weather was marvellously hot, even for the month of August. He had no sooner entered this room, than he said, 'These greens are very agreeable to me, for the day has been desperately hot.' When seated he conversed with sir Espaign du Lyon on the dogs that had best hunted; during which conversation his bastard-son sir Evan and sir Peter Cabestan entered the apartment, as the table had been there spread. He called for water to wash, and two squires advanced, Raymonet de Lasne and Raymonet de Copane: Ernaudon d'Espaign took the silver bason, and another knight, called sir Thibeaut, the napkin. The count rose from his seat, and stretched out his hands to wash; but no sooner had his fingers, which were handsome and long, touched the cold water, than he changed colour, from an oppression at his heart, and, his legs failing him, fell back on his seat, exclaiming, 'I am a dead man: Lord God, have mercy on me!' He never spoke after this, though he did not immediately die, but suffered great pain. The knights present and his son were much terrified: they carried him gently in their arms to another chamber, and laid him on a bed covering him well, thinking he was only chilled.

The two squires who had brought water to wash in the bason, said, to free themselves from any charge of having poisoned him, 'Here is the water: we have already drank of it, and will now again in your presence,' which they did, to the satisfaction of all. They put into his mouth bread, water, and spices, with other comforting things, but to no purpose, for in less than half an hour he was dead, having surrendered his soul very quietly. God, out of his grace, was merciful to him.

HEBERDEN

(William Heberden, 'A letter to Dr. Heberden, concerning the Angina Pectoris; and an account of the dissection of one, who had been troubled with this disorder. Read at the College, Nov. 17, 1772.' *Med. Trans. Coll. Physns Lond.*, 1785, **3**, 1–11.)

THIS paper, containing the 'Letter to Dr. Heberden' with his comments is little known and has been reprinted only once, in a paper by Harold N. Segall, 1945. We present it in full on account of the medical, historical, and human qualities displayed.

"Soon after the publication of the second volume of the *Medical Transactions* I received the following anonymous letter.

'SIR
Seeing, among the extracts from the Medical Transactions in the Critical Review of last month, your account of a disorder, which you term the *angina pectoris*, I found it so exactly correspond with what I have experienced of late years, that it determined me to give you such particulars, as I can recollect at those times to have felt; more especially as some sensations have frequently led me to think, that I should meet with a sudden death. I am now in the fifty-second year of my age, of a middling size, a strong constitution, a short neck, and rather inclining to be fat. My pulsations at a medium are about 80 in a minute; the extremes, when in a perfect state of health, beyond which I scarcely ever knew them, 72 and 90. I have enjoyed from my childhood so happy a state of health, as never to have wanted, nor taken, a dose of physic of any kind for more than twenty years: as well as I can recollect, it is about five or six years since, that I first felt the disorder which you treat of; it always attacked me when walking, and always after dinner, or in the evening. I never once felt it in a morning, nor when sitting, nor in bed. I never ride, and seldom use a coach, but it never affected me in one. The first symptom is a pretty full pain in my left arm a little above the elbow; and in

perhaps half a minute it spreads across the left side of my breast, and produces either a little faintness, or a thickness in my breathing; at least I imagined so, but the pain generally obliges me to stop. At first, as you observe, it went off instantaneously, but of late by degrees; and if, through impatience to wait its leaving me entirely, I resumed my walk, the pain returned. I have frequently, when in company, borne the pain, and continued my pace without indulging it; at which times it has lasted from five to perhaps ten minutes, and then gone off, as well as I can recollect, rather suddenly, as it came on, then lessening gradually. Sometimes I have felt it once a week; other times a fortnight, a month, or a longer time, may elapse without its once attacking me; but I think, I am more subject to it in the winter, than in the summer months. As, when the pain left me, I had no traces of having the least disorder within me of any kind, either from spitting blood, or any corrupted matter, nor ever entertained the least thought of any abscess being formed, I never troubled myself much about the cause of it, but attributed it to an obstruction in the circulation, or a species of the rheumatism.

I shall now proceed to acquaint you with those sensations, which to me seem to indicate a sudden death; but which, not being concomitant with the above mentioned disorder, I am ignorant whether they are to be attributed to it or not. I have often felt, when sitting, standing, and at times in my bed, what I can best express by calling it an universal pause within me of the operations of nature for perhaps three or four seconds; and when she has resumed her functions, I felt a shock at the heart, like that which one would feel from a small weight being fastened by a string to some part of the body, and falling from the table to within a few inches of the floor. At times it will return two or three times in half an hour; at other times not once a week; and sometimes I do not feel it for a long time; and I think I have been less subject to it for a year past, than for several former ones. As you have mentioned several, who within your knowledge have died suddenly, that were troubled with the *angina pectoris*, I suspect they were subject to what I have delineated, as I think that much more likely to occasion a sudden death, than either of the causes to which you attribute it. But be the cause, what it may, if it please God to take me away suddenly, I have left directions in my will to send an account of my death to you, with a permission for you to order such an examination of my body, as will shew the cause of it; and, perhaps, tend at the same time to a discovery of the origin of that disorder, which is the subject of this letter, and be productive of means to counteract and remove it.

I am, Sir, Yours,
UNKNOWN.'

London, April 16, 1772.

The foregoing letter seems to have been written in such a sensible and natural manner, that the writer would probably neither mistake his own feelings through fancy, nor misrepresent them through affectation; and therefore I judged it worthy to be communicated to the College, both in justice to the temper and judgement of the author, and as a just and original picture of this disorder.

In less than three weeks after he had sent this letter, I was informed, that in the midst of a walk, which he was taking after dinner, he leaned against a post, and begged a passenger to assist him, by whose help he reached a neighbouring house, where he vomited much; and was bled, but died in less than half an hour. At the same time I was acquainted, that, by a paper found in his will, if he died suddenly, he had desired, that I might immediately have notice of it, in order to have the body opened and examined. I used my best endeavours, that such a benevolent intention should not be frustrated, by procuring that experienced and accurate anatomist Mr. J. Hunter to open the body, which was done within 48 hours after his decease. But upon the most careful examination no manifest cause of his death could be discovered: the seat of the disease having been, as we may suppose, in some of those parts, the functions of which being not well understood in life, we can find no traces of their differences after death.

In general the viscera were well formed, and in a sound state, with marks of great robustness. The contents of the thorax were examined with peculiar attention, particularly the heart with its vessels and valves, and were all found to be in a natural condition, except some few specks of a beginning ossification upon the aorta, and some adhesions of the lungs to the pleura on the left side. The left ventricle of the heart was remarkably strong and thick, and as perfectly empty of blood, as if it had been washed. Nothing extraordinary could be perceived in the brain, unless that there was rather more water in the ventricles, than is common for such an age. It was very remarkable, that the blood was nowhere coagulated, and did not coagulate even after being more than two hours exposed to the air; but at the same time could not be called perfectly fluid; being of the consistence of thin cream; but there was no separation of any of its component parts.

This anatomical examination, for which I acknowledge myself much indebted to the manly sense and benevolent spirit of this worthy man, though it do not inform us, what the cause of the disease was, will however have its use by informing us what it was not. For since it was not owing to any mal-conformation, or morbid destruction of parts necessary to life, we need not despair of finding a cure: and as there were no appearances of inflammation or scirrhus or abscess, which in the former volume I mention as possible causes; we must not seek the remedy in bleeding and purging, and lowering the strength, but rather in the opposite class of medicines, which are usually called nervous and cordial, such as relieve and quiet convulsive motions, and invigorate the languishing principle of life.

The sensation, described in the letter, of an apparent suspension of life for a few seconds, is what I do not remember to have ever heard mentioned by any patient besides this; and though I say in the former paper upon this disorder, that I have seen it in twenty persons, I may truly say, that I have seen it in fifty. In this particular case, that universal pause of the vital actions is said to have been felt, when the patient was sitting, standing, and at times in his bed. Now as he was seized while he was walking with those symptoms, which ended in his death (which I remember to have happened to others of his fellow sufferers) it may seem probable, that he lost his life rather by an extraordinary aggravation of the *angina pectoris*, than of this particular sensation: but this must be decided by future experience."

VULPIAN

(Myocardial infarction as described and named by Vulpian in 1866, translated from the French, *L'Union Médicale*, 1866, n.s., **29**, 417–19.)

"SUMMARY of case 1. Old cerebral softening with speech disorder.—Recent cerebral softening.—Old clot in the left auricle.—Infarct of the left ventricular wall of the heart coincident with the presence of an old clot in one of the coronary arteries.—Rupture of this infarct into the cavity of the ventricle and into the pericardial cavity.—Haemorrhage into the pericardial cavity.

> Cases presented to the Medical Society of the Hospitals on 24th January 1866.
> By Monsieur Vulpian, physician to the Salpêtrière.

Case 1.—A female patient C., admitted to the Salpêtrière in the middle of the year 1865 [1864?] had, during the previous two years, suffered from a mild attack of apoplexy, which had resulted in slight weakness of the right upper and lower limbs, with complete loss of speech for a few moments. Although speech was regained, it remained difficult and the right hand showed signs of paralysis and numbness. On the 2nd of January 1865, she was admitted to the Infirmary, then being 75 years of age. She had just had a very severe attack of dizziness, without total loss of consciousness. She was still able to stand. The left arm was very limp, she was hardly able to move it. On the other hand, she was freely able to use her right arm, and only from information obtained from a member of the family did we know that this arm had been somewhat weak before this last attack. Speech was still more difficult than previously.

The next day she was much better. Her left arm had regained some of its strength and she was able to speak without too much difficulty. By the following day she had practically returned to her previous state. She had some difficulty in finding words, but in general, was able to speak quite well and make herself understood.

On the 7th January, about 6 o'clock in the morning, the nurse noticed that the patient was not sleeping naturally. She spoke to her and realized that she was in a profound coma. It was in this state that I found her at the moment of my arrival. There was complete paralysis of the left side. The left cheek was blown out at each expiration. Death took place the following night.

The post-mortem was carried out on the 9th of January 1865. Extensive areas of softening were found in the brain, dating from very different periods. I do not intend to enlarge on these findings. I will

only mention that among the early lesions there was extensive softening of the second and third convolution of the left side and among the
recent lesions, softening of the third convolution of the right side and
of the adjacent part of the convolutions of the insula.

I now come to the very remarkable lesion that I found in the heart.
On opening the pericardium, it was found to contain a large mass of
blackish, clotted blood, weighing 250 grams. There had apparently
been a rupture, either of the heart itself, or of the great vessels. At
first glance the site of this rupture could not be seen, but close examination showed, on the lateral wall of the left ventricle, just by the auriculo-
ventricular sulcus, a small pink spot, in the middle of which a slight
erosion could be seen. On pressing the ventricular wall below this
point between the fingers, a drop of half-coagulated black blood
emerged. This thus appeared to be the place from which the blood
had escaped. The ventricle was then opened but one could not immediately see, on the internal surface of the ventricle, the orifice of
communication between the above rupture and the ventricular cavity.
Only after lifting up a number of the trabeculae with the scissors,
could one recognize this internal orifice, at a level much lower than
that of the external opening. It was also very small and consisted,
just as the internal orifice, of an erosion of tissue. A probe could be
easily passed between the internal and external orifices, following
an oblique path extending more than two centimetres within the
ventricular wall. On opening the portion of the wall which was raised
by the probe, a flattened cavity could be seen hollowed out within the
ventricular wall. The walls of the cavity were constituted by the
muscular tissue of the heart; but here the tissue was softened and of a
brownish-reddish colour. With the back of the scalpel one could
remove the debris of the internal layer of this altered tissue.

The coronary arteries were carefully examined and the left artery
was found to contain a clot, evidently old, discoloured, and somewhat
granular in appearance. This was situated in a limited section of the
artery, where the vessel showed very marked atheromatous changes.
At this point the artery was completely obliterated for a distance of at
least half a centimetre. Above and below this point there were practically no changes in the vessel walls and the lumen was completely un-
obstructed.

In the left auricle there was an old clot of the size of a large nut
adherent to the endocardium. Most of this clot was decolorized and
was slightly softened and granular in appearance.

In this case conditions were thus favourable for the production of
arterial emboli. The arteries at the base of the brain were not examined

with sufficient care, so that we cannot say whether any important branches were obliterated.

As to the clot found in the coronary artery, I am not able to say whether this was due to an embolism, or whether it was a result of thrombosis or clotting on the spot. The atheromatous change in the section of the artery in contact with the clot is an argument in favour of the second mode of clot formation. But, in this actual case, it seems to me that the question does not allow of final solution.

In any case, the lesion of the heart wall appears to me to have been produced by the obliteration of this artery. There was very probably an infarct of the heart wall, which became softened and at a certain moment, perhaps during the last instants of life, due to powerful contractions of the heart, this focus, which was separated by a very fine layer of muscle tissue from the ventricular cavity and from the external surface, became opened at both these points: first into the ventricular cavity, then due to the pressure of the blood, into the pericardial cavity; thus giving rise to the haemorrhage within this cavity.

Microscopic examination of the softened tissue taken from the walls of this focus of softening in the heart showed torn muscle fibres, fatty granules and a few granular bodies."

List of Historical Surveys

A BIBLIOGRAPHY of surveys of the various topics in this volume, as far as could be traced in the literature (see third paragraph of our Preface).

Some are restricted in time coverage, while in others the subject matter is focused on a particular field, such as pathology, treatment or illustration. Also included are surveys on allied topics, such as arterial sclerosis or embolism in general. All these items have made some contribution to the history of coronary heart disease.

Items included in the main bibliography are marked by asterisks and presented in the form of short-title entries.

Benson, R. L. 'The present status of coronary artery disease.' *Arch. Path. Lab. Med.*, 1926, **2**, 876–916.

Brummer, P. 'Is angina pectoris a new disease?' *Nord. medhist. Årsb.*, 1968, 55–58.

Buess, Heinrich. 'Marksteine in der Entwicklung der Lehre von der Thrombose und Embolie.' *Gesnerus (Aarau)*, 1955, **12**, 157–89.

Cohn, Bernhard. *Klinik der Embolischen Gefässerkrankungen.* Berlin, A. Hirschwald, 1860. (Historical survey of embolism in general, pp. 1–39).

Cowdry, E. V. (Ed.). *Arterio-sclerosis, a Survey of the Problem.* London and New York, Macmillan, 1933.

*Danon, J. *The History of Angina Pectoris, etc.*, 1960.

Desportes, E. H. *Traité de l'Angine de Poitrine.* Paris, Crapelet, 1811.

*Dock, George. 'Historical notes etc.', 1939.

*Dock, William. 'Research in arteriosclerosis', 1958. 'Myocardial infarction, etc.', 1962.

*East, T. *The Story of Heart Disease*, 1958. (Lecture 3, The coronary circulation and its disorders, pp. 95–126.)

Gilbert, N. C. 'History of the treatment of coronary heart disease.' *J. Amer. med. Ass.*, 1952, **148**, 1372–76 (43 refs.).

*Herrick, J. B. *A Short History of Cardiology*, 1942.

*Huchard, H. *Traité clinique des Maladies du Coeur et de l'Aorte.* 3rd ed., 1899–1903, 3 vols. See II, 523–77.

Kahn, R. H. 'Zur Frage nach der Wirkung des Verschlusses der

Koronararterien des Herzens.' *Pflügers Arch. ges. Physiol.*, 1916, **163**, 506–10.

*Klemperer, P. 'The history of coronary sclerosis', 1960. (103 refs.)

*Kowal, S. J. 'Emotions and angina pectoris', 1960.

Krumbhaar, E. B. 'History of the Pathology of the Heart.' *In*: Gould, S. E. (Ed.), *Pathology of the Heart*, 2nd ed. Springfield, Ill., Thomas, 1960.

Laubry, C. *In*: 'Ce que la France a apporté à la Médecine depuis le Debut de XXe siècle.' (On cardiology: pp. 175–98, passim). Paris, Flammarion, 1943.

Levene, Arnold. 'Spontaneous rupture of the heart: a historical review.' *Postgrad. med. J.*, 1962, **38**, 334–37.

*Levine, Samuel A. *Coronary Thrombosis*, etc., 1929. (Historical data, pp. 2–7).

Lunedi, A. 'Considerazioni sulla sviluppo storico delle conoscenze nel campo delle cardiopatie dolorose da alterata circolazione coronarica. Lezione Prima. L'angina di petto ai tempi di Heberden nel cinquatennio 1768–1818.' *Riv. crit. clin. Med.*, 1964, **64**, 5–22.

Mattingly, Thomas W. 'Changing concepts of myocardial diseases (Chairman's Address).' *J. Amer. med. Ass.*, 1965, **191**, 33–37.

*Morgan, A. D. 'Some forms, etc.', 1968.

Mulcahy, R. 'The views of the nineteenth century Irish cardiologists on coronary artery disease.' *Irish J. med. Sci.*, 1963, ser. 6, No. 445, 35–44.

*Osler, W. *Lectures on Angina Pectoris*, etc., 1897. (History, pp. 1–8.)

Parrish, H. M. 'Has mankind always had coronary heart disease?' *J. Indiana med. Ass.*, 1962, **55**, 464–71.

Pazzini, A. 'Storia dell' infarto del miocardio.' *Pagine Storia Med.*, 1959, **3** (i), 5–9.

Rolleston, Humphry D. *History of Cardiovascular Diseases since Harvey's Discovery*, Cambridge Univ. Press, 1928. (passim).

— 'History of Angina Pectoris.' Ninth Finlayson Memorial Lecture. Repr. from *Glasgow med. J.*, Glasgow, 1937.

Royal College of Physicians: Pectoris Dolor. Catalogue of exhibition, prepared mainly by D. Evan Bedford. [1968.]

Schimert, G. *In*: *Handb. d. inn. Med.*, (Bergmann-Frey-Schwiegk), 4te Aufl., Bd.G (Herz u. Gefässe), Teil 3. Berlin-Göttingen-Heidelberg, 1960; pp. 653–57.

Schnebli, Margaret, 'Herzruptur und Herzinfarkt in historischer und aktueller Sicht.' *Schweiz. med. Wschr.*, 1957, **87**, 885–89.

Schott, A. 'Historical notes on the iconography of the heart.' *Cardiologia (Basel)*, 1956, **28**, 229–68.

*Schrenk, Martin. 'Die angina pectoris', 1967.

Smith, Thomas H. F. 'A chronology of atherosclerosis.' *Amer. J. Pharm.*, 1960, **132**, 390–405.

Snow, P. J. D. 'The early history of coronary disease.' *Manch. Univ. med. Sch. Gaz.*, 1955, **34**, 83–88.

Steven, J. L. 'Fibroid degeneration and allied lesions of the heart and their association with disease of the coronary arteries.' *Lancet*, 1887, **2**, 1153–56, 1205–8, 1255–57, 1305–57 (contains historical survey).

*Tiedemann, Friedrich. *Von der Verengung, etc.*, 1843. (See chapter on the history of arterial occlusion.)

Tortora, A. R. 'A brief history of the coronary vessels, coronary occlusion and the ECG.' (reprinted from) *N.Y. Phys.* 1958, March, (3 pp.).

Vierordt, Hermann. 'Todesursachen im Aerztlichen Stande' (passim). Stuttgart, Enke, 1926.

*Warburg, E. J. 'Ueber den Coronarkreislauf, etc.' 1930. (History, see pp. 439–59. Refs: see pp. 591–604.)

White, Paul D. 'The evolution of our knowledge about the heart and its diseases since 1928.' *Circulation* (*N.Y.*), 1957, **15**, 915–23.

Willius, F. A. 'Coronary Disease: certain significant contributions made during the last quarter century.' *Minn. Med.*, 1943, **26**, 33–40.

— 'The historic development etc.', 1945–46.

*Wrigley, P. F. M. 'Ischaemic heart disease etc.', 1965.

Bibliography

Abravanel, Isaac. *Commentary on the Earlier Prophets* (Hebr.), Pesaro, G. Soncino, *c.* 1511.

Adams, Robert. 'Cases of diseases of the heart accompanied with pathological observations.' *Dublin Hosp. Rep.*, 1827, 4, 353–453.

Aetius Amidenus. *Contractae ex Veteribus Medicinae Tetrabiblos*, [Latin translation by] Janus Cornarius. fol. Basle, H. Froben and N. Bischoff, 1542.

Ahrens, E. H. *Jr.* 'Nutritional factors and serum lipid levels.' *Amer. J. Med.*, 1957, 23, 928–52.

Aldabi, Meir. *Shevileh Emuna* (The Paths of Faith). Riva di Trento, Markeria for Madruzzo, 1559.

Alexander Trallianus, *Alexander von Tralles*. Original-Text und Uebersetzung von T. Puschmann [Greek and German text]. 2 vols. Vienna, W. Braunmüller, 1878–79. Reprinted Amsterdam, Hakkert, 1963.

Albertinus, H. F. 'Animadversiones Super Quibusdam Difficilis Respirationis Vitiis a Laesa Cordis, et Praecordiorum Structura Pendentibus'. *In: De Bononiensi Scientiarum et Artium Instituto atque Academia Commentarii*, tomus I, Bononiae, ex typ. Laelii a Vulpe, 1731, pp. 382–404. —Edited by M. H. Romberg, Berlin, A. Hirschwald, 1828.

Allbutt, T. C. *Diseases of the Arteries including Angina Pectoris*. 2 vols. London, Macmillan, 1915.

Amatus Lusitanus. *Curationum Medicinalium Centuria Sexta*, Venice, Valgrisius, 1560.

Anglo-Saxon Medical Manuscript, Wellcome MS. 46.

Anitschkow, N. and Chalatow, S. 'Ueber experimentelle Cholesterinsteatose.' *Zbl. allg. Path. path. Anat.*, 1913, 24, 1–9.

Aretaeus Cappadox. 'Αρεταιου καππα δοκον τα δωξομενα. Edited and translated by Francis Adams. London, Sydenham Society, 1856.

— *Traité des Signes, des Causes et de la Cure des Maladies aigues et chroniques.* Translated, with notes, by M. L. Renaud. Paris, Lagny, 1834.

Aristotle. *The Works of Aristotle.* Translated into English under the Editorship of W. D. Ross and J. A. Smith. Vol. IV. *Historia Animalium.* Translated by D'Arcy W. Thompson. Oxford, Clarendon Press, 1910.

Avicenna (Ibn Sina). *The Canon of Medicine.* [Arabic original] fol. Rome, Typographia Medicea 1593. Canon Libri i–v (translation into Latin by Gerard of Cremona); 1st ed. fol. Milan, Ph. de Lavagna, 1476. Hebrew translation by Nathan Meati and J. Lorki, fol. Naples, Gunzenhauser,

1491–92. English translation of the 1st book by O. C. Gruner, London, Luzac, 1930. Russian translation, Usbek S.S.R. Academy of Science, Tashkent, 1954–60.

Bailey, C. H. 'Atheroma and other lesions produced in rabbits by cholesterol feeding.' *J. exp. Med.*, 1916, **23**, 69–85.

Baillie, Matthew. *The Morbid Anatomy of some of the Most Important Parts of the Human Body.* London, J. Johnson & G. Nicol, 1793.

Baly, William. 'Rupture of the heart consequent on fatty degeneration, associated with softening of the brain.' *Trans. path. Soc. Lond.*, 1850–52, **3**, 264–69.

Baron, John. *The Life of Edward Jenner.* 2 vols. London, H. Colburn, 1838.

Bartoletti, F. *Methodus in Dyspnoeam.* Bologna, Tebaldini for Heirs of Dozza, 1633.

Basch, S. von. 'Ueber die Messung des Blutdrucks am Menschen.' *Z. klin. Med.*, 1880, **2**, 79–96.

— *Die Herzkrankheiten bei Arteriosklerose.* Berlin, A. Hirschwald, 1901 (see especially pp. 306–36).

Bauhinus, Caspar. *Theatrum Anatomicum.* Frankfurt, M. Becker, 1605.

Baumgarten, W. 'Infarction in the heart.' *Amer. J. Physiol.* 1899, **2**, 243–72.

Bäumler, Christian. 'Cases of partial and general idiopathic pericarditis.' *Trans. clin. Soc. Lond.*, 1872, **5**, 8–22.

Bayliss, W. M., and Starling, E. H. 'On the electromotive phenomena of the mammalian heart.' *Int. Mschr. Anat. Physiol.*, 1892, **9**, 256–81.

Bean, W. B. 'Clinical masquerades of acute myocardial infarction.' *J. Iowa St. med. Soc.*, 1962, **52**, 781–83.

Beck, Claude. 'Development of new blood supply to heart by operation.' *Ann. Surg.*, 1935, **102**, 801–13.

Bedford, D. Evan, see also Parkinson and Bedford.

— 'Coronary thrombosis.' *Practitioner*, 1933, **130**, 670–83.

— 'William Heberden's contribution to cardiology.' *J. roy. Coll. Physns Lond.*, 1968, **2**, 127–35.

— 'Harvey's third circulation. De circulo sanguinis in corde.' *Brit. med. J.*, 1968, **4**, 273–77.

Beith, Dr. 'Malformations and diseases of the heart and circulating organs. Rupture of the septum ventriculorum extending through the walls of the right ventricle.' *Trans. path. Soc. Lond.*, 1850–1852, **3**, 69–71. [Connection between obstruction of the coronary artery and local 'fatty degeneration'.]

Bell, Charles. *Engravings of the Arteries.* London, Longman, 1804.

Bellini, Lorenzo. *De Urinis et Pulsibus . . . de Morbis Capitis, et Pectoris, etc.* Bologna, Heirs of A. Pisarrius, 1683.

Belt, Elmer. *Leonardo the Anatomist.* Lawrence, Kansas, University of Kansas Press, 1955.

— 'Thirty-three anatomic firsts of Leonardo da Vinci.' *Spectrum*, (*Pfizer*), 1966, **14**, 79–81.

Benivieni, Antonio. *De Abditis Nonnulis ac Mirandis Morborum et Sanationum Causis*. [Facsimile reprint of the 1507 edition] translated by C. Singer, prefaced by E. R. Long. Springfield, Ill., Thomas, 1954.

Berengarius, Jacobus, *Carpensis*. *Isagoge Breves etc*. Bologna, B. Hectoris,1522.

— *A Short Introduction to Anatomy*. Translated by L. R. Lind. Chicago, Univ. of Chicago Press, 1959.

Bezold, Albert von. 'Von den Veränderungen des Herzschlages nach Verschliessung der Coronar-arterien.' *Unters. physiol. Lab. Würzburg*, 1867, **2**, 256–87.

Bichat, François Xavier. *Anatomie générale appliquée à la Physiologie et à la Médecine*. 4 vols. Paris, Brosson, Gabon et Cie, 1801.

Biernacki, E. 'Ueber die Beziehung des Plasmas zu den roten Blutkörperchen etc.' *Z. physiol. Chem.*, 1894, **19**, 179–224.

Bissing, F. W. von. *Denkmäler Aegyptischer Sculptur*. 3 vols. Munich, F. Bruckmann, 1914.

Black, Samuel. 'Case of angina pectoris, with remarks.' *Mem. med. Soc., Lond.*, 1795, **4**, 261–79.

— 'A case of angina pectoris, with a dissection [read in 1796].' *Mem. med. Soc. Lond.*, 1805, **6**, 41–49.

Blackall, John. *Observations on the Nature and Cure of Dropsies . . . to Which is Added an Appendix, containing Several Cases of Angina Pectoris, with Dissections*. London, Longman, 1813.

Blumer, George. 'Pericarditis epistenocardica.' *J. Amer. med. Ass.*, 1936, **107**, 178–81.

Bober, S. 'Coronary embolism' (letter to the Editor). *J. Amer. med. Ass.*, 1954, **155**, 775.

Bonet, T. *Sepulchretum, sive Anatomia Practica, ex Cadaveribus Morbo Denatis*. 3 vols. fol. Geneva, Chouët, 1679; 2nd ed. by Mangetus, Geneva and Lyons, Cramer and Perachon, 1700.

Booth, C. C. 'Dr. John Fothergill and the angina pectoris.' *Med. Hist.*, 1957, **I**, 115–22.

Bousfield, G. 'Angina pectoris. changes in the electrocardiogram during a paroxysm.' *Lancet*, 1918, **ii**, 457–58.

Bramwell, Byron. *Diseases of the Heart and Thoracic Aorta*. Edinburgh, Pentland, 1884.

Breasted, J. H. *The Edwin Smith Surgical Papyrus*. 2 vols. Chicago, University of Chicago Press, 1930.

Brown, K. W. *et al*. 'Coronary unit: an intensive-care centre for acute myocardial infarction.' *Lancet*, 1963, **ii**, 349–52.

Bruetsch, W. L. 'The earliest record of sudden death possibly due to atherosclerotic coronary occlusion.' *Circulation*, 1959, **20**, 438–41.

Brunton, T. Lauder. 'On the use of nitrite of amyl in angina pectoris.' *Lancet*, 1867, **ii**, 97–98.

Bryan, Cyril P. *The Papyrus Ebers*. Translated from the German version [of H. Joachim]. London, Bles, 1930.

Budge, E. A. Wallis. *Egyptian Magic*. London, Kegan Paul, 1899.

Burch, G. E. and De Pasquale, N. P. *A History of Electrocardiography*. Chicago, Year Book Medical Publishers, 1964.

Burchell, H. B., and Keys, T. E. 'The heart of George II of England.' *Bull. med. Libr. Ass.*, 1942, **30**, 198–202.

Burdon-Sanderson, J., and Page, F. J. M. 'Experimental results relating to the rhythmical and excitatory motions of the ventricle of the heart of the frog, and of the electrical phenomena which accompany them.' *Proc. roy. Soc. Lond.*, 1878, **27**, 410–14.

Burns, Allan. *Observations on some of the Most Frequent and Important Diseases of the Heart*. Edinburgh, T. Bryce, 1809.

Butter, William. *A Treatise on the Disease Commonly Called Angina Pectoris*. London, J. Johnson, 1791.

Cabanès, A. *Le Cabinet secret de l'Histoire*. 3rd ed. Paris, A. Michel, 1920.

Caelius Aurelianus. *On Acute Diseases and on Chronic Diseases*. Edited and translated by I. E. Drabkin, Chicago, University of Chicago Press, 1950.

Calabresi, M. 'J. M. Lancisi and "De Subitaneis Mortibus".' *In*: Essays in the History of Medicine, presented to Professor Arturo Castiglioni. Suppl. to *Bull. Hist. Med.* No. 3, 1944, 48–54.

Cariage, J. L. 'Les premières descriptions d'angine de poitrine: Lord Hyde, Comte de Clarendon, Nicolas-François Rougnon, William Heberden.' *J. Med. Lyon*, 1960, **41**, 437–50.

Cassius Felix. *De Medicina*. Ed. by Valentin Rose. Leipzig, Teubner, 1879.

Castellus, Bartholomaeus. *Totius Artis Medicae Methodo Divisiva Compendium et Synopsis*. Messina, P. Brea, 1597.

Celsus. *De Medicina*. Translated by W. G. Spencer (Loeb Classical Library), 3 vols. London, Heinemann, and Cambridge, Mass., Harvard University Press, 1935–38.

Chamberlaine, John. *Imitations of Original Designs by Leonardo da Vinci*. London, G. Nicol, 1796.

Chevalier, H. 'Blockpnoea on effort in emphysematous patients—a diagnostic challenge (Editorial).' *Amer. Heart J.*, 1967, **73**, 579–81.

Chirac, Pierre. *De Motu Cordis Adversaria Analytica*. Montpellier, J. Martel, 1698.

Clarendon, Edward Hyde, 1st Earl of. *The Life of Edward Earl of Clarendon, written by Himself*. Oxford, Clarendon Press, 1759.

Cohnheim, J., and v. Schulthess-Rechberg, A. 'Ueber die Folgen der Kranzarterienverschliessung für das Herz.' *Virchows Arch. path. Anat.*, 1881, **85**, 503–37.

Cohnheim, Julius. *Vorlesungen ueber Allgemeine Pathologie*, 2nd ed., 2 vols. Berlin, Hirschwald, 1882. English translation, London, New Sydenham Society, 1889.

— *Gesammelte Abhandlungen*, Berlin, Hirschwald, 1885.

Columbus, M. Realdus. *De Re Anatomica Libri XV*. Venice, Bevilacqua, 1559.

Corvisart, J. N. *Essai sur les Maladies et les Lesions organiques du Coeur et des Gros Vaisseaux*. Paris, Migneret, 1806.

Councilman, W. T. 'On the relations between arterial disease and tissue organs.' *Trans. Ass. Amer. Physns*, 1891, **6**, 179–99.

Cowper, William. 'Of ossifications and petrifactions in the coats of arteries, particularly in the valves of the great artery.' *Phil. Trans.*, 1705, **24** 1970–77.

Craigie, D. *Elements of General and Pathological Anatomy*. Edinburgh, A. Black, 1828.

Crell, Johann F. 'Dissertatio de Arteria Coronaria Instar Ossis Indurata Observatio' (1740). *In*: A. Haller, *Disputationes ad Morborum Historiam et Curationem Facientes*. Vol. II Ad Morbos Pectoris. Lausanne, Bousquet, 1757.

Cruveilhier, J. *Anatomie pathologique du Corps Humain*. 3 vols. Paris, J. B. Baillière, 1829–1842.

Czermak, J. N. 'Beschreibung und mikroskopische Untersuchung zweier ägyptischer Mumien.' *Sber. Akad. Wiss. Wien, Math.-naturw. Kl.*, 1852, **9**, 427–69.

Dahl-Iversen, E. 'Sir John Erichsen, a 19th century heart experimentalist.' *Acta chir. Scand.*, 1961, Suppl. 283, 1–7.

Danon, J. *The History of Angina Pectoris and Myocardial Infarction* [Hebrew with English summary]. Thesis, Jerusalem, 1960.

Day, H. W. 'The effectiveness of an intensive coronary care area.' *Amer. J. Cardiol.*, 1965, **15**, 51–54.

Deines, H. v., Grapow, H., Westendorf, W. 'Uebersetzung der Medizinischen Texte.' *In*: *Grundriss der Medizin der Alten Aegypter*, IV, 1. Berlin, Akademie-Verlag, 1955.

— 'Uebersetzung der Medizinischen Texte.' Erläuterungen, IV, 2, ibid. 1958.

Diversus, Petrus Salius. *De Febre Pestilenti Tractatus, et Curationes Quorundam Particularium Morborum, etc.* Frankfurt, Heirs of A. Wechel, 1586.

Dock, George. *Notes on the Coronary Arteries*. Ann Arbor, Michigan, The Inland Press, 1896;

— 'Historical notes on coronary occlusion: from Heberden to Osler.' *J. Amer. med. Ass.*, 1939, **113**, 563–68.

Dock, William. 'Research in arteriosclerosis—the first fifty years (Editorial).' *Ann. intern. Med.*, 1958, **49**, 699–705.

— 'Myocardial infarction becomes emeritus (Editorial).' *Circulation*, 1962, **26**, 481–83.

Donatus, Marcellus. *De Medica Historia Mirabili Libri Sex*. Venice, Valgrisius, 1588 (1st ed. 1586).

Dressler, William. 'The post-myocardial-infarction-syndrome.' *Arch. intern. Med.*, 1959, **103**, 28–42.

Dreyfuss, F. 'The incidence of myocardial infarction in various communities in Israel.' *Amer. Heart J.*, 1953, **45**, 749–55.

Du Bois-Reymond, E. *Untersuchungen ueber Thierische Elektricität*. 2 vols. Berlin, Reimer, 1848–84.

Düben, G. W. J., see Malmsten and Düben.

Dupuytren, G. *Leçons orales de Clinique chirurgicale*. vol. III, 2nd ed. Brussels Soc. Encylogr. des Sciences Méd., 1839.

Duretus, Ludovicus. *In*: Hollerius, Jacobus, *De Morbis Internis Liber, Auctoris Scholiis Illustratus, et L. Dureti Scolis [sic] . . . Auctus*. Paris, Ex off. Plantiniana. Apud A. Perrier, 1611.

East, C. F. Terence. *The Story of Heart Disease*. London, Dawson, *c.* 1958.

Ebbell, B. *The Papyrus Ebers, the Greatest Egyptian Medical Document*. Copenhagen, Munksgaard, 1937.

Ebers, G. *Papyros Ebers, das Hermetische Buch ueber die Arzneimittel der Alten Aegypter in Hieratischer Schrift*. Mit hieroglyphisch-lateinischem Glossar von Ludwig Stern (vol. II), 2 vols. Leipzig, Engelmann, 1875.

Ebner, A. 'Edme-Félix-Alfred Vulpian 1826–1887.' *Zürch. med. gesch. Abhandl.*, N.R. No. 49, Zürich, Juris, 1967.

Editorial: 'Testimony of the past.' *J. Amer. med. Ass.*, 1966, **197**, 723.

Ehrenfeld, E. N., Gery, I, and Davies, A. M. 'Specific antibodies in heart disease.' *Lancet*, 1961, **i**, 1138–41.

Einthoven, Willem. 'Ueber das normale menschliche Elektrokardiogramm und ueber die kapillar-elektrische Untersuchung einiger Herzkranken.' *Pflüg. Arch. ges. Physiol.*, 1900, **80**, 139–60.

— 'Die galvanometrische Registrierung des menschlichen Elektrokardiogramms, zugleich eine Beurteilung der Anwendung des Capillar-Elektrometers in der Physiologie.' *Pflüg. Arch. ges. Physiol.*, 1903, **99**, 472–80.

Engelmann, T. W. 'Ueber das elektrische Verhalten des thätigen Herzens.' *Pflüg. Arch. ges. Physiol.*, 1878, **17**, 68–99.

Enos, W. F., Holmes, R. H., and Beyer, J. 'Coronary disease among U.S. soldiers killed in action in Korea.' *J. Amer. med. Ass.*, 1953, **152**, 1090–1093.

Erichsen, John. 'On the influence of the coronary circulation on the action of the heart.' *Lond. med. Gaz.*, 1842, N.S., **2**, 561–64.

Esso, I. van. 'L'angine de poitrine est-elle mentionnée dans la Bible et le Talmud?' *Rev. Hist. méd. Hébr.*, 1954, **7**, 173–78.

Fåhraeus, R. 'The suspension-stability of the blood'. *Act. med. Scand.*, 1921, Supplement, **55**, 1–228.

Falconer, William. 'On morbus cardiacus.' *Mem. med. Soc. Lond.*, 1805, **6**, 1–40.

Falloppius, Gabriel. *Observationes Anatomicae*. Paris, B. Turrisanus, 1562. (1st edition, 1561.)

Fernel, Jean. *Universa Medicina*. Paris, A. Wechel, 1567.

Fishman, A. P., and Richards, D. W. (Eds.). *Circulation of the Blood: Men and Ideas*. New York, Oxford University Press, 1964.

Forbes, John, see Laënnec.

Forestus, Petrus. *Observationum . . . Liber* **17**, *De Cordis . . . Affectibus.* Leyden, Plantin, 1593.

Fothergill, John. 'Case of angina pectoris with remarks.' *Med. Obsns Inquir.*, 1776, **5**, 233–51.

— 'Farther account of the angina pectoris'. *Med. Obsns Inquir.*, 1776, **5**, 252–58.

Fox, R. Hingston. *William Hunter, Anatomist, Physician, Obstetrician (1718–1783).* London, Lewis, 1901.

Frati, Carlo. *Bibliografia Malpighiana.* Milan, 1897. [Photo-lithograph, Dawsons, London, 1960.]

Freind, John. *The History of Physick.* Part II, 2nd ed. London, J. Walthoe, 1727.

Froissart, John. *Chronicles of England, France, Spain, etc.* Translated from the French editions etc. by Thomas Johnes. 2 vols. London, Bohn, 1849.

Galen. Greek text with Latin translation by K. G. Kühn. 20 vols. (in 22), Leipzig, Cnobloch, 1821–1833.

— *De Anatomicis Administrationibus.* Translated into English by Charles Singer. London, Wellcome Historical Medical Museum, 1956.

— *On the Natural Faculties.* Translated into English by A. J. Brock, Loeb Classical Library, Heinemann, London, and Harvard University Press, 1916.

— *Oeuvres anatomiques-physiologiques et médicales de Galien.* Translated by Charles Daremberg, 2 vols. Paris, Baillière, 1854–1856.

— *Galen on the Usefulness of the Parts of the Body.* Translated by Margaret T. May, 2 vols., Cornell University Press, Ithaca, New York, 1968.

Gallavardin, M. Louis, 'Y-a-t-il un équivalent nondouloureux de l'angine de poitrine?' *Lyon méd.*, 1924, **133–34**, 345–58.

— 'Les syndromes d'effort dans les affections cardio-aortiques.' *J. Méd. Lyon*, 1933, **14**, 539–67.

Galvani, L. A. 'De Viribus Electricitatis in Motu Musculari Commentarius.' *In: De Bononiensi Scientiarum et Artium. Instituto atque Academia Commentarii*, tomus VII. Bologna, Typogr. Inst. Scientiarum, 1791, pp. 363–418.

Garengeot, R.-J.-C. 'Une observation singulière sur des parties musculeuses, ossifiées, ou sur un os trouvé dans le coeur.' *Histoire de l'Académie Royale des Sciences*, 1726, 24–25 (published in 1728).

Garrison, F. H. *An Introduction to the History of Medicine.* 4th edition. Philadelphia, Saunders, 1929.

Genty, M. 'Jean Cruveilhier.' *Rev. mensuelle illustr.*, 1934.

Ghalioungui, P. *Magic and Medical Science in Ancient Egypt.* London, Hodder & Stoughton, 1963.

Goble, A. J., Sloman, G., and Robinson, J. S. 'Mortality reduction in a coronary care unit.' *Brit. med. J.*, 1966, **i**, 1005–9.

Gorlin, R., Brachfeld, N., MacLeod, C., and Bopp, P. 'Effect of nitroglycerin on the coronary circulation in patients with coronary artery disease.' *Circulation*, 1959, **19**, 705–18.

Goss, C. M. 'On anatomy of veins and arteries by Galen of Pergamos.' *Anat. Rec.*, 1961, **141**, 355–66.

Grapow, H. *Ueber die Anatomischen Kenntnisse de Altägyptischen Aerzte.* Leipzig, J. C. Hinrichs, 1935.

— *Grundriss der Medizin der Alten Aegypter.* Vol. II, Berlin, Akademie-Verlag, 1955.

Grattan, J. H. G., and Singer, Charles. *Anglo-Saxon Magic and Medicine.* London, Wellcome Historical Medical Museum, 1952.

Groen, J., Tjong, B. K., Kamminga, C. E., and Willebrands, A. F. 'The influence of nutrition, individuality, and some other factors, including some forms of stress on the serum cholesterol; an experiment of nine months duration in 60 normal human volunteers.' *Voeding*, 1952, **13**, 556–87.

Gross, Louis. *The Blood Supply to the Heart in its Anatomical and Clinical Aspects.* New York and London, Hoeber, 1921.

Hales, Stephen. *Statical Essays.* (Vol. 2, containing Haemastaticks.) London, W. Innys & R. Manby, 1733.

Hall, G. H., Neale, G., and Young, D. M. 'Letter to the Editor on ventricular fibrillation.' *Lancet*, 1962, **i**, 1306–7.

Haller, Albrecht von. *Disputationes ad Morborum Historiam et Curationem Facientes.* Tomus II, Ad Morborum Pectoris [Hist. et Cur.]. Lausanne, Bousquet, 1757.

Hammer, Adam. 'Ein Fall von thrombotischem Verschlusse einer der Kranzarterien des Herzens.' *Wien. med. Wschr.*, 1878, **28**, 97–102.

Harvey, James. *Praesagium Medicum or The Prognostick Signs of Acute Diseases.* London, G. Strahan, 1706.

Harvey, William. *The Works* . . . Translated by R. Willis. London, The Sydenham Society, 1847.

— *Movement of the Heart and Blood in Animals.* Latin text and English translation by K. J. Franklin. Oxford, Blackwell, 1957.

— *Exercitationes Duae Anatomicae de Circulatione Sanguinis. Ad Joannem Riolanum Filium, etc.* Rotterdam, Arnold Leers, 1649.

— *The Circulation of the Blood.* Latin text, edited, annotated and translated by K. J. Franklin. Oxford, Blackwell, 1958.

— *Anatomical Studies on the Motion of the Heart and Blood.* Translated by C. D. Leake. Springfield, Ill., Thomas, 1928.

— *Prelectiones Anatomiae Universalis.* (1) Autotype Reproduction of the Original with Transliteration. By a Committee of the Royal College of Physicians of London. London, Churchill, 1886. (2) *Lectures on the Whole of Anatomy.* An Annotated Translation by C. D. O'Malley, F. N. L. Poynter and K. F. Russell. Berkeley, Univ. of California Press, 1961. (3) *The Anatomical Lectures of William Harvey.* Edited, translated and annotated by Gweneth Whitteridge, Edinburgh, Livingstone, 1964.

Heberden, William. 'Some account of a disorder in the breast.' *Med. Trans. Coll. Physns. Lond.*, 1772, **2**, 59–67.

— *Commentaries on the History and Cure of Diseases.* London, Payne, 1802.

— 'A letter to Dr. Heberden, concerning the angina pectoris; and an account of the dissection of one, who had been troubled with that disorder. Read at the College, Nov. 17, 1772.' *Med. Trans. Coll. Physns Lond.*, 1785, **3**, 1–11.

Hedley, O. F. 'Contributions of Edward Jenner to modern concepts of heart disease.' *Amer. J. publ. Hlth*, 1938, **28**, 1165–69.

Helmont, J. B. van. *Anfang der Artzney Kunst . . . in die Hochdeutsche Sprache.* uebersetzt. Sulzbach, printed for Endter by Holst, 1683.

Henle, Jacob. *Handbuch der Systematischen Anatomie des Menschen.* 3 vols. (vol. III: Gefässlehre). Braunschweig, Vieweg, 1855–1868.

Henschen, Folke. *The History of Diseases.* (English trans. by Joan Tate.) London, Longmans, 1966.

Herrick, J. B. *A Short History of Cardiology.* Springfield, Ill., Thomas, 1942. [Chapter 9: 'The Coronary Artery and its Diseases'].

— 'Clinical features of sudden obstruction of the coronary arteries.' *J. Amer. med. Ass.*, 1912, **59**, 2015–20.

— and Nuzum, F. 'Angina pectoris; clinical experience with two hundred cases.' *J. Amer. med. Ass.* 1918, **70**, 67–70.

— 'Thrombosis of the coronary arteries.' *J. Amer. med. Ass.*, 1919, **72**, 387–90.

— 'Some unsolved problems connected with acute obstruction of the coronary artery.' *Amer. Heart J.*, 1929, **4**, 633–40.

— 'Allen Burns, anatomist, surgeon and cardiologist (1781–1813).' *Bull Soc. med. Hist. Chicago*, 1935, **4**, 457–83.

— 'An intimate account of my early experience with coronary thrombosis.' *Amer. Heart J.*, 1944, **27**, 1–18.

— *Memories of Eighty Years.* Chicago, University of Chicago Press, 1949.

Hippocrates. Éditions used: Adams, Francis, *The Genuine Works of H.*, 2 vols. London, Sydenham Society, 1849. Littré, Emile, *Oeuvres Complètes d'H.* Traduction avec le texte Grec, 10 vols., Paris, Baillière 1839–1861. Jones, W. H. S. 'Works' with an English translation, 4 vols. London, Heinemann, and Cambridge, Mass., Harvard University Press, 1923.

Hirsch, August. *Biographisches Lexikon der Hervorragenden Aertze Aller Zeiten und Völker.* 5 vols. and Suppl. 2nd ed. Berlin and Vienna, Urban u. Schwarzenberg, 1929–35.

— *Handbuch der historisch-geographischen Pathologie.* 2 vols. 1st ed. Erlangen, 1859–1864; Engl. trans., New Sydenham Society, 1883–86.

Hochhaus, H. 'Zur Diagnose des plötzlichen Verschlusses der Kranzarterien des Herzens.' *Dtsch. med. Wschr.*, 1911, **17**, 2065–68.

Hodel, G., and Buess, H. 'Ernst Ziegler (1849–1905), ein grosser Forscher und Lehrer.' *Clio med.*, 1966, **1**, 303–18.

Hodgson, Joseph. *A Treatise on the Diseases of Arteries and Veins Containing the Pathology and Treatment of Aneurysms and Wounded Arteries.* London, T. Underwood, 1815.

Hoffmann, Friedrich. *Medicina Rationalis Systematica*, vol. III. Frankfurt, Varrentrapp, 1738.

— *Opera Omnium Physico-medicorum etc.*, 2nd supplement. Geneva, de Tournes, 1753.

Hoffman[n], Max. 'Die Lehre vom plötzlichen Tod in Lancisi's De subitaneis mortibus.' *Abh. Gesch. Med. Naturw.*, 1935, **6**, 1–62.

Hollman, Arthur. 'Coronary vasodilators.' *Med. Wld, Lond.*, 1963, **99**, 217–22.

Home, Everard. 'Life of John Hunter.' In: *John Hunter, A Treatise on the Blood*. London, G. Nicol, 1794.

Hood, Donald. ['Angina Pectoris immediately followed by Pericarditis.'] *Lancet*, 1884, **i**, 205.

Hooke, Robert. *Micrographia: or Some Physiological Descriptions of Minute Bodies made by Magnifying Glasses*. London, The Royal Society, 1665.

Huber, Karl. 'Ueber den Einfluss der Kranzarterienerkrankungen auf das Herz und die chronische Myocarditis.' *Virchows Arch. path. Anat.*, 1882, **89**, 236–58.

Huchard, Henri. *Traité clinique des Maladies du Coeur et de l'Aorte.* 3rd ed. 3 vols. Paris, Octave Duin, 1899–1903. [Vol. 2, pp. 523–77 deals with the period beginning at the end of the seventeenth century.]

Hunter, John. *A Treatise on the Blood, Inflammation and Gun-shot Wounds.* Ed. by E. Home. London, G. Nicol, 1794.

Hyrtl, Joseph. 'Beweis dass die Ursprünge der Coronar-Arterien . . . nicht bedeckt werden.' *Sber. Akad. Wiss. Wien, Math.-naturw. Kl.*, 1855, **14**, 373–85.

Ignatovski, A. I. 'Wirkung der tierischen Nahrung auf den Kaninchen-Organismus.' *Ber. Milit. -med. Akad. (St. Petersb.)*, (Izviest. imp. voyenno-med. Akad., St. Petersb.), 1908, **16**, 154–76. (French trans. in *Arch. med. experim.*, 1908, **20**, 1–20.)

Isidore of Seville. *Ethimologiarum Liber IV, De Medicina*. Masnou-Barcelona, Laboratorios del Norte de España, 1945. See Sharpe, W.

Jacobs, H. B., see Jenner E.

Jamin, F., and Merkel, H. *Die Koronararterien des Menschlichen Herzens in Stereoskopischen Röntgenbildern.* Jena, G. Fischer, 1907.

Jarcho, Saul. 'Latham on angina pectoris; excerpts from the Philadelphia edition, 1847.' *Amer. J. Cardiol.*, 1966, **17**, 879–84.

— (ed.) *Human Palaeopathology.* New Haven and London, Yale University Press, 1966.

Jenner, Edward. 'Letter to C. H. Parry.' In: *Parry, 1799*, p. 3–5, q.v.

— 'Letter to W. Heberden 1778' [possibly 1786, Le Fanu]. In: Jacobs, H. B., *Edward Jenner, a Student of Medicine, as Illustrated in his letters.* Contributions to Medical and Biological Research, Dedicated to Sir William

Osler, p. 740–55. New York, Hoeber, 1919. See also J. Baron's *Life of Edward Jenner* (1838).

— *An Inquiry into the Causes and Effects of the Variolae Vaccinae*. London, printed for the author by S. Law, 1798.

Joachim, H. *Papyros Ebers. Das Aelteste Buch Ueber Heilkunde*. Aus dem Aegyptischen zum Erstenmal Vollständig Uebersetzt. Berlin, Reimer, 1890.

Johnstone, James. 'Case of angina pectoris, from an unexpected disease in the heart.' *Mem. med. Soc. Lond.* 1792, **1**, 376–88.

Jokl, E. and Jokl, P. (eds.) *Exercise and Altitude*. Vol. I of series: Medicine and Sport. Basle, Karger, 1968.

Jonckheere, Frans. *Autour de l'Autopsie d'une Momie: le Scribe Royal Boutehamon*, Brussels, Fondation Égyptol. Reine Élisabeth, 1942.

— *Le Papyrus Médical Chester Beatty*. Brussels, Fondation Egyptol. Reine Élisabeth, 1947.

Jonnesco, T. 'Angine de poitrine guérie par la résection du sympathique cervicothoracique.' *Bull Acad. Méd. (Paris)*, 1920, **84**, 93–102.

Julian, Desmond G. 'Coronary care and the community.' *Ann. intern. Med.* 1968, **69**, 607–13.

Katz, A. M., and Katz, Ph.B. 'Diseases in the works of Hippocrates.' *Brit. Heart J.*, 1962, **24**, 257–64.

Keele, K. D. *Leonardo da Vinci On the Movement of the Heart and Blood*. Philadelphia, Lippincott, and London, Harvey and Blythe, 1952.

— 'John Hunter's contribution to cardio-vascular pathology.' *Ann. roy. Coll. Surg. Engl.*, 1966, **39**, 248–59.

Kellett, C. E. *Raymond de Vieussens' Experiments and Reflections*. Privately printed, 1961.

Kerckring, T. *Spicilegium Anatomicum, etc*. Amsterdam, Frisius, 1670.

Kernig, Vladimir. 'Behandlung der Angina pectoris.' *St. Petersb. med. Wschr.*, 1892, **17**, 177. Abstracted in the *Lancet*, 1892, **ii**, 438–39.

— 'Ueber objectiv Nachweisbare Veränderungen am Herzen, namentlich auch über Pericarditis nach Anfällen von Angina Pectoris.' *Berl. klin. Wschr.*, 1905, **43**, 10–14.

Keynes, G. *The Life of William Harvey*. Oxford, Clarendon Press, 1966.

Kirk, R. 'Pathology of the ancient Egyptian mummies.' *Proc. Alumni Ass. Malaya*, 1956, **9** (reprint: 11 pp.).

Klemperer, P. 'The history of coronary sclerosis.' *Amer. J. Cardiol.*, 1960, **5**, 94–107.

Kohn, Hans. 'Zur Geschichte der Angina pectoris; Heberden oder Rougnon.' *Z. klin. Med.*, 1927, **106**, 1–20.

Kölliker, A., and Müller, H. 'Nachweis der negativen Schwankung des Muskelstromes am natürlich sich contrahierenden Muskel.' *Verh. phys. -med. Ges.*, Würzburg, 1856, **6**, 528–33.

Kölster, R. 'Experimentelle Beiträge zur Kenntnis der myomalacia cordis.' *Skand. Arch. Physiol.*, 1892, **4**, 1–45.

Korotkow, N. [Note on the auscultatory method of blood pressure determination.] *Ber. milit. ärztl. Akad. (St Petersb.)*, 1905, **12**, 395. (See the paper by M. P. Multanowski, 'La méthode de Korotkow. Histoire de sa découverte, interprétation clinique et expérimentale et évaluation moderne.' 21st Intnat. Congr. Hist. Med., Siena, Pro-Memoria, 1968, summarized in Report, p. 109.)

Kowal, S. J. 'Emotions and angina pectoris, A historical review.' *Amer. J. Cardiol.*, 1960, **5**, 421–27.

Krehl, Ludolf. *Die Erkrankungen des Herzmuskels*. Vienna, A. Hölder, 1901.

Kreysig, F. L. *Die Krankheiten des Herzens*. 3 vols (in 4), Berlin, Maurer, 1814–1817.

Labat, R. *Traité Akkadien de Diagnostics et prognostics médicaux*. Leyden, Brill, 1951.

La Due, J. S., and Wroblewski, F. 'The significance of serum glutamic oxalacetic transaminase activity following acute myocardial infarction.' *Circulation*, 1955, **11**, 871–77.

Laënnec, R. T. H. *Traité de l'Auscultation Médiate*. 2 vols. Paris, J. A. Brosson & J. S. Chaude, 1819. 2nd ed. 1826. (English translation by John Forbes (1821 and several later editions) with annotations including observations on angina pectoris.)

— *A Treatise on the Diseases of the Chest . . . according to Diagnosis . . . by Means of Acoustick Instruments*. Translated by John Forbes. London, T. & G. Underwood, 1821.

Lancisi, G. M. *De Subitaneis Mortibus*. Rome, Buagni, 1707.

— *De Aneurysmatibus*. Latin text (1745 ed.) with English translation by W. C. Wright. New York, Macmillan, 1952.

Langer, K. 'Anastomosen der Kranzarterien.' *Sber. Akad. Wiss. Wien, math. -naturw. Kl.*, 1880.

Latham, Peter M. *Lectures on Subjects Connected with Clinical Medicine, Comprising Diseases of the Heart*. 2 vols. London, Longman, 1846.

— *The Collected Works*. 2 vols. London, The New Sydenham Society, 1876.

Laubry, C. and Mouquin, M. 'L'angine de poitrine et les affections cardioaortiques dans l'oeuvre de Morgagni.' *Presse méd*, 1950, **58**, 1–3.

Laufer, A., and Freund, M. 'A microscopic study of coronary atherosclerosis in Israel.' *J. Atheroscl. Res.*, 1962, **2**, 270–75.

Lawin, P. (Ed.), *Praxis der Intensivbehandlung*. Stuttgart, Thieme, 1968.

Leary, T. 'Atherosclerosis, the important form of arteriosclerosis, a metabolic disease.' *J. Amer. med. Ass.*, 1935, **105**, 475–81.

— 'Pathology of coronary sclerosis.' *Amer. Heart J.*, 1935, **10**, 328–37.

Leeson, T. S. 'Electron microscopy of mummified material.' *Stain Technol.*, 1959, **34**, 317–20.

Leeuwenhoek, A. van. *The Collected Letters* [Dutch and English]. Amsterdam, Swets & Zeitlinger, 1939–.

Le Fanu, W. R. *A Bibliography of Edward Jenner, 1749–1823*. London, Harvey & Blythe, 1951.

Lefebure, G. *Essai sur la Médecine Égyptienne a l'Epoque Pharaonique.* Paris, Presses Universitaires de France, 1956.

Leibowitz, J. O. 'Book of medical experiences ascribed to Abraham Ibn Ezra (1089–1164),' *Harofe Haivri (New York)* 1953, **26**, 151–59. [Hebrew with English summary.]

— 'Electroshock therapy in Ibn-Sina's Canon.' *J. Hist. Med.,* 1957, **12**, 71–72.

— 'The autopsy of King George II. A contribution to the history of myocardial infarction.' *Israel med. J.,* 1960, **19**, 264–66.

— 'Thrombo-embolic disease and heart block in Vesalius.' *Med. Hist.,* 1963, **7**, 258–64.

— 'The old age description in Ecclesiastes.' *J. Hist. Med.,* 1963, **18**, 283–284.

— 'J. U. Rumler and a letter of Vesalius.' *Med. Hist.,* 1964, **8**, 377–78.

— 'Early Attempts at Therapy in Coronary Disease.' *In: Current Problems in History of Medicine.* Proceedings of 19th Intern. Congr. Hist. Med., Basle 1964. Basle, Karger, 1966, 325–27.

— and Ullmann, D. T. 'Early references to heart block.' *J. Hist. Med.,* 1965, **20**, 43–51.

— 'Manuscript notes in a Rhazes-Maimonides incunable etc.' *Bull. Hist Med.,* 1965b, **39**, 424–33.

Leonardo da Vinci. *I Manoscritti di Leonardo da Vinci della Reale Biblioteca di Windsor. Dell'Anatomia, Fogli B.* Pubblicati da T. Sabachnikoff and G. Piumati, con traduzione in Lingua Francese. Turin, Roux & Viarengo, 1901.

— *Quaderni d'Anatomia.* Pubblicati da Vangensten, Fonahn, Hopstock. 6 vols. fol. Christiania Dybwad, 1911–18.

Lesky, Erna, see Rokintansky.

Levine, S. A. *Coronary Thrombosis; its Various Clinical Features.* Baltimore, Williams & Wilkins, 1929. [Historical data, pp. 2–7.]

Levine, S. A. and Tranter, C. L. 'Infarction of the heart simulating surgical abdominal conditions.' *Amer. J. med. Sci.,* 1918, **155**, 57–66.

Lewis, *Sir* Thomas. 'C. H. Parry, M.D., F.R.S., 1755–1822.' *Cardiff med. Soc. Proc.,* 1940–1941, **41**, 71–89.

— *Diseases of the Heart.* London, Macmillan, 1933.

— *Clinical Science. Illustrated by Personal Experience.* London, Shaw, 1934.

Leyden, E. 'Ueber die Sclerose der Coronar-Arterien und die davon abhangigen Krankheitszustände.' *Z. klin. Med.,* 1884, **7**, 459–86, 539–80.

Li, T. W., and Freeman, S. 'Experimental lipemia and hypercholesteronemia produced by protein depletion and by cholesterol-feeding in dogs.' *Amer. J. Physiol.,* 1946, **145**, 660–66.

Libman, Emanuel. 'Clinical varieties and therapy of precordial pain due to organic cardiovascular disease.' *Med. Rec.,* New York, 1916, **89**, 124.

Libman, E., and Sacks, B. 'Case illustrating the leucocytosis of progressive myocardial necrosis following coronary artery thrombosis.' *Amer. Heart J.,* 1927, **2**, 321–26.

Littré, Alexis. 'Observation sur une hydropsie particulière.' *Mém. Acad. roy. Sci.*, 1703, 90–94.

Lobstein, J. G. C. F. M. *Traité d'Anatomie pathologique.* 2 vols. Paris, F.-G. Levrault, 1829–33.

— *Lehrbuch der Pathologischen Anatomie. Deutsch bearbeitet von A. Neurohr.* 2 vols. Stuttgart, F. Brodhag, 1834–35.

Long, Allen R. 'Cardiovascular renal disease, report of three thousand years ago.' *Arch. Path. (Chicago)*, 1931, **12**, 92–94.

Louis, Antoine. *Lettres sur la Certitude des Signes de la Mort.* Paris, M. Lambert, 1752.

Lower, Richard. *Tractatus De Corde.* London, Redmayne, 1669. Facsimile edition prefaced by an introduction and translation by K. J. Franklin. (R. T. Gunther, *Early Science in Oxford*, vol. 9.) Oxford, for the subscribers, 1932.

MacBride, David. *A Methodical Introduction to the Theory and Practice of Physic.* London, W. Strahan, 1772. (cf. pp. 217 ff).

Mackenzie, James. *Angina Pectoris.* Oxford Medical Publications, 1923.

McMichael, J., and Parry, E. H. 'Prognosis and anticoagulant prophylaxis after coronary occlusion.' *Lancet*, 1960, **ii**, 991–98.

McMurrich, J. P. *Leonardo da Vinci, the Anatomist, 1452–1519.* Baltimore, Williams & Wilkins, 1930.

Maimonides (Moses ben Maimon). *Aphorismi Secundum Doctrinam Galeni.* [First Latin translation (anon.)], Bologna, Benedictus Hectoris, 1489. First printed Hebrew translation by Nathan Meati, Lemberg, Rosanes, 1834; latest Hebrew edition by S. Muntner, Jerusalem, Mosad Harav Kook, 1959.

— 'De accidentibus', translated and edited by A. Bar-Sela, H. E. Hoff and E. Faris. *Trans. Amer. philos. Soc.*, 1964, N.S. **54**, pt. 4.

Major, Ralph H., *Classic Descriptions of Disease.* Springfield, Ill., Thomas, 3rd ed., 1945.

Malinin, T. I. *et al.* 'Experimental coronary artery narrowing in swine. I. Morphological and histochemical myocardial changes.' *Johns Hopk. med. J.*, 1968, **122**, 102–11.

Malmsten, H. P., and Düben, G. W. J. 'Fall af ruptura cordis' [case of cardiac rupture]. *Hygiea*, 1859, **21**, 629–30. German translation in Warburg, E. J. 'Ueber den Coronarkreislauf und ueber die Thrombose einer Coronararterie.' *Acta med. Scand.*, 1930, **73**, 425–59, see pp. 448–50.

Malpighi, Marcello. 'De Polypo Cordis Dissertatio.' 1st ed. *In: De viscerum Structura Exercitatio Anatomica.* Bologna, G. Monti, 1666. Translated into English by J. M. Forrester, Uppsala, Almqvist & Wiksell, 1956; into Italian by L. Belloni, 1967, p. 193–216.

— *Opere Scelte, a cura di Luigi Belloni.* Torino, UTET, 1967.

— *Opere Omnia.* 3 vols. fol. London, Thomas Sawbridge, 1686.

Mann, G. 'Anatomische Sammlung Fredrik Ruysch's.' *Sudhoffs Arch. Gesch. Med.*, 1961, **45**, 176–78.

— 'The anatomical collections of Frederik Ruysch at Leningrad.' *Bull. Cleveland med. Libr.*, 1964, **11**, 10–13.

Marchand, F. 'Ueber Arteriosklerose.' *Verh. Kongr. inn. Med.*, 1904, **21**, 23–59.

Marie, René. *L'Infarctus du Myocarde et ses Conséquences*. Thèse de Paris, No. 88, 1896–1897.

Massa, Nicolaus. *Anatomiae Liber Introductorius*. Venice, Zilletus, 1559 (identical with the 1st ed., 1536).

Master, Arthur M. 'Anticoagulant therapy in the premonitory phase of acute coronary occlusion.' *Circulation*, 1961, **24**, 990–91.

Master, A., and Oppenheimer, E. 'A simple exercise tolerance test for circulatory efficiency with standard tables for normal individuals.' *Amer. J. med. Sci.*, 1929, **177**, 223–42.

Matteucci, C. 'Sur le courant électrique des muscles des animaux vivants ou récemment tués.' *C. r. Acad. Sci., Paris*, 1843, **16**, 197.

Meyenfeldt, F. H. van. *Het Hart (leb, lebab) in het Oude Testament*. Leiden, E. J. Brill, 1950.

Michaels, L. 'Aetiology of coronary artery disease: An historical approach.' *Brit. Heart J.*, 1966, **28**, 258–64.

Michelottus, Petrus Antonius. 'Epistola, Specimen complectens Universalis Morborum Sanguinis Ductuum.' *In: De Bononiensi Scientiarium et Artium Instituto atque Academia Commentarii*. Tomus I, Bologna, Laelius a Vulpe, 1731, pp. 418–82.

Miller, J. L., and Matthews, S. A. 'Effect on the heart of experimental obstruction of the left coronary artery.' *Arch. intern. Med.*, 1909, **3**, 476–484.

Mishnah, The. Translated by H. Danby. Oxford University Press, 1933.

Montagnana, Bartholomaeus. *Consilia Medica*, Lyons, J. Uyt, 1525 (earlier edition, Venice, B. Locatellus for O. Scotus, 1497).

Moodie, R. L. *Roentgenologic Studies of Egyptian and Peruvian mummies*. Chicago, Field Museum of National History, 1931.

Morand, S. F. 'Sur quelques accidents remarquables dans les organes de la circulation du sang.' *Mém. Acad. Sci. (Paris)*, 1732, 428–34.

Morgagni, G. B. *De Sedibus et Causis Morborum per Anatomen Indagatis Libri Quinque*. Padua, tipogr. Remondiana, 1761. (*The Seats and Causes of Diseases*. Translated by B. Alexander, 3 vols., London, Millar & Cadell, 1769; Abridged and elucidated by William Cooke, 2 vols. London, Longmans, 1822.)

Morgan, A. D. 'Some forms of undiagnosed coronary disease in nineteenth-century England.' *Med. Hist.*, 1968, **12**, 344–58.

— *Pathogenesis of Coronary Occlusion*. Springfield, Ill., Thomas, 1957.

Morris, J. N. 'Recent history of coronary disease.' *Lancet*, 1951, **i**, 69–73.

— Epidemiological surveys. *In*: 'Summary of Proceedings, B.M.A. Joint Annual Meeting, 1959. Section of Medicine and Cardiology.' *Brit. med. J.*, 1959, **ii**, 358.

Morris, J. N., and Crawford, M.D. 'Coronary heart disease and physical activity of work.' *Brit. med. J.*, 1958, **ii**, 1485–96.

Mundinus (Mondino de'Liucci). *Anothomia*. Padua, Cerdonis, 1484 (first ed., ibid., 1478).

— *Anatomia, Riprodotta da un Codice Bolognese*. (Photographic reproduction of a 15th-century Italian MS translation, original Latin text, and modern translation into Italian a cura del L. Sighinolfi, Bologna, Cappelli, 1930.)

Murrell, William. 'Nitro-glycerine as a remedy for angina pectoris.' *Lancet*, 1879, **i**, 80–81, 113–15, 151–52, 225–27.

Myasnikov, A. L. 'Influence of some factors on the development of experimental cholesterol atherosclerosis.' *Circulation*, 1958, **17**, 99–113.

Naunyn, B. *Erinnerungen, Gedanken und Meinungen*. Munich, J. F. Bergmann, 1925.

Neuburger, Max. 'Die Entwicklung der Lehre von den Herzkrankheiten.' *Wien. med. Wschr.*, 1928, **78**, 79–81, 122–26.

Nicolai, G. F., and Simons, A. 'Zur Klinik des Elektrokardiogramms.' *Med. Klin.*, 1909, **5**, 160–67.

Nicholls, Frank. 'Observations concerning the Body of his late Majesty [King George II], October 1760.' *Phil. Trans.* 1761, 52, pt. 1, 265–75.

Obrastzow, W. P., and Straschesko, N. D. 'Zur Kenntnis der Thrombose der Koronararterien des Herzens.' *Z. klin. Med.*, 1910, **71**, 116–32. Russian original in *Russk. Vrach*, 1910; reproduced in *Klin. Med.* (*Mosk.*), 1949, **27**, 15.

O'Malley, C. D. *Andreas Vesalius of Brussels, 1514–1564*. Berkeley and Los Angeles, University of California Press, 1964.

— and Saunders, J. B. de C. M. *Leonardo da Vinci on the Human Body*. New York, Schuman [1952].

Oppenheimer, E. H., and Esterly, J. R. 'Some aspects of cardiac pathology in infancy and childhood. II: Unusual coronary endarteriitis with congenital cardiac malformations.' *Bull. Johns Hopk. Hosp.*, 1966, **119**, 343–54.

Oribasius. *Oeuvres: Texte Grec, Traduit en Français par Bussemaker et Daremberg*. 6 vols. Paris, Imprimerie Nationale, 1851–76.

Orth, J. 'Die Lokalisation der Infarkte und Schwielen der Herzmuskulatur und ihre Beziehung zu der Gefässversorgung des Herzens.' *Berl. klin. Wschr.*, 1909, **46**, 614–15.

Osler, William. *Lectures on Angina Pectoris and Allied States*. Edinburgh and London, Pentland, 1897. New York, Appleton, 1897.

— 'The Lumleian Lectures on angina pectoris.' *Lancet*, 1910, **i**, 697–702, 839–44.

Pagel, Walter. *Paracelsus; an Introduction to Philosophical Medicine in the Era of the Renaissance*. Basle and New York, Karger, 1958.

Panum, P. L. 'Experimentelle Beiträge zur Lehre von der Embolie.' *Virch. Arch. path. Anat.*, 1862, **25**, 308–38, 433–530.

Paracelsus, Theophrastus. Works edited by K. Sudhoff. 14 vols. Munich and Berlin, R. Oldenburg, 1922–33.

Pardee, H. E. B. 'An electrocardiographic sign of coronary artery obstruction.' *Arch. intern. Med.*, 1920, **26**, 244–57.

— 'Heart disease and abnormal electrocardiograms, with special reference to the coronary T wave.' *Amer. J. med. Sci.*, 1925, **169**, 270–83.

Paré, Ambroise. *The Workes . . . translated out of Latine and compared with the French*, by Th. Johnson. London, T. Cotes and R. Young, 1634.

Parkinson, J., and Bedford, D. E. 'Cardiac infarction and coronary thrombosis.' *Lancet*, 1928, **i**, 4–11.

— 'Successive changes in the electrocardiogram after cardiac infarction (coronary thrombosis).' *Heart*, 1928, **14**, 195–239.

Parry, Caleb Hillier. *An Inquiry into the Symptoms and Causes of the Syncope Anginosa, Commonly called Angina Pectoris, Illustrated by Dissections.* Bath and London, R. Crutwell, 1799.

Paulus Aegineta. *The Seven Books.* Translation and Commentary by Francis Adams. 3 vols., London, Sydenham Society, 1844–1847.

Payne, J. F. 'Two cases of sudden death from affection of the heart, examined in post mortem theatre.' *Brit. med. J.*, 1870, **i**, 130–31.

Peacock, T. B. 'Aneurysm of the left coronary artery.' *Trans. path. Soc. Lond.*, 1846–48, **1**, 227–30.

Peete, D. C. *Psychosomatic Genesis of Coronary Artery Disease.* Springfield, Ill., Thomas, 1955.

Percival, T. 'A case of angina pectoris, with a dissection.' *Med. philos. Comment.*, 2nd ed., 1784, **3**, 180–82.

Pettigrew, T. J. *History of Egyptian Mummies.* London, Longman, 1834.

Philipp, J. 'R. Vieussens' and J. M. Lancisi's Verdienste um die Lehre von den Krankheiten des Herzens.' *Janus (Breslau)*, 1847, **2**, 580–98; 1848, **3**, 316–26.

— *Die Kenntnis von den Krankheiten des Herzens im Achtzehnten Jahrhundert.* Berlin, Hirschwald, 1856.

Pickering, George. 'Pathogenesis of myocardial and cerebral infarction. Nodular arteriosclerosis.' *Brit. med. J.*, 1964, **i**, 517–29.

Pissinus, Sebastianus. *De Cordis Palpitatione Cognoscenda, et Curanda Libri Duo.* Frankfurt, C. Marnius and heirs of J. Aubrius, 1609.

Platter, Felix. *Observationum . . . Libri Tres.* Basle, Waldkirch for König, 1614.

— *Observationes.* Krankheitsbeobachtungen in drei Büchern. 1. Buch übersetzt von G. Goldschmidt, bearbeitet von H. Buess. Berne, Huber, 1963.

Pliny. *Natural History.* With an English translation by H. Rackham and others. Loeb Classical Library, 10 vols. London, Heinemann, and Cambridge, Mass., Harvard University Press, 1938–63.

Porter, Ian H. 'The nineteenth-century physician and cardiologist Thomas Bevill Peacock (1812–82).' *Med. Hist.*, 1962, **6**, 240–54.

15

Pratt, F. H. 'The nutrition of the heart through the vessels of Thebesius and the coronary veins.' *Amer. J. Physiol.*, 1898, **1**, 86–103.

— 'Swedenborg on the Thebesian blood flow of the heart.' *Ann. med. Hist.*, 1932, 434–39.

Prendergast, J. 'Galen's view of the vascular system in relation to that of Harvey.' *Proc. roy. Soc. Med., Section of Hist. Med.*, 1928, **22**, 1839–1847.

Quain, Richard, 'On fatty diseases of the heart.' *Med. chir. Trans.*, 1850, **33**, 121–96.

— Dilatation of the arch of the aorta, and plugging and obliteration of the left coronary artery.' (Read by C. T. Williams). *Trans. path. Soc. Lond.*, 1872, **23**, 57–59.

Radcliffe, C. B. 'A case of acute uncomplicated myocarditis in which the disease was diagnosed during life.' *Brit. med. J.*, 1866, **i**, 132–33; *Lancet*, 1866, **i**, 124.

Ratcliffe, H. L. 'Phylogenetic considerations in the etiology of myocardial infarction.' *In*: *The Etiology of Myocardial Infarction*. Ed. James, T. N., and Keys, J. W., pp. 61–89. Boston, Mass., Little, Brown & Co., 1963.

Rhazes. *A Treatise on the Smallpox and Measles*. Translated into English by W. A. Greenhill. London, New Sydenham Society, 1848.

Riad, Naguib. *La Médecine au Temps des Pharaons*. Paris, Maloine, 1955.

Riva-Rocci, S. 'Un nuovo sfigmomanometro.' *Gazz. med. Torino*, 1896, **47**, 981.

Robb-Smith, A. H. T. *The Enigma of Coronary Heart Disease*, London, Lloyd-Luke, 1967.

Robinson, J. S. 'Coronary care unit versus hospital mortality in acute myocardial infarction.' (Abstract of paper read at the 4th Asian Pacific Congress of Cardiology held in Jerusalem and Tel Aviv, 1–7 September, 1968). *Israel J. med. Sci.*, 1968, **4**, 1114.

Rokitansky, Carl. *Manual of Pathological Anatomy*. Trans. by G. Day. London, New Sydenham Society, 1852. [German original 1841–46.]

— *Selbstbiographie und Antrittsrede*. Eingeleitet, herausgegeben u. mit Erläuterungen versehen von Erna Lesky. *Sber. Akad. Wiss. Wien, philos.-hist. Kl.*, 234 Bd., *3* Abh., Vienna, Böhlau, 1960.

Rolleston, Humphry D., 'The history of angina pectoris.' *Glasg. med. J.*, 7th ser., 1937, **9**, 205–25.

Romberg, Ernst. *Lehrbuch der Krankheiten des Herzens und der Blutgefässe*. Stuttgart, Enke, 1909.

Rosenbloom, J. Letter to the Editor [Earl of Clarendon case.] *Ann. med. Hist.*, 1922, **4**, 210–11.

Roth, M. *Andreas Vesalius Bruxellensis*. Berlin, Reimer, 1892.

Rougnon, N. F. *Lettre à M. Lorry*. Besançon, Charmet, 1768.

— *Considerationes Pathologico-semioticae*. 2 vols. Besançon, 1786–88.

Rowling, J. Thompson. Pathological changes in mummies. *Proc. roy. Soc. Med., Hist. Med. Sect.*, 1961, **54**, 409–15.

Royal College of Physicians of London. *Dolor Pectoris*. Catalogue of an Exhibition illustrating the History of Angina Pectoris. London, 1968.

Rudius, Eustachius. *De Pulsibus Libri Duo*. Frankfurt, J. Spiers and heirs of R. Beatus, 1602.

Ruffer, Marc A. 'Histological studies on Egyptian mummies.' *Mém. Inst. Egypt.*, 6, fasc. 3, Cairo, Diemer, 1911.

— 'On arterial lesions found in Egyptian mummies (158 B.C.–A.D. 525).' *J. Path. Bact.*, 1911, 15, 453–62.

— 'Studies in palaeopathology in Egypt.' *J. Path. Bact.*, 1913, 17, 149–62.

— *Studies in the Palaeopathology of Egypt*. Edited by R. L. Moodie. University of Chicago Press, 1921.

Rufinus. *The Herbal of Rufinus*. Edited by L. Thorndike and F. S. Benjamin. University of Chicago Press, 1946.

Rufus of Ephesus: *Oeuvres: texte collectionné sur les manuscrits traduit en français, avec une introduction par C. Daremberg*. Paris, Imprimerie nationale, 1879.

Ruysch, Frederik. *Thesaurus Anatomicus Quartus*. Amsterdam, J. Wolters, 1704.

Ryle, J. A., and Russell, W. T. 'Natural history of coronary disease.' *Brit. Heart J.*, 1949, 11, 370–89.

Samuelson, B. 'Ueber den Einfluss der Coronar-Arterien-Verschliessung auf die Herzaktion.' *Z. klin. Med.*, 1881, 2, 12–33.

Sandison, A. T. 'The histological examination of mummified material.' *Stain Technol.*, 1955, 30, 277–83.

— 'Preparation of large histological sections of mummified tissues.' *Nature (Lond.)*, 1957, 179, 1309–10.

— 'Degenerative vascular disease in the Egyptian mummy.' *Med. Hist.*, 1962, 6, 77–81.

— 'A pathologist looks at Egyptian mummies.' *Proc. Scot. Soc. Hist. Med.*, 1961–63, 8–14.

— 'The study of mummified and dried human tissues.' *In*: Brothwell, D., and Higgs, E. (eds). *Science in Archaeology*, 413–25. London, Thames & Hudson, 1963.

Saunders, J. B. de C. M. *The Transitions from Ancient Egyptian to Greek Medicine*. Lawrence, University of Kansas Press, 1963.

Saxonia, Hercules. *De Pulsibus*. Frankfurt am Main, Palthenius, 1604.

— *Prognoseon Practicarum*. Vicenza, Bolzetta, 1620.

Scarpa, Antonio. *Sull'Aneurisma. Riflessioni ed Osservazioni Anatomico-chirurgiche*. Pavia, Bolzani, 1804.

— *A Treatise on Aneurism*. Translated into English from the Italian by J. H. Wishart, 2nd ed., Edinburgh, Stirling and Slade, 1819.

Scherf, D. and Schott, A. *Extrasystoles and Allied Arrhythmias*. London, Heinemann, 1953.

Scherk, G. 'Zur Klinik der Arteriothrombosen.' *Dtsch. med. Wschr.*, 1933, 59, 921–23.

Schierbeck, A. *Measuring the Invisible World; the Life and Works of Antoni van Leeuwenhoek, F.R.S.* London, Abelard-Schuman, [1959].

Schrenk, Martin. 'Die Angina pectoris.' *Sudhoff's Arch., Gesch. Med.*, 1967, **51**, 165–83.

Seegmiller, J. E. Discussion at the symposium on Allopurin, Heberden Society, Roy. Coll. Physns. Lond. 1966. *Ann. rheum. Dis.*, supplement to vol. **25**, 1966.

Segall, Harold N. 'The first clinico-pathological case history of angina pectoris: self-diagnosis by an anonymous physician; autopsy by John Hunter: reported by William Heberden in 1772.' *Bull. Hist. Med.*, 1945, **18**, 102–8.

Sénac, J. B. de. *Traité de la Structure du Coeur, de son Action et de ses Maladies.* 2 vols. Paris, J. Vincent, 1749.

— *Traité des Maladies du Coeur*, 2nd ed. [1st ed. 1781]. 2 vols. Paris, Méquignon the elder, 1783.

Seneca. *Epistulae Morales.* 3 vols. The Loeb Classical Library, London, Heinemann, and Cambridge, Mass., Harvard University Press, 1925.

Sharpe, W. 'Isidore of Seville.' *Trans. Amer. philos. Soc.*, 1964, N.S. **54**, pt. 2, 1–75.

Shattock, S. G. 'A report upon the pathological condition of the aorta of King Mereptah, traditionally regarded as the Pharaoh of the Exodus.' *Proc. roy. Soc. Med., Path. Sect.*, 1909, **2**, 122–27.

— 'Microscopic sections of the aorta of King Mereptah.' *Lancet*, 1909, **i**, 319.

Siegel, R. E. 'Description of circulatory collapse and coronary thrombosis in the fifth century A.D. by Caelius Aurelianus.' *Amer. J. Cardiol.*, 1961, **7**, 427–31.

— 'Discovery of coronary sclerosis as a cause of angina pectoris.' *Arch. intern. Med.*, 1963, **112**, 647–51.

— *Galen's System of Physiology and Medicine.* Basle and New York, S. Karger, 1968.

Sigerist, Henry E. *A History of Medicine.* Vol. I: *Primitive and Archaic Medicine.* New York, Oxford University Press, 1951.

Singer, C., and Rabin, C. *A Prelude to Modern Science.* London, Wellcome Historical Medical Museum, 1946.

Smith, Fred M. 'The ligation of coronary arteries with electro-cardiographic study.' *Arch. intern. Med.*, 1918, **22**, 8–27.

Smith, G. Elliot. *The Royal Mummies.* Service des Antiquités de l'Égypte. Catalogue Générale des Antiquités Égyptiennes du Musée du Caire, vol. 59, Cairo, 1901, and Cairo, 1912.

Smith, G. Elliot, and Dawson, W. R. *Egyptian Mummies.* London, G. Allen & Unwin, 1924.

Smith, John. *King Solomon's Portraiture of Old Age.* London, J. Hayes for S. Thomson, 1666.

Snapper, I. *Chinese lessons to Western Medicine.* New York, Interscience Publ. Inc., 1941.

— 'Diet and atherosclerosis: truth and fiction.' *Amer. J. Cardiol.*, 1963, **11**, 283–89.

Snell, W. E. 'Nathan Drake, M.D.: a literary practitioner and his illness.' *Proc. roy. Soc. Med., Sect. Hist. Med.*, 1965, **58**, 263–66.

Sobernheim, J. F. *Praktische Diagnostik der Inneren Krankheiten mit Vorzüglicher Rücksicht auf Pathologische Anatomie.* Berlin, A. Hirschwald, 1837.

Sones, F. M. *Jr.*, and Shirey, E. K. 'Cine-coronary arteriography.' *Mod. Conc. Cardiov. Dis.*, 1962, **31**, 735–38.

Souques, A. 'La douleur dans les livres hippocratiques.' *Bull. Hist. Méd.* (Paris), 1937, **31**, 209–44; 1938, **32**, 178–86; 1939, **33**, 131–44; 1940, **34**, 53–59; (no more published).

Spalteholz, W. 'Die Koronararterien des Herzens.' *Verh. anat. Ges.*, 21-te Vers., 1907.

Sprague, Howard B. 'Environment in relation to coronary artery disease.' *Arch. environm. Hlth*, 1966, **13**, 4–12.

Stannard, J. 'Benedictus Crispus, an eighth-century poet.' *J. Hist. Med.*, 1966, **21**, 24–46.

Steeves, G. W. 'Medical allusions in the writings of Francis Bacon.' *Proc. roy. Soc. Med., Sect. Hist. Med.*, 1912–13, **6**, 76–96.

Stensen, Niels (Steno, Nicolaus). *De Musculis et Glandulis Observationum Specimen.* Amsterdam, P. Warnaer for P. le Grand, 1664.

Stenzel, Christian Gottfried. 'Dissertatio de Steatomatibus Aortae, 1723.' [Reproduced in:] A. v. Haller, *Disputationes ad Morborum Historiam, etc.*, I, 562. Lausanne, Bousquet, 1757.

Sternberg, Josef. 'Ueber Erkrankungen des Herzmuskels im Auschluss an Störungen des Coronararterien-Kreislaufes.' [Thesis] Marburg, G. Schirling, 1887.

Sternberg, Maximilian. 'Pericarditis epistenocardica.' *Wien. med. Wschr.*, 1910, **60**, 14–23.

— *Das Chronische-Partielle Herzaneurysma.* Leipzig and Vienna, Deuticke, 1914.

Steuer, R. O. and Saunders, J. B. de C. M. *Ancient Egyptian and Cnidian Medicine.* Berkeley and Los Angeles, University of California Press, 1959.

Steuer, Robert O. 'Wḥdw, Aetiological principle of pyaemia in ancient Egyptian medicine.' *Bull. Hist. Med.*, Suppl. No. 10, Baltimore, 1948.

Stuckey, N. W. 'Ueber die Veränderungen der Kaninchen-Aorta bei der Fütterung mit verschiedenen Fettsorten.' *Zbl. allg. Path. path. Anat.*, 1912, **23**, 910–11.

Sudhoff, K. 'Die gedruckten mittelalterlichen medizinischen Texte in germanischen Sprachen. Eine literarische Studie.' *Sudhoff's Arch. Gesch. Med.*, 1910, **3**, 273–303.

Swedenborg, E. *Oeconomia Regni Animalis.* London and Amsterdam, Changuion, 1740–41.

— *Regnum Animale*, 3 pts. Hagae Comitum, A. Blyvenburg, 1744–45.

Talmud, Babylonian. Translated into English with Notes under the Editorship of I. Epstein, 34 vols. London, Soncino, 1935–52.

Temkin, O. [Book review.] 'The Papyrus Ebers, translated by B. Ebbell.'
    Isis, 1938, **28**, 126–31.

Testa, Antonio G. *Delle Malattie del Cuore*. Edited by N. U. Sormani.
    2 vols. Milan, Schilpathi, Truffi, Fusi, 1813 [1st ed. Bologna, 1810–11].

Thebesius, Adam Christian. *Dissertatio Medica de Circulo Sanguinis in Corde*.
    Leyden, J. A. Langerak, 1716 [1st ed. 1708].

Thurman, John. 'On aneurisms of the heart; with cases.' *Med.-chir. Trans.*,
    1838, **21**, 187–265.

Tiedemann, Friedrich. *Von der Verengung und Schliessung der Pulsadern in
    Krankheiten*. Heidelberg and Leipzig, K. Groos, 1843.

Toor, M., Katchalsky, A. *et al.* 'Serum lipids and atherosclerosis among
    Yemenite immigrants in Israel.' *Lancet*, 1957, **i**, 1270–73.

Truex, R. C., Nolan, F. G., Truex, R. C. Jr., Schneider, H. P., and Perl-
    mutter, H. I. 'Anatomy and pathology of the whale heart with special
    reference to the coronary circulation.' *Anat. Rec.*, 1961, **141**, 325–53.

Ungar, H., and Laufer, A. 'Necropsy studies of atherosclerosis in the Jewish
    population of Israel.' *Path. Microbiol. (Basle)*, 1961, **24**, 711–17.

Ungar, H., Laufer, A., and Ben-Ishay, Z. 'Atherosclerosis and Myocardial
    Infarction in Various Groups in Israel.' *In: The Genetics of Migrant and
    Isolate Populations*. Edited by E. Goldschmidt. Baltimore, Williams &
    Wilkins, 1963, pp. 120–27.

Varignana, Bartolomeo. Commentaries on Galen Avicenna a.o. in Vatican
    Library MSS 4451, 4452 and 4454.

Vassé, Loys. *In: Anatomen Corporis Humani Tabulae Quatuor*. Paris, Foucherius,
    1540.

Vesalius, Andreas. *De Humani Corporis Fabrica Libri Septem*. 2nd ed. Basle,
    Oporinus, 1555.

— *Anatomicarum Gabrielis Falloppii Observationum Examen*. Venice, Franciscis,
    1564. 2nd ed. Hanau, Typ. Wechelianis, 1609.

Vierordt, Hermann. *Medizinisches aus der Geschichte*. 3rd ed. Tübingen,
    Laupp, 1910.

Vieussens, Raymond de. *Novum Vasorum Corporis Humani Systema*. Amster-
    dam, P. Marret, 1705.

— *Nouvelles Découvertes sur le Coeur, etc.* Paris, L. d'Houry, 1706.

— *Traité Nouveau de la Structure et des Causes du Mouvement naturel du
    Coeur*. Toulouse, Guillemette, 1715.

Vineberg, A. M. 'Development of anastomosis between the coronary vessels
    and a transplanted internal mammary artery.' *Canad. med. Ass. J.*, 1946,
    55, 117–19.

Virchow, Rudolf. 'Ueber die Verstopfung der Lungenarterie.' *Froriep's
    Notizen Geb. Natur. Heilk.*, 1846, January.

— 'Thrombose und Embolie 1846–56.' Edited and prefaced by Rud. Beneke.
    In: Sudhoff's Klassiker der Medizin, vol. 7–8. Leipzig, A. Barth, 1910.

— *Gesammelte Abhandlungen zur Wissenschaftlichen Medizin*. Frankfurt am
    Main, Meidinger, 1856.

— *Die Cellularpathologie in ihrer Begründung auf Physiologische und Pathologische Gewebelehre.* Berlin, Hirschwald, 1858.

Vital, Hayim, Shaarei Kedushah [Hebr., *Gates of Holiness*]. Aleppo, Sason, 1865 [1st ed. Amsterdam, 1715].

Volta, A. 'An account of some discoveries made by Mr. Galvani, with experiments and observations on them.' *Phil. Trans.*, 1793, **83**, 10–44.

Vulpian, E. F. A. [case report from the Salpêtrière] 'Ramollissement cérébral ... Caillot ancien dans l'auricle gauche. Infarctus de la paroi du ventricule gauche du coeur coincidant avec l'existence d'un caillot ancien dans l'une des arterès coronaires etc.' *Un. méd.*, (Paris), 1866, N.S. **29**, 417–19.

Wall, John. 'A Letter to Dr. Heberden on the angina pectoris.' *In his*: *Medical Tracts*. Oxford, D. Prince & J. Cooke, 1780 [see pp. 324–35].

— 'On angina pectoris.' *Med. Trans. roy. Coll. Physns*, 1785, **3**, 12–24.

Waller, Augustus D. 'A demonstration on man of electromotive changes accompanying the heart's beat.' *J. Physiol.*, 1887, **8**, 229–34.

Walpole, Horace. *Memoirs of the Reign of King George the Second*, ed. Lord Holland. London, Colburn, 1846.

Warburg, E. J. 'Ueber den Coronarkreislauf und über die Thrombose einer Coronararterie.' *Acta med. Scand.*, 1930, **73**, 425–59, 545–604; [History 439–59]; References 591–604.

Warren, John. 'Remarks on Angina pectoris.' *New Engl. J. Med. Surg.*, 1812, **I**, 1–11. Reprinted in *New Engl. J. Med.*, 1962, **266**, 3–7.

Warren, John Collins. *Cases of Organic Diseases of the Heart with Dissections and Some Remarks to point out the Distinctive Symptoms of these Diseases.* Boston, T. B. Watt, 1809.

Waterston, D. 'Sir James Mackenzie's heart.' *Brit. Heart J.*, 1939, **I**, 237–48.

Wedel (Wedelius), 'Georg Wolfgang. 'De Pulsu Intercurrente.' *In*: *Ephemeridum Medico physicarum Germanicarum Academiae Imperialis Leopoldinae Naturae Curiosorum*, 1684.

Weigert, Carl. 'Ueber die pathologischen Gerinnungsvorgänge.' *Virchow's Arch. path. Anat.*, 1880, **79**, 87–123.

Wenckebach, K. F. 'A lecture on angina pectoris, etc.' *Brit. med. J.*, 1924, **i**, 809–15.

Wepfer, Johann Jakob. *Observationes Medico-practicae de Affectibus Capitis Internis et Externis.* Schaffhausen, J. A. Ziegler, 1727.

West, Samuel. 'Complete obliteration of one coronary artery; sudden death; remarks upon the anastomosis of the coronary arteries.' *Trans. path. Soc. Lond.*, 1882–83, **34**, 66–67.

White, Paul D. *Heart Disease.* 4th ed. New York, Macmillan, 1951.

— and Donovan, Helen. *Hearts, their Long Follow-up.* Philadelphia and London, Saunders, 1967.

Wiggers, C. J. 'The functional consequences of coronary occlusion.' *Ann. intern. Med.*, 1945, **23**, 158–69.

Williams, Charles J. B. *The Pathology and Diagnosis of Diseases of the Chest.* 4th ed. London, Churchill, 1840.

Williams, Herbert U. 'Gross and microscopic anatomy of two Peruvian mummies.' *Arch. Path. (Chicago)*, 1927, **4**, 26–33.

Willis, Thomas. *Pharmaceutice Rationalis.* English trans. by Samuel Pordage. London, Dring, Harper and Leigh, 2 vols. 1679–81.

— *Opera Omnia.* Amsterdam, H. Wetstenius, 1682.

Willius, F. A. 'The historic development of knowledge relating to the coronary circulation and its diseases.' *Proc. Mayo Clin.*, 1945, **20**, 103–6, 155–56, 326–36; 1946, **21**, 77–90, 185–91.

Willius, F. A., and Keys, Thomas E. *Cardiac Classics.* London, Henry Kimpton, 1941.

Wilson, F. N. *et al. The Distribution of the Currents of Action and of Injury Displayed by Heart Muscle and Other Excitable Tissues.* Ann Arbor, University of Michigan Press, 1933.

Wilson, John A. 'Medicine in ancient Egypt.' *Bull. Hist. Med.*, 1962, **36**, 114–28.

Wilson, L. G., 'Erasistratus, Galen and the pneuma.' *Bull. Hist. Med.*, 1959, **33**, 293–314.

Wolferth, C. C. and Wood, F. C. 'The electrographic diagnosis of coronary occlusion by the use of chest leads.' *Amer. Heart J.*, 1932, **7**, 404.

Wolferth, C. C., see also Wood, F. C.

Wood, F. C., Wolferth, C. C., and Livezey, M., 'Angina pectoris.' *Arch. Intern. Med.*, 1931, **47**, 339–65.

Wood, F. C., and Wolferth, C. C. 'Experimental coronary occlusion: inadequacy of the three conventional leads, etc.' *Arch. Intern. Med.*, 1933, **51**, 771–88.

Wood, Paul. *Paul Wood's Diseases of the Heart and Circulation.* 3rd ed., rev. and enl. London, Eyre & Spottiswoode, 1968.

— 'The erythrocyte sedimentation rate in diseases of the heart.' *Quart. J. Med.*, 1936, N.S. **5**, 1–19.

Wooster, D. *Diseases of the Heart.* San Francisco, H. H. Bancroft, 1867.

Wright, I. S., *et al.* 'Report of the committee for evaluation of anticoagulants in the treatment of coronary thrombosis with myocardial infarction.' *Amer. Heart J.*, 1948, **36**, 801.

Wrigley, P. F. M. 'Ischaemic heart disease in the nineteenth century.' *Oxford Med. School Gaz.*, 1965, 158–73.

Ziegler, E. *Lehrbuch der allgemeinen und speciellen pathologischen Anatomie.* 2 vols. Jena, G. Fischer, 1881–1885.

— *A Textbook of Pathological Anatomy and Pathogenesis.* Translated and edited by D. MacAlister. 2nd ed. 2 vols. New York, W. Wood, 1885–97.

— 'Ueber myomalacia cordis.' *Virchow's Arch. path. Anat.*, 1882, **90**, 211.

Index

Abigail, *wife of Nabal*, 39–40
Abravanel, Isaac, 40
Abscess, heart, 52, 79, 108, 109
Adams, Francis, 27, 29, 31, 38, 176
Adams, Robert, 110–11
— 'Cases of diseases of the heart accompanied with pathological observations', 110–11
Aetius, 41
Age factor in coronary heart disease, 26, 75, 91, 122, 154, 168–69, 174
Ahrens, E. H., 167
Aldabi, Meir, 48
Alexander of Tralles, 41
Alexander, B., 69, 74, 77, 78, 143
Allbutt, *Sir* Clifford T., 69, 78, 100, 143–44
— *Diseases of the Arteries including Angina Pectoris*, 143
Amatus Lusitanus, 2, 55–57, 61, 66, 176
— *Curationum medicinalium centuria sexta*, 55–57
Amyl nitrite, 170
Anaemia, 46, 152
Anastomoses, coronary, 67, 152–54
— — capillary, 153
— — wide, 153
— — *see also* Circulation, collateral
Anatomical Society of Paris, 133
Anatomy, coronary, 4, 33, 34, 47, 48, 50, 51, 67, 73, 74, 75, 178
— *see also* Pathology
Aneurysm, 3, 7, 17, 24, 57, 75, 107
— aortic, 54, 75, 78, 79, 82, 106, 107, 125
— cardiac, 4, 9, 53, 77, 103, 110, 111, 113, 115, 130, 137, 139, 140, 145
— coronary artery, 115
Angina pectoris, xv, 3, 5, 6, 7, 11–12, 13, 22, 39, 50, 63, 65, 70, 73, 77–78, 83, 84–106, 110–113, 118–122,
16

134, 139, 140, 141, 143–44, 158, 159, 160, 161, 165, 180, 181, 183
— medical therapy in, 31, 32, 42, 43, 119–20, 169–71, 183
— surgical intervention in, 171–72
Anglo-Saxon magic and medicine, 42–43, 169
Animals, 40–41, 45
Anitschkow, N., 166
'Anonymous', *Dr.*, *see* Haygarth, *Dr.*
Anticoagulant drugs, 172
Antipater, 69, 126, 127
Antiquity of C.H.D., 14, 25, 172–76
Apopléxie du cœur, 111, 139, Pl. 1
Aretaeus, 30–32, 37, 38, 45, 147, 163–64, 169, 174
— *Causes and Symptoms in Acute Diseases*, 31
— *Therapeutics*, 31, 32
Aristotle, 28, 35, 154
— *Historia animalium*, 28
Arnold, Thomas, 9, 117–23, 143, 175
—, Case-history of, 119–22
Arteriosclerosis, xv, 1, 7, 8, 17, 18, 50, 57, 90, 92, 98, 102, 104, 106, 107, 108, 109–10, 122, 125, 128, 137, 138, 139, 152, 160, 163, 187
— effect of diet on, 40, 93, 165, 166–68, 169, 174
— in Egyptian mummies, 15–19
Atheroma, 7, 8, 16, 17, 18, 76, 77, 108, 121, 123, 128, 129, 130, 143, 168, 173, 185
Atherosclerosis, 7, 18, 24, 108, 123, 128, 166, 167
Asclepiades, 37
Avicenna, 41, 44–46, 48, 154, 164
— *Canon*, 44–46
— *De Viribus Cordis*, 164

Bacon, Francis, 58, 59
— Essay on 'Friendship', 58
Bailey, C. H., 166
Baly, William, 114
Bamberger, Heinrich von, 135
Baron, J., 93
— Life of Edward Jenner, 93
Bartoletti, F., 69, 75, 148
— Methodus in Dyspnoeam, 69
Basch, Samuel von, 161
Basle, Switzerland, 43, 61
Bath, Somerset, 93, 94, 97
Bauhin, Caspar, 54
— Theatrum anatomicum, 54
Bäumler, Christian, 140, 142
Baylac, Joseph, 161
Bayliss, W. M., 155
Bean, W. B., 13, 173–74
— 'Clinical masquerades of acute myo-
    cardial infarction', 173–74
Beck, Claude, 171
Bedford, D. Evan, 13, 31, 65, 91, 158,
    159, 161
Bell, Sir Charles, 105
Bellini, Lorenzo, 3, 71, 74, 76
— De Urinis et Pulsibus, 71
Belloni, Luigi, 68
Belt, E., 50, 51
Benedictus Crispus, 43
Benivieni, Antonio, 2, 51–52, 109
— De abditis nonnulis ac mirandis morborum
    et sanationum causis, 51–52
Berengarius, Jacobus, Carpensis, 52, 177
— Isagoge Breves
Berlin, Germany, 125, 137, 155
Besançon, France, 100
Bezold, Albert von, 9, 114, 131, 137, 153
Bible, The, 2, 39–40, 164
— Ecclesiastes, 40, 82
— Ezekiel, 40
— Genesis, 39
— Jeremiah, 39
— Samuel Bk. I (case-history of Nabal),
    39–40, 164
Bichat, François Xavier, 109
— Anatomie générale, 109
Biernacki, E., 162
Birmingham, Warwickshire, General
    Hospital and Eye Infirmary, 119
Bissing, F. W. von, 24

Black, Samuel, 6, 96–97, 98, 105, 140
Blackall, John, 65
— Observations on the Nature and Cure of
    Dropsies, 65
'Blockpnée', 101
Blood, see Coagulation, Circulation,
    Laboratory aids to diagnosis
— 'heaping up of corpuscles', 37, 70
— non-coagulability of, 60, 78, 87, 89–
    90, 93, 103, 182
Blumer, G., 140
Bober, S., 137
Boerhaave, Herman, 80
Bologna, Italy, 47, 154
Bonaccorsi, Cardinal, 109
Bonet, Théophile, 3, 54, 68, 70, 76, 107,
    124, 127
— Sepulchretum, 3, 54, 68, 70–71
Booth, C. C., 93
Bousfield, G., 13, 158
Bradley, S. E., 36
Bramwell, Byron, 141
Breasted, J. H., 21
British Heart Journal, 168
Brock, A. J., 36, 178
Bruetsch, W. L., 24
Brunswick, Duchess of, 81
Brunton, T. Lauder, 170
— 'On the use of nitrite of amyl in
    angina pectoris', 170
Bryan, C. P., 21
Bucknill, S., 119–22
Bucknill, S. B., 119–22
Budge, E. A. Wallis, 19
Buess, H., 62, 138
Buffalo University School of Medicine,
    U.S.A., 18
Burch, G. E., 157
Burchell, H. B., 82
Burdon-Sanderson, J., 155
Burns, Allan, 6–7, 98, 104–5, 160
— Observations on some of the most fre-
    quent and important Diseases of
    the Heart, 6, 104–5
Butter, William, 97
Bylebyl, J. J., 55
Byzantine medicine, 41

Caelius Aurelianus, 2, 3, 5, 8, 31, 37–38,
    84, 110, 127

Calabresi, M., 75

Calcification, *see* Ossification

Caldani, Leopoldo Marco Antonio, 153

Canadian Journal of Medical Sciences, 135

Cardia, 22. See *also* Heart, different meanings of the word

Cardiac insufficiency, 4, 5, 6, 10, 63, 93, 96, 99, 139, 140, 142, 148, 149

'Cardiac passion', 37

Cardialgia, 1, 26–27, 168

Cardimona, 34

Cardiogmos, 26–27, 37, 75

Cardiology, 4, 45, 60, 81, 82, 159

— text-books and theses, 4, 10, 60, 128, 141, 144, 145

Cardiomalacia, 8, 110

Cariage, J. L., 99–100, 101

Cassius Felix, 38–39

Celsus, 37, 108, 169

Chalatov, S., 166

Chamberlaine, John, 50

Champollion, Jean François, 19

Charles V, *Emperor* [Charles I of Spain], 52

Charles, M., 100

Cheyne-Stokes respiration, 122

Chicago, U.S.A., 149

Chirac, Pierre, 8–9, 71–72, 114, 130, 152–53

— *De Motu Cordis Adversaria Analytica*, 71–72

Cholesterol, 128, 166–68

Choulant, L., 50

Circulation, collateral, coronary, 9, 10, 67, 113, 123, 129, 132, 139, 146, 150, 152–54, 171

Circulation, coronary, 6, 7, 34, 52, 67, 82, 114, 147

—, systemic [general], 1, 3, 21, 60, 63, 65, 81, 181

—, 'Third', 2, 34, 65, 177

Clarendon, Edward, *Earl of*, Lord High Chancellor, 65–66

Cleveland, Ohio, U.S.A., 171

Clift, William, 88, 103

Coagulation of blood, 3, 8, 24, 28, 29, 57, 60, 68, 69, 70, 75, 81, 87, 89–90, 112, 127, 128, 129, 136

Cohnheim, Julius, 9, 67, 105, 114, 129, 131–32, 137, 153, 166

—, *Lectures on General Pathology*, 132, 137

Coiter, V., 79

Collapse, circulatory, 2, 6, 23, 31, 37, 45, 58, 59, 134, 136, 139

Columbus, M. Realdus, 52, 55, 74, 80, 177

— *De re anatomica*, 55

Cooke, W., 82

Coronary artery, anomalies of, 121, 123

— — disease, xv, xvi, 1, 2, 7, 8, 9, 10, 13, 39, 73, 93, 99, 114, 144, 151, 167

— calcification, *see* ossification

— heart disease

    abdominal manifestations, 148, 149, 151, 152, 162, 174

    bedside diagnosis, 135, 137, 144, 148–49, 160, 161

    etiology, 38, 42, 70, 93, 98, 108, 125, 163–69, 173

    heredity, 108, 122, 169, 171, 174

    incidence, 13, 91, 99, 167, 168, 171–76

    sudden death, 2, 6, 10, 12, 13, 24, 26, 35, 47, 58, 59, 60, 61, 69, 73, 74, 75, 86, 102, 117, 129, 130, 139, 141, 146, 150, 151, 153, 165, 171, 175, 176, 180–81

    theories of, 6, 7, 8, 10, 12, 14, 78, 93, 97, 102, 105, 106, 112, 143, 144, 160

    See *also:* Anatomy, Angina pectoris, Coronary artery disease, Coronary vessels, Dietary influences on, Dyspnoea, Emotional factors, Ischaemic heart disease, Laboratory aids, Myocardial infarction, Obstruction, Occlusion, Pain, Pathology, Physiology, Syncope, Therapy, Thrombosis

— vasodilators, 170–71

— vessels, 2, 3, 4, 5, 6, 17, 33, 34, 47, 48, 50, 51, 52, 65, 67, 74, 75, 89, 94, 177, 178

Corvisart, Jean Nicholas, *Baron*, 83, 165

Councilman, W. T., 123

Cournand, A., 36

Cowper, William, 113

Cracow, Poland, University of, 137

Craigie, D., 108
— *Elements of General and Pathological Anatomy*, 108
Crawford, M. D., 168
Crell, Johann F., 76–77, 94, 107
— *Dissertatio de arteria coronaria instar ossis indurata*, 76
Cruveilhier, Jean, 46, 111, 130, 139, 153, Pl. 1, Pl. 14
— *Anatomie pathologique du corps humain*, 111
Czermak, J. N., 15–16

Dahlerup, *Dr.*, 130
Dahl-Iversen, E., 114
Danon, Joseph, xvi, 40
Darcy, *Sir* Robert, 63, 116, 164
Daremberg, Charles, 33, 34, 35, 36, 79, 177
David, *King of Israel*, 39, 40
Davison, M. H. Armstrong, 67
Day, G., 125
Deines, H. V., 22
De Langen, C. D., 167
DePasquale, N. P., 157
Dietary influences on coronary heart disease, 93, 108, 163, 166–69, 174
Diversus, Petrus Salius, 2, 58, 60, 75, 87, 126, 127
— *De Affectibus particularibus*, 58–59
Dock, George, 10, 142–43, 145, 152
— 'Notes on the coronary arteries', 142
— 'Historical notes on coronary occlusion from Heberden to Osler', 142
Dock, William, 9, 137, 167
Donato, Marcello, 64
Donbrow, P., xvi
Donovan, H., 173
Drabkin, I. E., 8, 37, 127
Drelincourt, Carolus, 70, 76
Dressler, William, 142
Dreyfuss, F., 166
Düben, G. W. J., 9, 64, 115–17, 133
Dublin Medical Press, 117
Du Bois-Reymond, E., 155
Dupuytren, G., *Baron*, 54
Duretus, Ludovicus, 61
Dyscrasia, 125. *See also* Heart, dyscrasias of,

Dyspnoea, 5, 6, 53, 69, 75, 77, 78, 82, 86, 87, 95, 101, 134, 136, 139, 140, 142, 143, 147–48, 149, 170, 181

East, T., 28, 118
— *The Story of Heart Disease*, 118
Ebbell, B., 21
Ebers, G., 20
— *See also* Papyrus Ebers.
Ebner, E., 133
Egypt, Ancient, 1, 15–24
— — Chester Beatty papyrus, 23
— — Ebers papyrus, 1, 20–24
— — Edwin Smith surgical papyrus, 21
— — mummies: degenerative diseases in, 1, 15–19
— — — examination of coronary vessels and myocardium by A. R. Long, 17–18
Electrocardiography, 13–14, 135, 141, 150, 152, 154–160
Einthoven, Willem, 13, 154, 155–57, Pl. 15
— 'On the normal human electrocardiogram and on the capillar-electrometric examination of some heart patients', 156
— 'The galvanometric registration of the human electrocardiogram . . .', 156
Embolism, coronary, 141, 147
— pulmonary, 8, 62, 127, 128
Embolization, 8, 16, 125, 127, 128, 133, 137, 159, 172, 185, 187
Emotional factors in coronary heart disease, 40, 44, 64, 92–93, 103, 115, 147, 163–66
End-arteries, 9, 131, 132
—, functional, 132
Engelmann, T. W., 155
Enos, W. F., *et al.*, 'Coronary disease among United States soldiers killed in action in Korea,' 168–69
Epidemic Encephalitis Economo, 1
Erasistratus, 36, 38, 84
Erichsen, John, 9, 114, 130, 153
— 'On the influence of the coronary circulation on the action of the heart', 114

Erythrocyte sedimentation rate, 14, 162
Esso, I. van, 39
Esterly, J. R., 169
Ethnological variations, 163, 166–67
Experimental arteriosclerosis, 166–68
— coronary artery occlusion, 130–32, 163
— embolism, 130–31, 137
— ligation of coronaries, 8–9, 13, 71–72, 114, 130–31, 137, 152–53, 158, 171
— — — pulmonary vein, 114

Fåhraeus, R., 162
— 'The suspension-stability of the blood', 162
Falloppius, Gabriel, 54
— Observationes anatomicae, 54
Fantoni, J., 70
Fatty degeneration, 125, 138, 139, 143, 168, 186
Fenger, Dr., 130
Fernel, Jean, 109
— Pathologia, 109
Fever, see Temperature measurement
Finke, L. L., 167
Fishman, A., 36
— (Ed.), Circulation of the Blood, 36
Foix, de, Count, 66–67, 179–180, Pl. 4
Forbes, J., 139
Forestus, Petrus, 74
Fothergill, John, 6, 89, 92, 93, 97, 102, 103, 105, 165
— 'Case of an Angina pectoris, with Remarks', 92
— 'Farther account of the angina pectoris', 92, 165
Fox, R. H., 50
Franklin, Kenneth J., 63, 64, 65, 67
Frati, Carlo, 68
— Bibliografia Malpighiana, 68
Freeman, S., see Li, T. W., and Freeman, S.
Freind, John, 59
— History of Physic, 59
Froissart, Sir John, 66, 179–80
— Chronicles, 66, 179–80
Fulton, John F., 156

Gairdner, Prof., 100

Galen, 2, 3, 4, 8, 11, 27, 32–36, 40, 41, 45, 46, 55, 56, 58, 61, 62, 65, 67, 69, 72, 78, 79, 114, 126–27, 131, 154, 163, 177–78
— On Anatomical Procedures, 33, 34, 36, 72, 114
— On Diseases, 34
— On the Affected Parts, 35, 36, 62, 69, 78–79
— On the Natural Faculties, 36, 178
— On the Usefulness of the Parts of the Body, 33, 34, 177–78
— Praesagium de pulsibus, 35, 58
Gallavardin, L., 101
Galvani, L. A., 154
Garengeot, R.-J.-C., 81
Garrison, F. H., 45, 101
Gaskell, E., xvi
Gasser, Achilles, 54, 79
Genty, M., 111
George II, 82–83, 96, 176
Geographical pathology, 167
Gerard of Cremona, 45
Gerard, John, Herbal, 64
Goble, A. J., et al., 'Mortality reduction in a coronary care unit', 171
Gorlin, R., 171
Grant, Dr., 160
Grapow, H., 1, 21–22
— Grundriss der Medizin der alten Aegypter, 21–24
Grattan, J. H. G., 42, 169
Greece, Ancient, 1–2, 25–39
Groen, J., 167
Gross, Louis, The Blood Supply of the Heart, 152–154
Gunter, surgeon, 95

Hales, Stephen, 161
Hall, G. H., 59
Haller, Albrecht von, 107, 123, 153, Pl. 12
Hammer, Adam, 9, 135–37, 149
— 'A case of thrombotic occlusion of one of the coronary arteries of the heart', 135
Harvey, William, 2, 3, 5, 34, 40, 54, 60, 63–65, 67, 76, 82, 85, 93, 102, 116, 131, 132, 164, 165, 177, Pl. 3
— De motu cordis, 64, 131

— 'First Disquisition to John Riolan', 64–65
— 'Second Disquisition to John Riolan', 63–64, 65, 164
— Praelectiones, 54
Haygarth, Dr. ['Dr. Anonymous'], 60, 83, 87–90, 93, 94, 125, 127, 171, 180–82
Heart, 158
Heart as a muscle, 30, 33, 34, 67, 177
—, dyscrasias of the, 35–36, 46–47
—, different meanings of the word, 1–2, 20, 22, 26, 27, 31, 37
Heart-block, 52, 53, 61, 110, 131, 137, 140, 157
'Heartburn', 1
Hebb, Christopher Henry, 83
Heberden, William, 4–5, 6, 7, 22, 28, 38, 42, 50, 53, 60, 63, 73, 78, 83–92, 93, 94, 95, 97, 98, 99, 100, 101, 102, 104, 105, 117, 122, 125, 127, 142, 144, 157, 164, 169, 170, 171, 175, 180–83, Pl. 9
— 'Some account of a disorder of the breast, 4, 83 ff.
    Commentaries, 5, 38, 84–89, 92, 170
Heberden, William, Jr., 84
Hebrew University Medical School, Jerusalem, xvi, xvii
Hedley, O. F., 94
Heidelberg, Germany, 123, 155
Helmont, J. B. van, 166
Henle, Jacob, 153
Herbert, General, 103
Herophilus, 38
Herrick, James B., 11, 12, 13, 28, 42, 104, 141, 146, 147, 148, 149–52, 154, 158, 161, 173, 175
— 'Clinical features of sudden obstruction of the coronary arteries, 149–50
— 'Intimate account of my early experience with coronary thrombosis, 150
— Memories of Eighty Years, 150
— Short History of Cardiology, 141
Hippocrates, 2, 25–30, 34, 35, 37, 46, 56, 57, 61, 75, 126, 168, 176
— Ancient Medicine, 176

— Aphorisms, 26, 27, 47, 54, 75, 168
— Coan Prenotions, 25–26, 75
— On Diseases, 34
— On the Heart, 30
— Prognostics, 28
— Regimen in Acute Diseases, 27, 28–30
Hirsch, August, 124, 167
Histoire de l'Académie Royale des Sciences, 81
Hochhaus, H., 149, 161
— 'Diagnosis of sudden occlusion of the coronary arteries', 149
Hodel, C., 138
Hodgson, Joseph, 112–13, 119–22
— Treatise on the diseases of arteries and veins, 112–13
Hoffmann, Friedrich, 82, 98, 144
— Medicina rationalis systematica, 82
— Opera omnium physico-medicorum etc., suppl. secundum, 82
Hoffmann, M., 75
Hollerius, J., 61
Hollman, Arthur, 170
Home, Sir Everard, 102, 103, 165
— Life of John Hunter, 103
Hood, Donald, 141
Hooke, Robert, 116
— Micrographia, 116
Huber, Karl, 9
Huchard, Henri, 10, 12, 82, 86, 106, 141, 144, 148
— Traité clinique des maladies du cœur et de l'aorte, 144
Hunter, John, 50, 88, 89, 90, 92, 93, 94, 95, 102–3, 162, 165, 182
— MS. account of dissections of morbid bodies, 88, 103
— Treatise on the Blood, Inflammation and Gunshot Wounds, 90
Hunter, William, 50
Hygiea, 115
Hyrtl, Joseph, 153
Hysteria, 62

Ibn Ezra, Abraham, 43
Ibn Haitam, Abd al Rahman, 43
Ignatovski, A. I., 166
— 'On the influence of animal food on the tissues of the rabbit', 166
Imersel, Dominus de, 52–54, 164

Infarct, use of the word, 54, 64, 127
Infarction, myocardial, *see* Myocardial infarction
International Society of Geographical Pathology, 9th Conference, 167
Intensive coronary care units, 171
Ischaemic heart disease, 4, 5, 14, 19, 53, 81, 83, 105, 116, 118, 122, 140, 158, 171
Isidore of Seville, 42
— *Etymologiae*, 42
Izak, G., 90

Jacob, 36
Jacobi, Abraham, 135
Jacobs, H. B., 93
James I[James VI of Scotland], 39
Jamin, F., 153
Jarcho, Saul, 15, 79, 123
— (Ed.) *Human palaeopathology*, 15
Java, 167
Jenner, Edward, 6, 50, 89, 93–95, 97
Jerusalem, Israel, xvi, 166
Jewish University and National Library, xvi
Joachim, H., 20
Johnes, Thomas, 179–80
Johns Hopkins Institute of the History of Medicine, xvi
Johnson, Samuel, 83
Johnstone, James, 82, 95–96, 105, 107
Jokl, E. and P., 84
Jonckheere, F., 23
Jones, W. H. S., 26, 27
Jonnesco, T. H., 171
Journal des Sçavans, 99
Journal of the American Medical Association, 175
Judah ha-Nassi, 40

Karplus, H., 90
Katchalsky, A., 166–67
Katz, H. M., 28
Katz, Ph. B., 28
Keele, K. D., xvi, 27, 50, 51, 88, 89, 103
Kerckring, T., 68
Kernig, Vladimir, 14, 76, 141, 142, 161
— Kernig's sign, 141
— 'Treatment of angina pectoris', 141
Keynes, *Sir* Geoffrey, 40

—, *Life of William Harvey*, 40
Keys, S. T., 82, 109
Kiev, U.S.S.R., 147, 149
— University, 148
Klemperer, P., 28, 69, 173
Kock, W., 115
Kohn, H., 100
Kölliker, A., 155
Kölster, R., 153
Korczinski, Edward, 137
Korean War, 168, 169, 176
Korotkov, N., 161
Kowal, S. J., 165
Krehl, L., 13, 146–47, 149, 150, 151, 154
— *Die Erkrankungen des Herzmuskels*, 146–47
Kreysig, F. L., 106
Kühn, K. G., 8, 33, 34, 35, 36, 58, 126
Kussmaul, Adolf, 135

Labat, R., 25
Laboratory aids to diagnosis, 14, 160–63
— erythrocyte sedimentation rate, 14, 162
— leucocytosis, 14, 159, 161–62
— serum transaminase, 162–63
La Due, J. S., 14, 163
Laënnec, R. T. H., 8, 111–12
— *Traité de l'ausculation médiate*, 8, 111–12
Lancet, 141, 158
Lancisi, G. M., 3–4, 74–75, 107, 176
— *De aneurysmatibus*, 3, 75
— *De subitaneis mortibus*, 3, 74–75
Langdon-Brown, *Sir* Walter, 172
Langer, K., 153
Latham, Peter M., 9, 11, 117–18, 119–23, 152, 165
— *Lectures on subjects connected with clinical medicine*, 117
Laubry, C., 77
Laufer, A., 167
Leake, Chauncey D., 131
Leary, T., 166
Leeson, T. S., 15
Leeuwenhoek, A. van, 116
LeFanu, W. R., 94
Leibowitz, J. O., 40, 43, 44, 54, 61, 82, 164, 169
Leipzig, Germany, 108
— University Library, 20

Leonardo da Vinci, 2, 49–51, 74, 109

Lesky, Erna, 125

Leucocytosis in coronary thrombosis, 14, 159, 161–62

Levene, A., 64, 117

Levine, S. A., 14, 144, 159, 161–62

Lewis, Sir Thomas, 12, 94, 99, 159, 160

— Clinical Signs illustrated by Personal Experiences, 160

— Diseases of the Heart, 160

Leyden, E. von, 9–10, 64, 96, 129, 137–40, 148

— 'On the sclerosis of the coronary arteries and the morbid states arising from them', 137

Leyden, The Netherlands, 167

— University, Physiological Institute, 156

Li, T. W., and Freeman, S., 'Experimental lipemia and hypercholesterolemia produced by protein depletion and by cholesterol-feeding in dogs', 167

Libman, Emanuel, 14, 159, 161, 162

Lieber, Elinor, xvi

Lieutaud, Joseph, 107

Ligation, see Experimental

Lind, L. R., 52

Lipids, blood, 90, 108, 167

Lipothymia, 2, 6, 59

Lippmann, Gabriel, 155

Lister, Lord, 114

Littré, Alexis, 127, 128

Littré, Emile, 25–30, 34, 57, 126

Lobstein, J. G. C. F. M., 7, 8, 109–10, 123, 138

— Traité d'Anatomie pathologique, 7, 109–10

London, 16, 155

London Hospital, The, 173

Long, A. R., 17–18

Long, E. R., 51

Lorry, A.-Ch., 99, 100

Los Angeles County Medical Association, U.S.A., 142

Louis, Antoine, 55

'Love-pulse', 163

Lower, Richard, 67–68, 74

— Tractatus de Corde, 67–68

Lumleian Lectures (1910), 11

Macalister, D., 138

Mackenzie, Sir James, 12, 143, 159

— Angina pectoris, 159

McMichael, Sir John, 172

McMurrich, J. P., 50

Maimonides, 46–47, 126, 164

— Aphorisms, 46–47

— De Accidentibus, 164

Major, R. H., 119, 135

— Classic Descriptions of Disease, 119, 135

Malinin, T. I., 131

Malmsten, H. P., 9, 64, 115–17

Malpighi, Marcello, 3, 67, 68–69, 109, 116

— De Polypo Cordis, 68

— De viscerum structura, 68

— Opera omnia, 68

— Opera scelte, 68

Mann, G., 73

Marchand, F., 108, 123

Marcus, S., 43

Marie, René, 10, 14, 145, 161

— 'L'infarctus du myocarde et ses conséquences . . .', 10, 145

Massa, Nicholas, 109

— Anatomiae liber introductorius, 109

Master, A. M., 158, 172

Matteucci, Carlo, 154–55

Matthews, S. A., 153

May, M. T., 33, 34, 177

Medical Transactions of the College of Physicians of London, 4, 180

Mejopragia cordis, 148

Mering, F. F., 148

Mering, J. von, 148

Merkel, H., 153

Merneptah, Pharaoh, 16

Metabolites, 132

Metropolitan Museum of Art, New York, 18

Meyenfeldt, F. H. van, 39

Michaelis, G. H., 82

— Biblia Hebraica, 82

Michaels, L., 173, 175

Michelotti, P. A., 127–28

— Tractatus Universalis Morborum Sanguinis Ductuum, 127–28

Michigan University, U.S.A., 142, 158

Microscopy, 9, 16, 113, 116, 129, 133, 138, 139

Miller, J. L., 153
Minkowski, O., 148
Minnesota University, U.S.A., 171
Mishnah, The, 40
Mitral stenosis, 73, 126
Montagnana, Bartholomaeus, 59
— Consilia Medica, 59
Moodie, R. L., 17
Morand, S. F., 81, 82, 96, 107
'Morbus cardiacus', 2, 38, 169
Morgagni, Giovanni Battista, 4, 54, 68–69, 71, 74, 76, 77–81, 82–83, 85, 97, 107, 124, 143, 144, 153
— The Seats and Causes of Diseases investigated by Anatomy, 4, 77–81
Morgan, A. D., 113
Morris, J. N., 168, 173
Moscow, U.S.S.R., 147
— University, 147
Mouquin, M., 77
Muir, Robert, 168
Müller, E. A., 144
Müller, H., 155
Mundinus, 47–48
— Anothomia, 47
Murrell, William, 170
Myasnikov, A. L., 166
— 'Influence of some factors on the development of experimental cholesterol atherosclerosis', 166
Myocardial infarction, xv, 1, 2, 3, 6, 7, 8, 9, 10, 11, 12, 13, 14, 30, 40, 46, 52, 55, 58, 59, 60, 62, 63, 64, 69, 75–76, 79, 82, 85, 90, 95, 97, 98, 99, 101, 103, 104, 105, 109, 111, 112, 113, 115, 118, 127, 130, 131, 132, 133, 134, 135, 137, 139, 142, 143, 144, 145, 158, 161, 163, 168, 171, 172, 174, 183 ff.
— necrosis, 8, 9, 64, 81, 111, 112, 113, 114, 116, 138, 148, 161, 162, 163
— scars, 4, 17, 18, 79–80, 92, 102, 103, 114, 153, 169
Myocarditis, chronic, 9, 18, 35, 79, 129, 130, 134, 139
Myocardium, 3, 5, 6, 10, 11, 17–18, 81, 85, 91, 93, 97, 98, 99, 111, 113, 143, 144, 146, 147, 172

Myomalacia cordis, 8, 46, 117, 138–39, 142

Nabal, 39–40, 164
Nasse, H., 162
Naunyn, B., 153
Neale, G., 59
Neuburger, Max, 60, 79
New England Journal of Medicine, 105
New York, U.S.A., 135, 142
Nicholls, Frank, 82–83, Pl. 8
Nicolai, G. F., 158
Nitroglycerine, 170–71

Obrastzow, W. P., 11, 12, 141, 147–49, 152, 161
Obstruction, idea of, xv, 2, 6, 19, 23, 24, 25, 26, 28, 46, 55–58, 66, 75, 88, 125, 126, 175, 181
'Obstruction in the heart', xv, 3, 8, 36, 41, 71, 97, 110, 113, 127, 149, 150
'Obstruction in the lung', 19, 41
Obstruction, vascular, 2, 29, 45, 46, 58, 59, 101, 170
Occlusion, coronary, 3, 9, 24, 71, 79, 81, 82, 94, 124, 125, 128, 131–33, 135–37, 139, 140, 146, 148, 149, 150, 151–53, 161, 172, 175, 185
— of the pulmonary artery, 126
O'Malley, C. D., 50, 54
Oppenheimer, E. H., 158, 169
Oribasius, 41
Osler, Sir William, 11, 13, 95, 99, 100, 118, 122, 123, 130, 141, 142, 145, 150, 165, 168
— Lectures on angina Pectoris and Allied States, 11, 118, 130, 165
Ossification and calcification, coronary, 3, 6, 7, 18, 70, 71, 74, 76, 77, 92–93, 94, 96, 97, 98, 105, 106, 110, 113, 114, 115, 123, 125, 134–35, 138
'Ox-heart', 3, 64

Padua, Italy, 47, 55, 61
Page, F. J. M., 155
Pagel, Walter, 57, 109
— Paracelsus, 57
Pain, anginal, 1, 2, 12, 27, 39, 41, 43, 78, 84–88, 91, 98, 101, 112, 143, 160

— — *See also* Angina pectoris
— —, absence of, 11, 137, 151, 174
'Pain in the heart', 39, 41, 42, 43, 45, 51,
     53, 62
— precordial, 1, 2, 3, 4, 19, 25, 29,
     42–43, 53, 54, 62, 70, 75, 82,
     86, 115, 142, 179, 180
—— *see also* Dyspnoea
Pain versus dyspnoea, 69, 75, 87, 99, 101,
     148, 174
Palaeopathology, *see* Egypt, Peru
Panum, P. L., 9, 114, 130–31, 137, 153
Papyrus Chester Beatty, 23
Papyrus Ebers, 1, 20–24
Papyrus Edwin Smith, 21
Paracelsus, Theophrastus, 57
— *Tartarus cordis*, 57
Pardee, H. E. B., 13, 158
Paré, Ambroise, 57–58
Paris, France, 133, 145, 155, 161, 184
Parkinson, Sir John, 91, 158, 159, 161
Parry, Caleb Hillier, 6, 7, 10, 31, 64, 93,
     94, 95, 97–99, 105–6, 140, 148,
     160
— *An Inquiry into the Symptoms and
     Causes of the Syncope Anginosa
     . . .*, 97–99
Parry, E. H., 172
Pathology, coronary, 4, 9, 10, 18, 47–48,
     51–52, 54, 60, 74–76, 77–83,
     89, 92–93, 94, 96–98, 100, 103,
     105, 110, 113, 115, 116, 123–30,
     133, 134, 136, 137, 143
Paul of Aegina, 38, 41
Pavia, Italy, 154
Pavinsky, 141
Payne, J. F., 127, 134–35
Paytherus, *surgeon*, 6, 94
Peacock, Thomas B., 115
Peete, D. C., 39
Pelvet, N., 138
Peptic ulcer, 3, 64, 172
Percival, T., 97, 105
Pericardial effusion, 35, 46, 96
Pericarditis epistenocardica, 142
—, secondary, 76, 113, 140–41, 142, 143,
     151, 152, 161
Pericardium, 60, 77, 78, 79, 82, 97, 116,
     143, 153, 171, 184
Periodicals, medical, 95, 101, 150

Peru, pathological examination of mum-
     mies from, 16, 17, 19
Petrov, B. D., 147
Philipp, J. J., 75
Physiology, coronary, 36, 47–48, 52,
     55, 64–65, 67, 98, 102, 105, 123,
     138, 150, 177
— *see also* Pathology
Pickering, *Sir* George, 17, 123, 168
Pisa, Italy, 154
Pissinus, Sebastianus, 59
Plato, 2, 154
— Menon dialogue, 154
Platter, Felix, 61–62, 74
— *Observationes*, 61–62
Pliny, 108
Polypus, cardiac, 53, 68, 69, 70, 75, 78,
     81, 101, 127
Porter, Ian H., 115
Post-myocardial-infarction-syndrome,
     142
Potain, P. C., 138, 161
Pottier, Jacques, 75
Poynter, F. N. L., xvi
Prague, Physiological Institute, 15
Pratt, F. H., 74
Prendergast, G., 37
Prevention, 93
Prognosis, 13, 25, 26, 32, 35, 60–61,
     138–39, 146, 150, 152, 162, 173
Pulmonary oedema, 86, 100, 121, 139
— thrombosis, 8
Pyloric stenosis, 3, 64

Quain, Richard, 113–14, 138
— 'On fatty diseases of the heart', 113
Radcliffe, C. B., 133–34
Ragusa, Yugoslavia, 55
Ratcliffe, H. L., 40
Rhazes, 42
Rhythm, cardiac, anomalies of, 37,
     58–60, 89, 90, 91, 127, 130, 131,
     132, 134–35, 157, 159, 160, 171,
     181, 183
Riolan, Jean, 2, 63–65, 102
Riva-Rocci, S., 161
Robb-Smith, A. H. T., 168
— *The enigma of coronary heart disease*, 168
Robert, J., 75
Rokitansky, Carl, 124–25

— *Autobiography*, 125
— *Manual of Pathological Anatomy*, 125
Rolleston, *Sir* Humphry D., 99, 112
Romberg, Ernst, 149
Rome, Ancient, 25–32
Rose, V., 38
Roselaar, M., 97
Rosenbloom, J., 65
Ross, Herefordshire, 94
Roth, M., 54
—, *Andreas Vesalius Bruxellensis*, 54
Rougnon, N. F., 93, 96, 99–101, 103, 148
— *Considerationes pathologico-semeioticae*, 101
Rowling, J. Thomson, 19
Royal College of Physicians, London, xvi, 4, 83, 143
— *Medical Transactions*, 4, 83
Royal College of Surgeons of England, 103
Royal Society, London, 67, 82
Royal Society of Medicine, London, xvi
— Pathological Section, 16
Rudius, E., 59
Ruffer, *Sir* Marc Armand, 16–17, 18
Rufinus, 44
Rupture, cardiac, 3, 4, 63, 64, 77, 81, 82, 96, 110, 113, 115–17, 132–33, 138, 145, 184–86
Russell, W. T., *see* Ryle, J. A., and Russell, W. T.
Russian Congress of Internal Medicine (1909), 147
Ruysch, Fredrik, 73, 74
Ryle, J. A., and Russell, W. T., 'Natural history of coronary disease', 168

Sacks, B., 159, 162
St. George's Hospital, London, 102, 165
St. Louis, Missouri, U.S.A., 135
St. Petersburg, Russia, 104, 166
St. Petersburg Medical Weekly, 141
Salpêtrière, Paris, 133, 184
Samuelson, B., 153
Sandison, A. T., 17, 18–19
Saul, *King of Israel*, 39
Saunders, J. B. de C. M., 24, 50
Saussure, Horace Benedict de, 84

Saxonia, Hercules, 54, 61, 62, 132, 133, 164
— *De Pulsibus*, 61, 62, 132
— *Prognoseon practicarum lib.* II, 54
Scarpa, Antonio, 7, 8, 17, 82, 83, 103, 106–9, 113, 125, 168, 169, Pl. 10, Pl. 11
— *Sull' Aneurisma . . .*, 106–7
Scherf, D. and Schott, A., 59
Scherk, Gerhard, 14, 162
Schierbeck, A., 118
Schrenk, M., 166
Schulthess-Rechberg, A. von., 131
Sclerosis, coronary, 1, 10, 51, 76–77, 91, 92, 110, 138–40, 142–43, 152, 166
Scribonius Largus, 154
Seegmiller, J. E., 97
Segall, Harold N., 80, 90, 180
Sénac, J. B. de, 4, 8, 60, 75–76, 79, 97, 109, 142, 153
— *Traité des Maladies du Coeur*, 75–76
— *Traité sur la Structure du Coeur . . .*, 75
Senckenberg Foundation, Frankfurt-on-Main, 129
Seneca, 97
Sharpe, W. D., 39, 42
Shattock, S. G., 16
Shock, cardiogenic, 2, 37–38, 60, 82, 90, 103, 130, 151, 169, 174, 175
Siegel, R. E., 36, 37, 97
Sigerist, H. E., 18
Simons, A., 158
Singer, Charles, 33, 34, 42, 50, 51, 72, 114, 169
Smith, Fred. M., 13, 152, 158, 171
Smith, *Sir* Grafton Elliot, 16, 17, 19, 21
Smith, John, 40
Sobernheim, J. F., 79
Snapper, I., 167
— *Chinese Lessons to Western Medicine*, 167
— 'Diet and atherosclerosis: truth and fiction', 167
Social and occupational influences on coronary heart disease, 164–65, 168
Sones, F. M., *Jr.*, 172
Soranus, 37

Souques, A., 26
Spalteholz, W., 153
Sphygmomanometry, 14, 131, 148, 151, 152, 159, 161
Sprague, H. B., 174–75
Stannard, J., 43
Starling, E. H., 155
'Status anginosus', 14, 86, 96, 147, 161
Steatomatous [fatty] degeneration, 7, 107–8, 113, 138
Steeves, G. W., 59
Steno, Nicolaus, 30
Stenzel, C. G., 107, 108, Pl. 13
— Dissertatio de steatomatibus aortae, 107
Stern, L., 20
Sternberg, J., 147
    'On diseases of the myocardium following disturbances in the coronary circulation', 147
Sternberg, M., 76, 142
Steuer, R. O., 24
Stokes, William, 23, 138
Stokes–Adams syndrome, 23, 110
Strasbourg, 109, 135
Straschesko, N. D., 11, 141, 147–49
Stuckey, N. W., 166
Sudhoff, K., 43, 57
— Klassiker der Medizin, 128
Surgery as therapeutical measure in coronary heart disease, 171, 172
Surveys, list of, xv, 187
Sweating Sickness (sudor anglicus), 1
Swedenborg, E., 74
Symons, H. J. M., 77
Syncope, cardiac, 2, 3, 25, 31–32, 36, 38–39, 55–56, 59, 60, 61, 62, 68, 71, 75, 86, 98, 135, 147, 161, 163, 169, 174, 175
— anginosa, 6, 97–98, 99, 104, 112

Talma, F. J., 130
Talmud, Babylonian, 2, 19, 39–41, 45
— — Tractate Hulin, 41
— — Tractate Sabbath, 41
Temkin, O., xvi, 21, 35
Temperature measurement, 14, 38, 148, 159, 161–62
Testa, A. G., 82
Thebesian valves, veins, 74

Thebesius, Adam Christian, 3, 73–74, 76, 153, 154, Pl. 6, Pl. 7
— Dissertatio medica de circulo sanguinis in corde, 73–74
Therapy, 42–44, 169–71
— amyl nitrite, 170
— intensive care units, 171
— nitroglycerine, 170–71
— opium, 43, 120
— surgical procedures, 172
Thorvaldsen, B., 130, 176
Thrombo-embolism, 30, 52–54, 68, 86, 127, 164
Thrombosis, concept of, 6, 7, 8, 26, 118, 126, 128–29, 142
— coronary, 6, 8, 9, 10, 11, 12, 13, 14, 30, 35, 37, 52, 60, 87, 91, 94, 101, 112, 113, 115, 117–18, 128, 129, 132, 134–35, 139, 140, 144, 145, 147–48, 149, 150, 152, 161, 172, 173, 185
— —, anticoagulant drugs in, 172
— —, laboratory aids to diagnosis, 14, 160–63
— general, xv, 25, 41, 54, 68, 74, 79, 104, 111, 122, 125, 127, 128, 132, 173
Thrombus, 6, 8, 17, 36, 53, 54, 57, 60, 70, 76, 81, 103, 111, 113, 123, 126, 127, 136, 141, 143, 151, 162, 183
— recanalized, 94, 116, 150
Thurnam, John, 103
Tiedemann, F., 123–24, 138, 139
— Von der Verengung und Schliessung der Pulsadern in Krankheiten, 124
Toor, J., 166–67
Toronto, Canada, 135
Transaminase, serum, 14, 163
Tranter, Ch. L., 162
Traube, L., 137

Ullmann, D. T., 61, 164
Ungar, H., 90, 167
Uterus, 'suffocation' of, 62
Utrecht, The Netherlands, 155

Varignana, Bartolomeo, 47
Vassé, Loys, 29–30
Ventricular fibrillation, 59, 90

Vesalius, Andreas, 49, 50, 51, 52, 55, 68, 79, 127, 132, 135, 149, 164, 176
— Anatomicarum Gabrielis Falloppii Observationum Examen, 54
— Fabrica, 50, 51, 52–54, 132
— Tabulae anatomicae, 50
Vesling, Johann, 80
Veterinary medicine, coronary manifestations in, 40–41, 45
Vienna, Austria, 135
Vierordt, H., 130
Viets, Henry R., 156
Vieussens, Raymond, 4, 73, 74
— Novum vasorum corporis humani systema, 73
Vineberg, A. M., 172
Virchow, Rudolf, 6, 8, 30, 123, 124–26, 127, 128–29
— Die Cellularpathologie, 126, 128
— Gesammelte Abhandlungen zur wissenschaftlichen Medizin, 128
— 'Occlusion of the pulmonary artery', 126
— On Thrombosis and Embolism, 128
Vital, Rabbi Hayim, 58
— Shaare Kedushah, 58
Volta, A., 154
Vulpian, E. F. A., 116, 132–33, 184–86

Wall, John, 97, 98
Waller, A. D., 155
— 'A demonstration on man of electromotive changes accompanying the heart's beat', 155
Walpole, Horace, 82
—Memoirs of the Reign of King George II, 82
Warburg, E. J., 69, 115, 117
Warren, John, 105–6, 123
— 'Remarks on angina pectoris', 105–6
Warren, John Collins, 7, 105–106, 118
— Cases of Organic Diseases of the Heart, with Dissections, 106
Waterston, D., 'Sir James Mackenzie's Heart', 159–60
Wedel, G. W., 127
Weigert, Carl, 9, 116, 118, 129–30, 133, 175

'Uber die pathologischen Gerinnungs-Vorgänge', 129–30
Wellcome Institute of the History of Medicine, xvi, 143
— Manuscript, 43
Wenckebach, K. F., 143
Wepfer, Johann Jakob, 109
— Observationes medico-practicae de affectibus capitis internis et externis, 109
Westendorf, W., 22
Westergren method, 162
White, Paul D., xvi, 13, 150, 171, 173
— Heart Disease, xvi, 137, 159
— Hearts, their long follow-up, 173
Wiggers, C. J., 153
Williams, Charles J. B., 113, 142
— Pathology and Diagnosis of Diseases of the Chest, 113
Williams, H. U., 17
Willis, Robert, 63
Willis, Thomas, 69–70, 74, 170
— Pharmaceutice Rationalis, 69–70
Willius, F. A., 28, 77, 119, 173
— Cardiac Classics, 119
Wilson, F. N., 158
Wilson, John A., 1, 21
Wilson, L. G., 36
Windsor Castle, 50
Wishart, J. H., 7, 106
Wolferth, C., 158
Wood, F., 158
Wood, Paul, 86, 128, 137, 142, 162
— Diseases of the Heart and Circulation, 86, 128, 137, 142
Wooster, D., 165
Wright, I., 172
Wright, W. C., 75
Wrigley, P. F. M., 118
Wroblewski, F., 14, 163
Würzburg, Germany, 155

Yemen, 166
Young, D. M., 59
Young, Thomas, 19

Ziegler, E., 8, 46, 110, 138–39